SURGICAL OPTIONS FOR THE TREATMENT OF HEART FAILURE

Developments in Cardiovascular Medicine

VOLUME 225

The titles published in this series are listed at the end of this volume.

Surgical Options for the Treatment of Heart Failure

edited by

ROY G. MASTERS, MD FRCSC

Division of Cardiac Surgery,
University of Ottawa Heart Institute,
Ottawa, Ontario, Canada

SPRINGER-SCIENCE+BUSINESS MEDIA, B.V.

A C.I.P. Catalogue record for this book is available from the Library of Congress

ISBN 978-94-017-4142-2 ISBN 978-0-585-29191-8 (eBook)
DOI 10.1007/978-0-585-29191-8

Printed on acid-free paper

Table of Contents

List of Contributors

Vinay Badhwar
McGill Uniiversity, Division of Cardiovascular and Thoracic Surgery, Montreal General Hospital, Montreal, Canada

Leah E. Bennett
ISHLT Registry, Richmond, VA, U.S.A.

Farah N.K. Bhatti
Papworth Hospital, Papworth, Everard, Cambridge, United Kingdom

Robert O. Bonow
Northwestern University Medical School, Division of Cardiology, Chicago, IL, U.S.A.

Mark M. Boucek
ISHLT Registry, Richmond, VA, U.S.A.

Ray C-J Chiu
McGill Uniiversity, Division of Cardiovascular and Thoracic Surgery, Montreal General Hospital, Montreal, Canada

Umer Darr
Yale University, Cardiothoracic Surgery, New Haven, Connecticut, U.S.A.

Naranjan S. Dhalla
University of Manitoba, Institute of Cardiovascular Sciences, St.Boniface General Hospital Research Center, Winnipeg, Canada

Joh . A. Elefteriades
Yale University, Cardiothoracic Surgery, New Haven, Connecticut, U.S.A.

Bennie Fiol
ISHLT Registry, Richmond, VA, U.S.A.

David Francsichelli
Medtronic Inc., Minneapolis, Minnesota, U.S.A.

Xiaobing Guo
University of Manitoba, Institute of Cardiovascular Sciences, St.Boniface General Hospital Research Center, Winnipeg, Canada

Joe Helou
University of Ottawa, Ottawa Heart Institute, Ottawa, Canada

Paul J. Hendry
University of Ottawa, Ottawa Heart Institute, Ottawa, Canada

Jeffrey D. Hosenpud
ISHLT Registry, Richmond, VA, U.S.A.

Richard J. Kaplon
Department of Thoracic and Cardiovascular Surgery, Cleveland Clinic Foundation, Cleveland, Ohio, U.S.A.

Berkeley M. Keck
ISHLT Registry, Richmond, VA, U.S.A.

Wilbert J. Keon
University of Ottawa, Ottawa Heart Institute, Ottawa, Canada

Robert Kormos
University of Pittsburgh, Pittsburgh, Pennsylvania U.S.A.

Roy G. Masters
University of Ottawa, Ottawa Heart Institute, Ottawa, Canada

Patrick M. McCarthy
Department of Thoracic and Cardiovascular Surgery, Cleveland Clinic Foundation, Cleveland, Ohio, U.S.A.

Tofy Mussivand
University of Ottawa, Ottawa Heart Institute, Ottawa, Canada

Richard Novick
ISHLT Registry, Richmond, VA, U.S.A.

Habib Samady
Yale University, Cardiothoracic Surgery, New Haven, Connecticut, U.S.A.

Lloyd C. Semelhago
McMaster University, McMaster Clinical Unit, Hamilton, Canada

Lynne Warner Stevenson
Harvard Medical School, Brigham and Women's Hospital, Boston, MA, U.S.A.

George Tellides
Yale University, Cardiothoracic Surgery, New Haven, Connecticut, U.S.A.

John Wallwork
Papworth Hospital, Papworth, Everard, Cambridge, UK

Jingwei Wang
University of Manitoba, Institute of Cardiovascular Sciences, St.Boniface General Hospital Research Center, Winnipeg, Canada

Franz J. Th. Whackers
Yale University, Cardiothoracic Surgery, New Haven, Connecticut, U.S.A.

Meher Yepremyan
Yale University, Cardiothoracic Surgery, New Haven, Connecticut, U.S.A.

Barry Zaret
Yale University, Cardiothoracic Surgery, New Haven, Connecticut, U.S.A.

Introduction

Despite the significant decline in heart disease mortality rates over the last 25 years, heart failure has remained a significant problem. We are now confronted with large numbers of terminally ill patients for whom conventional therapies for heart failure have been exhausted and for whom repeated hospital visits are necessary.

There now is a major thrust towards a management strategy which embraces a comprehensive approach including vigorous preventive measures and earlier surgical interventions. This book outlines the major surgical options for the treatment of heart failure and brings together a very broad base of opinions with contributions from several outstanding individuals.

With the improved knowledge and techniques to control rejection, transplantation has become the central pillar in the surgical management of this group of patients. Unfortunately, because of limited donor supply the technique cannot be applied to large numbers of patients. A great deal of excitement, however, exists in the potential for xenotransplantation as a supplement to homotransplantation. The use of cardiac assist devices has become a reality with several hundred LVADS and BiVADS implanted throughout the world and cardiac replacement with total artificial hearts continues to be used successfully as a bridge to transplantation. We are on the threshold of the broad application of assist devices to provide prolonged relief of heart failure and restore patients to an ambulatory home environment and hopefully return to the work force in significant numbers. The renewed interest in ventricular remodelling, early mitral valve repair, improved techniques for dealing with ventricular aneurysms and early revascularization during acute ischemic episodes has opened the doors to significant improvements in cardiac function in large numbers of heart failure patients. This represents yet another opportunity to prolong the lives and relieve the suffering of heart failure patients and leave the door open for ultimate cardiac replacement with either transplantation or devices should this be necessary.

This book is a timely and useful contribution to the overall knowledge of the management of the heart failure patient and provides a useful and worthwhile read for every cardiac surgeon of the day.

Wilbert J. Keon
University of Ottawa Heart Institute
Ottawa, Canada

1. PATHOPHYSIOLOGY OF CONTRACTILE DYSFUNCTION IN HEART FAILURE

Naranjan S. Dhalla, MD, Jingwei Wang, and Xiaobing Guo

Introduction

Heart failure is a clinical syndrome in which the cardiac output is inadequate to meet the metabolic needs of the body.[1] Essentially, it is a pathological state in which impaired cardiac pump activity decreases ejection of the blood and impedes venous return. The pathologic stimuli for the occurrence of heart failure can be categorized as follows: (a) conditions which lead to the development of pressure or volume overload (b) conditions which produce abnormal cardiac muscle contraction and relaxation and (c) conditions which limit ventricular filling.[2] A wide variety of diseases (Table 1) including valvular heart disease, ischemic heart disease, cardiomyopathy, septal defects, hypertension and pericardial disease can result in heart failure.[3-6]

The occurrence of heart failure is about one to three per cent of the population in Western countries and the incidence and prevalence are increasing.[7-9] Thus a better understanding of the pathophysiologic mechanisms involved in the genesis of heart failure is necessary for a clearer rationale for pharmacologic treatment and development of new agents and procedures to increase survival and improve quality of life.

The sequence of the main pathophysiological processes (Figure 1) which contribute to the development of heart failure include neurohumoral activation and ventricular chamber remodeling.[10] Accordingly, these processes will be discussed to gain some insight into the remodeling of the extracellular matrix and the subcellular organelles such as myofibrils, sarcolemma (SL) and sarcoplasmic reticulum (SR) in the failing heart.

Neurohumoral activiation

The activation of the sympathetic nervous system is the first response to left ventricular dysfunction. Sympathetic activation initially compensates for the loss of cardiac output by increasing heart rate and venous return. However, it may also contribute to myocardial cell loss and fibrosis in the chronic phase of heart failure.[11,12] Additionally, high levels of plasma catecholamines for a prolonged period of time can attenuate the function of the β-adrenergic receptor pathway. The failing heart shows a reduced response to adrenergic

Roy Masters (editor), Surgical Options for the Treatment of Heart Failure, 1-13.

Type of Failure	*Causes*
Pressure overload	Aortic stenosis Systemic arterial hypertension
Volume overload	Aortic or mitral regurgitation Congenital heart disease Thyrotoxicosis
Primary myocardial disease	Cardiomyopathy Myocarditis
Secondary myocardial abnormalities	Ischemia (coronary heart disease) Inflammation Infiltrative diseases
Impaired ventricular filling	Constrictive pericarditis Restrictive

stimulation resulting in alterations in the β-adrenergic signal transduction pathway. Such changes include downregulation of β_1-adrenoceptors, uncoupling of β-adrenoceptor from adenylyl cyclase, and an increase in the functional activity of inhibitory guanine nucleotide-binding proteins (G_i-proteins).[13,14] The density of β-adrenoceptors has been shown to be decreased in congestive heart failure due to idiopathic cardiomyopathy, ischemic cardiomyopathy, as well as myocardial infarction and the degree of downregulation is related to the severity of failure.[15,16] The decrease in β_1-receptor density and β-adrenoceptor downregulation probably account for much of the decrease in inotropic potential in the failing heart.[17] On the other hand, the density of β-adrenoceptors was increased in congestive heart failure due to aortic constriction in guinea pigs.[18] Furthermore, some investigators have reported both an increase and a decrease in the density of α-adrenoceptors in a hamster model of congestive heart failure due to genetic cardiomyopathy.[19, 20] Finally, other studies have shown either an increase or no change in the density of β-adrenoceptors in congestive heart failure in cardiomyopathic hamsters and in patients with heart failure of various etiologies.[21 - 23] The results from these studies suggest that the changes in adrenergic receptors in the myocardium may depend both on the etiology of congestive heart failure and the stage of the heart failure.

The activation of the sympathetic nervous system is accompanied by the activation of the renin-angiotensin-aldosterone system and the release of vasopressin leading to vasoconstriction, retention of sodium, increase of body fluid and formation of edema.[24 - 26] Angiotensin II can increase catecholamine synthesis and produce ventricular hypertrophy and it also has vasoconstrictive properties that may expand the ischemic area. Furthermore, it has been reported that chronically elevated endothelin-1 levels and subsequent activation of its receptor may play a role in the progression of heart failure.[27,28] In addition, atrial natriuretic peptide is released in the circulation in congestive heart failure and this has diuretic , vasodilatory and aldosterone secretion inhibitory effects which are beneficial to heart failure.[14]

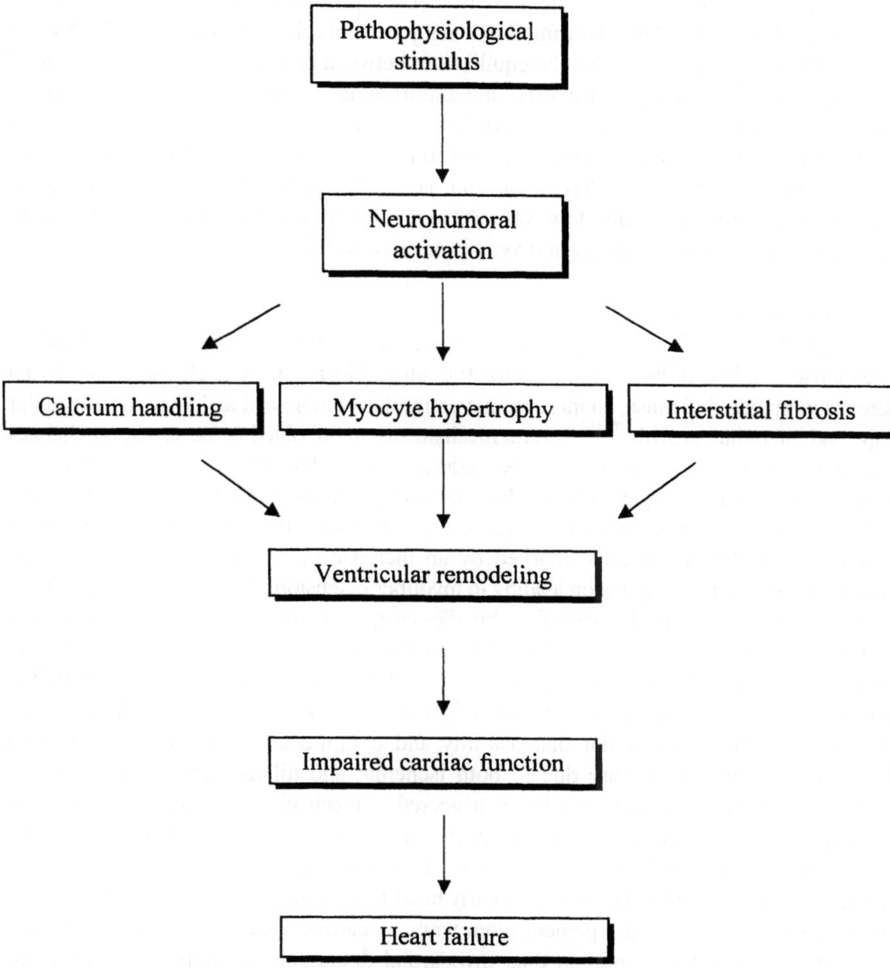

Figure 1. *Factors influencing myocardial remodeling in heart failure*

Cardiac remodelling

Extracellular matrix changes

The extracellular matrix is a flexible, supporting structure that surrounds the cell.[2, 29] The changes in the extracellular matrix during the development of heart failure include increases in fibronectin, laminin and vimentin contents, as well as deposition of collagen fibers I, III, VI, and IV in the myocardium.[30,31] There is an increase in collagen tissue concentrations in the rat ventricular free wall after myocardial infarction and fibrosis remote from the infarct site is regarded as "the major cause of ventricular remodeling" in ischemic cardiomyopathy.[32, 33] Such an increase in extracellular matrix proteins promotes myocardial stiffness and thus impairs contractile activity.[34] Disruption and discontinuity in collagen fibers have also been observed during the development of dilated cardiomyopathy both in animal models and in patients and the equilibrium between proteinase, which is capable of breaking down the extracellular matrix, and antiproteinase is also altered following heart failure.[35-37] In addition, Zellner et al. have found a reduction in myocyte attachment to the basement membrane proteins laminin, fibronectin and collagen IV in tachycardia-induced heart failure.[38] All these extracellular matrix changes can lead to a loss of force transmission via the ventricular free wall and to an alteration in cardiomyocyte alignment which would cause fiber slippage and ventricular free wall thinning.[39]

Ventricular remodeling

Myocardial hypertrophy is an important cardiac compensatory mechanism in heart failure in response to a loss of functioning contractile units. Heart failure is characterized by an increase in myocardial mass, an increase in ventricular volume and a change in ventricular shape and interstitial growth.[40,41] Several mechanisms are involved in the structural changes in cardiac remodeling. Cardiac muscle undergoes remodeling by increasing its length (dilatation) or volume (hypertrophy) rather than increasing the cell numbers.[42] Since adult cardiac myocytes cannot divide to increase their numbers, heart chamber enlargement occurs by hypertrophy of cells, marked by an increase in the number of intracellular sarcomeres; sarcomeric expansion leading to myofiber extension. Ventricular dilatation can be due to myocyte slippage between fiber bundles as in cardiomyopathy and in non-infarcted segments after myocardial infarction, being produced by activation of collagenase that disrupts the collagen myocyte supports.[43,44] Ultimately, collagen growth including deposition of new collagen and expansion of pre-existing collagen occurs. This collagen overgrowth reduces ventricular distensibility and compliance. Myocardial interstitial fibrosis occurs in heart failure due to both ischemic and dilated cardiomyopathies.[45] Ventricular remodeling is considered to be triggered by mechanical and biochemical factors, including the neurohormones norepinephrine, angiotensin II and vasopressin, cardiac growth factors and fibroblast growth factors as a consequence of intracellular second messengers cyclic AMP and calcium. In early heart failure, dilatation may increase cardiac performance but chronic enlargement often worsens cardiac function. Although cardiac hypertrophy is a better adaptation than myocardial dilatation for improving ventricular contraction, severe cardiac hypertrophy lasting for a long period results in a loss of contractility. Several surgical treatments have been employed to arrest or reverse the ventricular remodeling. Partial ventriculectomy is performed to remove a substantial portion of the lateral wall to make the dilated heart smaller.[46] Left ventricular assist devices have been shown to unload the failing ventricle, improve systemic blood supply and thereby decrease neurohumoral activation.[47] Lastly, dynamic cardiomyoplasty by wrapping the heart with skeletal muscle has been reported to limit cardiac dilation.[48]

Recently, the role of programmed cell death (apoptosis) in ventricular remodeling and the development of heart failure have gained much attention.[49, 50] Olivetti et al. in a study of human heart tissue showed that necrosis and apoptosis both cause cell death in patients with ischemic and idiopathic heart failure [12]. Reduced coronary blood flow and increased wall stress are the potential triggers of apoptosis in the failing heart.[14] However, the role of apoptosis is usually questioned on the basis of the fact that the number of myocytes so affected (0.2 to 3.0%) at any given time is too low to account for the impairment of cardiac performance seen in heart failure. Nonetheless, myocardial remodeling is initially compensatory but finally myocardial structure is changed so that the pumping efficiency of the heart is further impaired and the contractility is decreased. Accordingly, cardiac remodeling is critical to the development of progressive heart failure.[4] In advanced cardiac failure secondary to both ischemia and dilated cardiomyopathy, myocyte loss is a feature of the myopathic process and may occur by either necrosis or apoptosis.[51] Apoptosis involves cell shrinkage, condensation of chromatin and fragmentation of chromosomal DNA.[52] Recent studies have demonstrated that apoptosis occurred in constituent myocytes of failed explanted human hearts and in animal hearts with induced heart failure. As well, cardiac myocytes in acute myocardial infarction, in the hypertrophied heart and in the aging heart, also undergo apoptosis.[53] Furthermore, p53, a gene involved in apoptosis, is involved in the failing heart and the cytokine tumor necrosis factor-α, an inducer of apoptosis, is increased in heart failure.[40]

Subcellular Remodeling

There is a general agreement that the Ca^{2+} handling by cardiomyocytes is altered both in failing human hearts as well as in animal models of heart failure. Abnormal intracellular Ca^{2+} handling is one of the major causes of both systolic and diastolic dysfunction.[54, 55] The mechanisms of this abnormal Ca^{2+} handling are still unclear, however possible factors include alterations in SL L-type Ca^{2+} channels, SL Na^+/Ca^{2+} exchange, SL Ca^{2+}-pump, SR Ca^{2+}-pump and SR Ca^{2+} release channels, all of which participate in the regulation of Ca^{2+} movements. Studies have shown decreased SR Ca^{2+} uptake in a variety of animal models of heart failure models and in humans, abnormal Ca^{2+} release from SR in dilated cardiomyopathy and prolonged duration of intracellular Ca^{2+} transients in hypertrophied myocytes.[56 - 58] However, other investigators have found either no change or upregulation in SR Ca^{2+} uptake.[59, 60] Thus, several other factors such as defects in SL membranes may contribute to the abnormalities of calcium homeostasis in failing myocardium.[61] Finally it has been suggested that the contractile dysfunction in failing hearts may actually be due to attenuated sensitivity of myofibrils to Ca^{2+}.

Myofibrils in failing hearts

In heart failure the alterations in the contractile proteins appear to include an initial increase in protein synthesis in response to ventricular overload and a shift to fetal forms of myosin with an ultimate reduction in protein synthesis. A shift in myocardial isozyme content from V_1 (αα, fast, high ATPase activity) to V_3 (ββ, slow, low ATPase activity) has been documented in different models of experimental heart disease and is believed to occur at the transcriptional level.[62 - 65] In response to stimulation of α_1-adrenoceptors in neonatal rat cardiomyocytes evidence has indicated that hypertrophy in these cells is characterized by selective upregulation of early developmental contractile protein isogenes, including those for β-myosin heavy chain.[66] This shift is not important in humans, since human ventricles contain primarily the ββ isoform. However, a shift from αα to ββ does occur in the human atrium in heart failure.[67, 68] Several of the functional changes occurring in the failing heart can be explained by an increase in the synthesis of V_3 myosin isozyme with a characteristic derived from ATP used for the depressed rate of myocardial contraction may be beneficial to the failing heart.[69] In addition, changes of contractile proteins are not confined to the myosin heavy chains because in human heart failure, a marked decrease in the myosin light chain content has also been reported.[70, 71] However, the atrial form of myosin light chain-1 has been shown to increase in other investigations.[72] Morano et al. have demonstrated that in the isolated human myocardium, force development and calcium responsiveness were profoundly affected by the interaction between myosin light chain and actin.[73] Therefore, alterations in myosin light chain in heart failure may be of functional consequence for contractile activation.[74] Furthermore, an abnormal troponin-T isoform (T2) is produced in advanced heart failure but its significance is unclear so far.[75] Of more importance in heart failure is a reduction of contractile protein production. A marked loss of myofibrillar protein was observed in electron micrographs of the failing human heart and this reduction of contractile units seems to form the basis for the depression of both systolic function and ejection fraction and the prognosis of heart failure.[76]

Sarcolemma (SL) in failing hearts

The status of the Ca^{2+} channels may depend on the type of heart failure.[5] Reports of increased density of Ca^{2+} channels from genetic cardiomyopathic hamster hearts imply that intracellular Ca^{2+} overload through augmented sarcolemma Ca^{2+} influx may be the mechanism of pathological alterations in these hearts.[77 - 79] However, in ischemic heart disease induced by global ischemic or hypoxia-reoxygenation injury, it has been shown that calcium channel binding densities are reduced.[80, 81] Likewise, the density of L-type calcium channels is decreased in congestive heart failure in rats following myocardial infarction and in dogs with myocardial failure following intracoronary microembolization.[82 - 84] In addition, a significant decrease in mRNA encoding Ca^{2+} channels has been reported in the left ventricle of patients with heart failure due to dilated and ischemic cardiomyopathy.[85 - 87] Finally, in one study the number of Ca^{2+} channels in the hypertrophied right ventricle of rats with congestive heart failure secondary to a large left ventricular myocardial infarction was not changed compared with control values.[82]

Alterations in sarcolemmal Na^+/Ca^{2+} exchange and Ca^{2+}-pump activities have been observed in several experimental animal models of heart failure and decreased Na^+/Ca^{2+} exchange and Ca^{2+}-pump activities have been seen in 120-280 day old cardiomyopathic hamsters.[88, 89] These findings suggest that a depression in Na^+/Ca^{2+} activity may result in a reduced Ca^{2+} efflux from the myocardium, which may contribute to the occurrence of intracellular Ca^{2+} overload. Many studies have investigated the status of SL Na^+/K^+ ATPase enzyme in both human and experimental heart failure. Na^+/K^+ ATPase activity has been observed to be reduced in the failing human heart, in UM-X7.1 cardiomyopathic hamster hearts, in rabbit hearts with left ventricular hypertrophy, in rat hearts with ischemia-reperfusion injury and in the viable left ventricle of rats with congestive heart failure due to myocardial infarction.[54,90 - 93] These observations have revealed that a reduction in SL Na^+/K^+ ATPase in heart failure is important for contractile dysfunction, generation of arrhythmia and for the effectiveness of digoxin treatment.[94] However, increased Na^+/K^+ ATPase activity has been observed in the BIO 14.6 strain of cardiomyopathic hamsters and in canine hearts with volume or pressure overload.[95 - 97] Further, SL Ca^{2+}-pump activity was not altered in the failing hearts due to myocardial infarction.[93] Therefore, the biochemical changes in heart failure reflecting remodeling of the SL membrane seem to depend on the etiology of the disease.

Sarcoplasmic Reticulum (SR) in failing hearts
The SR plays the most important role in regulating cytoplasmic Ca^{2+} during cardiac contraction and relaxation. Calcium is released through the Ca^{2+}-release channel (ryanodine receptor) whereas calcium is taken up by the SR via Ca^{2+}-pump which is regulated by phospholamban. The calcium inside the lumen of the SR is stored in combination with calsequestrin. The ATP-dependent Ca^{2+} sequestration rate is reduced in the animal model of the failing heart from a variety of etiologies including hypertrophy, ischemia, pacing-induced, genetic, diabetic and drug-induced.[55, 98 - 105] The status of SR Ca^{2+} ATPase has been studied in different animal models of myocardial failure. A decrease in SR Ca^{2+} ATPase protein level was observed in failing guinea pig hearts following banding of the descending aorta as compared to an age-matched sham group and the attenuation in SR Ca^{2+} ATPase activity was more than the reduction in protein levels.[98, 106] Decreased gene expression of SR Ca^{2+} ATPase in Syrian hamsters with hereditary cardiomyopathy has also been observed.[107] In a rat model of myocardial infarction, SR Ca^{2+} ATPase mRNA and protein levels decreased in parallel to the severity of congestive heart failure and in the left ventricular myocardium from rats with ascending aortic banding, a decrease in SR Ca^{2+} ATPase mRNA level occurred in failing animals.[108] Furthermore, it has been reported that mRNA levels of SR Ca^{2+} ATPase is reduced in the failing as compared to the non-failing human heart.[109, 110] However, in one report SR Ca^{2+} ATPase mRNA level did not change significantly from the baseline, despite development of pacing tachycardia-induced heart failure.[111]

There are indications that ryanodine receptor function may be altered in heart failure. The density of ryanodine receptors was decreased in a rat model of pressure overload cardiac hypertrophy whereas a normal ryanodine protein level was maintained in the failing human heart.[112, 113] Both reduction and no change in mRNA levels have been observed in dilated cardiomyopathy.[114, 115] The results concerning mRNA levels in failing human hearts are somewhat contradictory and appear to be related to the etiology of heart failure. The mRNA and protein levels of phospholamban have also been found to be decreased in human heart failure and only one study showed a small decrease in phospholamban protein levels relative to total protein in the failing heart due to dilated cardiomyopathy.[116 - 119] A decrease in phospholamban could be a compensatory change that would relieve inhibitory on the SR Ca^{2+} ATPase in the failing hearts. A reduced phosphorylation of phospholamban could decrease the rate at which calcium is resequestered by the SR, and thus result in prolonged calcium transients and delayed relaxation in the failing heart.[120, 121] In left ventricular biopsies from dogs with tachycardia-induced heart failure, no change in phospholamban mRNA levels was observed at the onset of clinical heart failure compared to the baseline.[111] The calsequestrin content of the heart appears to be unchanged in heart failure.[122 - 126] Studies in the failing human myocardium consistently showed unchanged mRNA and protein levels calsequestrin as compared to the nonfailing myocardium.[85, 113, 118, 125] These observations show a great deal of specificity in terms of remodeling of the SR membrane during the development of heart failure. However, virtually nothing is known regarding the relationships among SR, SL, myofilament and extracellular matrix remodeling during the development of heart failure.

Summary

Heart failure is a clinical syndrome which is associated with impaired cardiac function, decreased ejection fraction and impeded venous return. Studies on the human heart and experimental animal models of heart failure have suggested that the mechanisms involved in contractile dysfunction in heart failure may include neurohumoral activation, alterations in calcium handling by SL and SR, and reduced sensitivity of myofilaments to Ca^{2+}. Although changes in extracellular matrix are generally considered to account for ventricular remodeling and subsequent heart failure, the remodeling of subcellular organelles such as SL, SR and myofibrils may also play a critical role in the genesis of cardiac dysfunction in the failing heart. Extensive research is needed for understanding the relationship between extracellular matrix remodeling and subcellular remodeling in order to improve our knowledge on the pathophysiology of contractile dysfunction in heart failure.

Acknowledgements

The research reported in this article was supported by a grant from the Medical Research Council of Canada (MRC Group in Experimental Cardiology).

References

1. Katz AM. Evolving concepts of heart failure: cooling furnace, malfunctioning pump, enlarging muscle. Part II: Hypertrophy and dilatation of the failing heart. J Card Fail 1998;4:67-81.
2. Piano MR, Bondmass M, Schwertz DW. The molecular and cellular pathophysiology of heart failure. Heart Lung 1998;27:3-19.
3. Calkins ME. Pathophysiology of congestive heart failure in ESRD. Am Nephrol Nurs Assoc J 1996;23:457-63.
4. Patterson JH and Adams KF, Jr. Pathophysiology of heart failure: changing perceptions. Pharmacotherapy 1996;16:27S-36S.
5. Dhalla NS, Afzal N, Beamish RE, Naimark B, Takeda N, Nagano M. Pathophysiology of cardiac dysfunction in congestive heart failure. Can J Cardiol 1993;9:873-87.
6. Rich MW. Epidemiology, pathophysiology, and etiology of congestive heart failure in older adults. J Am Geriatr Soc 1997;45:968-74.
7. Nicholls MG. Hypertension, hypertrophy, heart failure. Heart 1996;76:92-7.
8. Schocken DD, Arrieta MI, Leaverton PE, Ross EA. Prevalence and mortality rate of congestive heart failure in the United States. J Am Coll Cardiol 1992;20:301-6.
9. Birks EJ and Yacoub MH. The role of nitric oxide and cytokines in heart failure. Coron Artery Dis 1997;8:389-402.
10. Parmley WW. Pathophysiology of congestive heart failure. Am J Cardiol 1985;55:9A-14A.
11. Anversa P, Kajstura J, Olivetti G. Myocyte death in heart failure. Curr Opin Cardiol 1996;11:245-51.
12. Olivetti G, Abbi R, Quaini F, et al. Apoptosis in the failing human heart. N Engl J Med 1997;336:1131-41.
13. Dhalla NS, Wang X, Sethi R, Das PK, Beamish RE. Beta-adrenergic linked signal transduction mechanisms in failing hearts. Heart Failure Reviews 1997;2:55-65.
14. Moser DK. Pathophysiology of heart failure update: the role of neurohumoral activation in the progression of heart failure. Am Assoc Clin Nurs Clin Issues 1998;9:157-71.
15. Bristow MR, Ginsburg R, Minobe W, et al. Decreased catecholamine sensitivity and beta-adrenergic-receptor density in failing human hearts. N Engl J Med 1982;307:205-11.
16. Denniss AR, Colucci WS, Allen PD, Marsh JD. Distribution and function of human ventricular beta adrenergic receptors in congestive heart failure. J Mol Cell Cardiol 1989;21:651-60.
17. Bristow MR. Pathophysiologic and pharmacologic rationales for clinical management of chronic heart failure with beta-blocking agents. Am J Cardiol 1993;71:12C-22C.
18. Karliner JS, Barnes P, Brown M, Dollery C. Chronic heart failure in the guinea pig increases cardiac alpha 1- and beta-adrenoceptors. Eur J Pharmacol 1980;67:115-8.
19. Karliner JS, Alabaster C, Stephens H, Barnes P, Dollery C. Enhanced noradrenaline response in cardiomyopathic hamsters: possible relation to changes in adrenoceptors studied by radioligand binding. Cardiovasc Res 1981;15:296-304.
20. Kagiya T, Hori M, Iwakura K, et al. Role of increased alpha 1-adrenergic activity in cardiomyopathic Syrian hamster. Am J Physiol 1991;260:H80-8.
21. Sen L, Liang BT, Colucci WS, Smith TW. Enhanced alpha 1-adrenergic responsiveness in cardiomyopathic hamster cardiac myocytes. Relation to the expression of pertussis toxin-sensitive G protein and alpha 1-adrenergic receptors. Circ Res 1990;67:1182-92.
22. Bristow MR, Minobe W, Rasmussen R, Hershberger RE, Hoffman BB. Alpha-1 adrenergic receptors in the nonfailing and failing human heart. J Pharmacol Exp Ther 1988;247:1039-45.
23. Vago T, Bevilacqua M, Norbiato G, et al. Identification of alpha 1-adrenergic receptors on sarcolemma from normal subjects and patients with idiopathic dilated cardiomyopathy: characteristics and linkage to GTP-binding protein. Circ Res 1989;64:474-81.
24. Middlekauff HR. Mechanisms and implications of autonomic nervous system dysfunction in heart failure. Curr Opin Cardiol 1997;12:265-75.
25. Esler M, Kaye D, Lambert G, Esler D, Jennings G. Adrenergic nervous system in heart failure. Am J Cardiol 1997;80:7L-14L.
26. Sigurdsson A and Swedberg K. The role of neurohormonal activation in chronic heart failure and postmyocardial infarction. Am Heart J 1996;132:229-34.
27. Sakai S, Miyauchi T, Kobayashi M, Yamaguchi I, Goto K, Sugishita Y. Inhibition of myocardial endothelin pathway improves long-term survival in heart failure. Nature 1996;384:353-5.
28. Spinale FG, Walker JD, Mukherjee R, Iannini JP, Keever AT, Gallagher KP. Concomitant endothelin

receptor subtype-A blockade during the progression of pacing-induced congestive heart failure in rabbits. Beneficial effects on left ventricular and myocyte function. Circulation 1997;95:1918-29.
29. Buck CA and Horwitz AF. Cell surface receptors for extracellular matrix molecules. Annu Rev Cell Biol 1987;3:179-205.
30. Schaper J and Speiser B. The extracellular matrix in the failing human heart. Basic Res Cardiol 1992;87:303-9.
31. Beltrami CA, Finato N, Rocco M, et al. Structural basis of end-stage failure in ischemic cardiomyopathy in humans. Circulation 1994;89:151-63.
32. McCormick RJ, Musch TI, Bergman BC, Thomas DP. Regional differences in LV collagen accumulation and mature cross-linking after myocardial infarction in rats. Am J Physiol 1994;266:H354-9.
33. Weber KT. Extracellular matrix remodeling in heart failure: a role for de novo angiotensin II generation. Circulation 1997;96:4065-82.
34. Dixon IM, Ju H, Jassal DS, Peterson DJ. Effect of ramipril and losartan on collagen expression in right and left heart after myocardial infarction. Mol Cell Biochem 1996;165:31-45.
35. Cannon RO, Butany JW, McManus BM, et al. Early degradation of collagen after acute myocardial infarction in the rat. Am J Cardiol 1983;52:390-5.
36. Tyagi SC, Kumar SG, Haas SJ, et al. Post-transcriptional regulation of extracellular matrix metalloproteinase in human heart end-stage failure secondary to ischemic cardiomyopathy. J Mol Cell Cardiol 1996;28:1415-28.
37. Tyagi SC. Extracellular matrix dynamics in heart failure: a prospect for gene therapy. J Cell Biochem 1998;68:403-10.
38. Zellner JL, Spinale FG, Eble DM, Hewett KW, Crawford FA, Jr. Alterations in myocyte shape and basement membrane attachment with tachycardia-induced heart failure. Circ Res 1991;69:590-600.
39. Weber KT and Brilla CG. Pathological hypertrophy and cardiac interstitium. Fibrosis and renin-angiotensin-aldosterone system. Circulation 1991;83:1849-65.
40. Baig MK, Mahon N, McKenna WJ, et al. The pathophysiology of advanced heart failure. Am Heart J 1998;135:S216-30.
41. Pouleur H G, Konstam M A, Udelson J E, Rousseau M F. Changes in ventricular volume, wall thickness and wall stress during progression of left ventricular dysfunction. The SOLVD Investigators. J Am Coll Cardiol 1993;22:43A-8A.
42. Francis GS and Chu C. Post-infarction myocardial remodelling: why does it happen? Eur Heart J 1995;16:31-6.
43. Caulfield JB and Borg TK. The collagen network of the heart. Lab Invest 1979;40:364-72.
44. Schwartz K, Chassagne C, Boheler KR. The molecular biology of heart failure. J Am Coll Cardiol 1993;22:30A-33A.
45. Beltrami CA, Finato N, Rocco M, et al. The cellular basis of dilated cardiomyopathy in humans. J Mol Cell Cardiol 1995;27:291-305.
46. Batista RJ, Santos JL, Takeshita N, Bocchino L, Lima PN, Cunha MA. Partial left ventriculectomy to improve left ventricular function in end-stage heart disease. J Card Surg 1996;11:96-7.
47. Levin HR and Weisfeldt ML. Deep thoughts on tin men. Fact, fallacy, and future of mechanical circulatory support. Circulation 1997;95:2340-3.
48. Kass DA. Surgical approaches to arresting or reversing chronic remodeling of the failing heart. J Card Fail 1998;4:57-66.
49. Bing OH. Hypothesis: apoptosis may be a mechanism for the transition to heart failure with chronic pressure overload. J Mol Cell Cardiol 1994;26:943-8.
50. Kajstura J, Cheng W, Reiss K, et al. Apoptotic and necrotic myocyte cell deaths are independent contributing variables of infarct size in rats. Lab Invest 1996;74:86-107.
51. Davies C H, Harding S E, Poole-Wilson P A. Cellular mechanisms of contractile dysfunction in human heart failure. Eur Heart J 1996;17:189-198.
52. Kerr J F, Wyllie A H, Currie A R. Apoptosis: a basic biological phenomenon with wide-ranging implications in tissue kinetics. Br J Cancer 1972;26:239-57.
53. Sabbah H N and Sharov V G. Apoptosis in heart failure. Prog Cardiovasc Dis 1998;40:549-62.
54. Lindenmayer GE, Sordahl LA, Harigaya S, Allen JC, Besch HR, Jr., Schwartz A. Some biochemical studies on subcellular systems isolated from fresh recipient human cardiac tissue obtained during transplantation. Am J Cardiol 1971;27:277-83.
55. Afzal N and Dhalla NS. Differential changes in left and right ventricular SR calcium transport in congestive heart failure. Am J Physiol 1992;262:H868-74.
56. Kimura S, Bassett AL, Saida K, Shimizu M, Myerburg RJ. Sarcoplasmic reticulum function in skinned fibers of hypertrophied rat ventricle. Am J Physiol 1989;256:H1006-11.

57. Whitmer JT, Kumar P, Solaro RJ. Calcium transport properties of cardiac sarcoplasmic reticulum from cardiomyopathic Syrian hamsters (BIO 53.58 and 14.6): evidence for a quantitative defect in dilated myopathic hearts not evident in hypertrophic hearts. Circ Res 1988;62:81-5.
58. Gwathmey JK, Copelas L, MacKinnon R, et al. Abnormal intracellular calcium handling in myocardium from patients with end-stage heart failure. Circ Res 1987;61:70-6.
59. Movsesian MA, Colyer J, Wang JH, Krall J. Phospholamban-mediated stimulation of Ca^{2+} uptake in sarcoplasmic reticulum from normal and failing hearts. J Clin Invest 1990;85:1698-702.
60. Kuramochi T, Honda M, Tanaka K, et al. Contrasting effects of an angiotensin converting enzyme inhibitor and a calcium antagonist on calcium transients in isolated rat cardiac myocytes. Cardiovasc Res 1994;28:1407-13.
61. Musat S and Dhalla NS. Alteration in cardiac sarcolemmal ATP receptors by oxyradicals. Ann N Y Acad Sci 1996;793:1-12.
62. Rupp H, Elimban V, Dhalla NS. Diabetes-like action of intermittent fasting on sarcoplasmic reticulum Ca^{2+}-pump ATPase and myosin isoenzymes can be prevented by sucrose. Biochem Biophys Res Commun 1989;164:319-25.
63. Afzal N, Pierce GN, Elimban V, Beamish RE, Dhalla NS. Influence of verapamil on some subcellular defects in diabetic cardiomyopathy.Am J Physiol 1989;256:E453-8.
64. Mercadier JJ, Lompre AM, Wisnewsky C, et al. Myosin isoenzyme changes in several models of rat cardiac hypertrophy. Circ Res 1981;49:525-32.
65. Chevalier B, Callens F, Charlemagne D, et al. Signal and adaptational changes in gene expression during cardiac overload. J Mol Cell Cardiol 1989;21:71-7.
66. Simpson PC, Long CS, Waspe LE, Henrich CJ, Ordahl CP. Transcription of early developmental isogenes in cardiac myocyte hypertrophy. J Mol Cell Cardiol 1989;21:79-89.
67. Swynghedauw B. Developmental and functional adaptation of contractile proteins in cardiac and skeletal muscles. Physiol Rev 1986;66:710-71.
68. Mercadier JJ, Bouveret P, Gorza L, et al. Myosin isoenzymes in normal and hypertrophied human ventricular myocardium. Circ Res 1983;53:52-62.
69. Alpert NR and Mulieri LA. Increased myothermal economy of isometric force generation in compensated cardiac hypertrophy induced by pulmonary artery constriction in the rabbit. A characterization of heat liberation in normal and hypertrophied right ventricular papillary muscles. Circ Res 1982;50:491-500.
70. Hirzel HO, Tuchschmid CR, Schneider J, Krayenbuehl HP, Schaub MC. Relationship between myosin isoenzyme composition, hemodynamics, and myocardial structure in various forms of human cardiac hypertrophy. Circ Res 1985;57:729-40.
71. Margossian SS, White HD, Caulfield JB, Norton P, Taylor S, Slayter HS. Light chain 2 profile and activity of human ventricular myosin during dilated cardiomyopathy. Identification of a causal agent for impaired myocardial function. Circulation 1992;85:1720-33.
72. Sutsch G, Brunner UT, von Schulthess C, et al. Hemodynamic performance and myosin light chain-1 expression of the hypertrophied left ventricle in aortic valve disease before and after valve replacement. Circ Res 1992;70:1035-43.
73. Morano I, Ritter O, Bonz A, Timek T, Vahl CF, Michel G. Myosin light chain-actin interaction regulates cardiac contractility. Circ Res 1995;76:720-5.
74. De Tombe PP. Altered contractile function in heart failure. Cardiovasc Res 1998;37:367-80.
75. Anderson PA, Malouf NN, Oakeley AE, Pagani ED, Allen PD. Troponin T isoform expression in humans. A comparison among normal and failing adult heart, fetal heart, and adult and fetal skeletal muscle. Circ Res 1991;69:1226-33.
76. Hammond EH, Menlove RL, Anderson JL. Predictive value of immunofluorescence and electron microscopic evaluation of endomyocardial biopsies in the diagnosis and prognosis of myocarditis and idiopathic dilated cardiomyopathy. Am Heart J 1987;114:1055-65.
77. Wagner JA, Reynolds IJ, Weisman HF, Dudeck P, Weisfeldt ML, Snyder SH. Calcium antagonist receptors in cardiomyopathic hamster: selective increases in heart, muscle, brain. Science 1986;232:515-8.
78. Finkel MS, Marks ES, Patterson RE, Speir EH, Steadman KA, Keiser HR. Correlation of changes in cardiac calcium channels with hemodynamics in Syrian hamster cardiomyopathy and heart failure. Life Sci 1987;41:153-9.
79. Kobayashi A, Yamashita T, Kaneko M, Nishiyama T, Hayashi H, Yamazaki N. Effects of verapamil on experimental cardiomyopathy in the BIO 14.6 Syrian hamster. J Am Coll Cardiol 1987;10:1128-38.
80. Matucci R, Bennardini F, Sciammarella ML, et al. [^{3}H]-nitrendipine binding in membranes obtained from hypoxic and reoxygenated heart. Biochem Pharmacol 1987;36:1059-62.
81. Nayler WG, Dillon JS, Elz JS, McKelvie M. An effect of ischemia on myocardial dihydropyridine binding

sites. Eur J Pharmacol 1985;115:81-9.
82. Dixon IM, Lee SL, Dhalla NS. Nitrendipine binding in congestive heart failure due to myocardial infarction. Circ Res 1990;66:782-8.
83. Gopalakrishnan M, Triggle DJ, Rutledge A, Kwon YW, Bauer JA, Fung HL. Regulation of K^+ and Ca^{2+} channels in experimental cardiac failure. Am J Physiol 1991;261:H1979-87.
84. Gengo PJ, Sabbah HN, Steffen RP, et al. Myocardial beta adrenoceptor and voltage sensitive calcium channel changes in a canine model of chronic heart failure. J Mol Cell Cardiol 1992;24:1361-9.
85. Takahashi T, Allen PD, Lacro RV, et al. Expression of dihydropyridine receptor (Ca^{2+} channel) and calsequestrin genes in the myocardium of patients with end-stage heart failure. J Clin Invest 1992;90:927-35.
86. Barry WH and Bridge JH. Intracellular calcium homeostasis in cardiac myocytes. Circulation 1993;87:1806-15.
87. Fabiato A. Calcium-induced release of calcium from the cardiac sarcoplasmic reticulum. Am J Physiol 1983;245:C1-14.
88. Wagner JA, Weisman HF, Snowman AM, Reynolds IJ, Weisfeldt ML, Snyder SH. Alterations in calcium antagonist receptors and sodium-calcium exchange in cardiomyopathic hamster tissues. Circ Res 1989;65:205-14.
89. Makino N, Jasmin G, Beamish RE, Dhalla NS. Sarcolemmal Na^+-Ca^{2+} exchange during the development of genetically determined cardiomyopathy. Biochem Biophys Res Commun 1985;133:491-7.
90. Panagia V, Singh JN, Anand-Srivastava MB, Pierce GN, Jasmin G, Dhalla NS. Sarcolemmal alterations during the development of genetically determined cardiomyopathy. Cardiovasc Res 1984;18:567-72.
91. Yazaki Y and Fujii J. Depressed Na-K-ATPase activity in the failing rabbit heart. Jpn Heart J 1972;13:73-83.
92. Balasubramanian V, McNamara DB, Singh JN, Dhalla NS. Biochemical basis of heart function. X. Reduction in the Na^+-K^+-stimulated ATPase activity in failing rat heart due to hypoxia. Can J Physiol Pharmacol 1973;51:504-10.
93. Dixon IM, Hata T, Dhalla NS. Sarcolemmal calcium transport in congestive heart failure due to myocardial infarction in rats. Am J Physiol 1992;262:H1387-94.
94. Bundgaard H and Kjeldsen K. Human myocardial Na,K-ATPase concentration in heart failure. Mol Cell Biochem 1996;163-164:277-83.
95. Sulakhe PV and Dhalla NS. Alterations in the activity of cardiac Na^+-K^+-stimulated ATPase in congestive heart failure. Exp Mol Pathol 1973;18:100-11.
96. Khatter JC and Prasad K. Myocardial sarcolemmal ATPase in dogs with induced mitral insufficiency. Cardiovasc Res 1976;10:637-41.
97. Prasad K, Khatter JC, Bharadwaj B. Intra- and extracellular electrolytes and sarcolemmal ATPase in the failing heart due to pressure overload in dogs. Cardiovasc Res 1979;13:95-104.
98. Zarain-Herzberg A, Afzal N, Elimban V, Dhalla NS. Decreased expression of cardiac sarcoplasmic reticulum Ca^{2+}-pump ATPase in congestive heart failure due to myocardial infarction. Mol Cell Biochem 1996;163-164:285-90.
99. Qi M, Shannon TR, Euler DE, Bers D M, Samarel AM. Downregulation of sarcoplasmic reticulum Ca^{2+}-ATPase during progression of left ventricular hypertrophy. Am J Physiol 1997;272:H2416-24.
100. Zarain-Herzberg A, Rupp H, Elimban V, Dhalla NS. Modification of sarcoplasmic reticulum gene expression in pressure overload cardiac hypertrophy by etomoxir. FASEB J 1996;10:1303-9.
101. O'Brien PJ, Ianuzzo CD, Moe GW, Stopps TP, Armstrong PW. Rapid ventricular pacing of dogs to heart failure: biochemical and physiological studies. Can J Physiol Pharmacol 1990;68:34-9.
102. Panagia V, Lee SL, Singh A, Pierce GN, Jasmin G, Dhalla NS. Impairment of mitochondrial and sarcoplasmic reticular functions during the development of heart failure in cardiomyopathic (UM-X7.1) hamsters. Can J Cardiol 1986;2:236-47.
103. Tahiliani AG and McNeill JH. Diabetes-induced abnormalities in the myocardium. Life Sci 1986;38:959-74.
104. Tomlinson CW, Godin DV, Rabkin SW. Adriamycin cardiomyopathy: implications of cellular changes in a canine model with mild impairment of left ventricular function. Biochem Pharmacol 1985;34:4033-41.
105. Movsesian MA and Schwinger RH. Calcium sequestration by the sarcoplasmic reticulum in heart failure. Cardiovasc Res 1998;37:352-9.
106. Kiss E, Ball NA, Kranias EG, Walsh RA. Differential changes in cardiac phospholamban and sarcoplasmic reticular Ca^{2+}-ATPase protein levels. Effects on Ca^{2+} transport and mechanics in compensated pressure-overload hypertrophy and congestive heart failure. Circ Res 1995;77:759-64.
107. Kuo TH, Tsang W, Wang KK, Carlock L. Simultaneous reduction of the sarcolemmal and SR calcium ATPase activities and gene expression in cardiomyopathic hamster. Biochim Biophys Acta 1992;1138:343-

9.
108. Feldman AM, Weinberg EO, Ray PE, Lorell BH. Selective changes in cardiac gene expression during compensated hypertrophy and the transition to cardiac decompensation in rats with chronic aortic banding. Circ Res 1993;73:184-92.
109. Hasenfuss G, Reinecke H, Studer R, et al. Relation between myocardial function and expression of sarcoplasmic reticulum Ca^{2+}-ATPase in failing and nonfailing human myocardium. Circ Res 1994;75:434-42.
110. Limas CJ, Olivari MT, Goldenberg IF, Levine TB, Benditt DG, Simon A. Calcium uptake by cardiac sarcoplasmic reticulum in human dilated cardiomyopathy. Cardiovasc Res 1987;21:601-5.
111. Williams RE, Kass DA, Kawagoe Y, et al. Endomyocardial gene expression during development of pacing tachycardia-induced heart failure in the dog. Circ Res 1994;75:615-23.
112. Naudin V, Oliviero P, Rannou F, Sainte Beuve C, Charlemagne D. The density of ryanodine receptors decreases with pressure overload-induced rat cardiac hypertrophy. FEBS Lett 1991;285:135-8.
113. Schillinger W, Meyer M, Kuwajima G, Mikoshiba K, Just H, Hasenfuss G. Unaltered ryanodine receptor protein levels in ischemic cardiomyopathy. Mol Cell Biochem 1996;160-161:297-302.
114. Go LO, Moschella MC, Watras J, Handa KK, Fyfe BS, Marks AR. Differential regulation of two types of intracellular calcium release channels during end-stage heart failure. J Clin Invest 1995;95:888-94.
115. Brillantes AM, Allen P, Takahashi T, Izumo S, Marks AR. Differences in cardiac calcium release channel (ryanodine receptor) expression in myocardium from patients with end-stage heart failure caused by ischemic versus dilated cardiomyopathy. Circ Res 1992;71:18-26.
116. Linck B, Boknik P, Eschenhagen T, et al. Messenger RNA expression and immunological quantification of phospholamban and SR-Ca^{2+}-ATPase in failing and nonfailing human hearts. Cardiovasc Res 1996;31:625-32.
117. Flesch M, Schwinger RH, Schnabel P, et al. Sarcoplasmic reticulum Ca^{2+}-ATPase and phospholamban mRNA and protein levels in end-stage heart failure due to ischemic or dilated cardiomyopathy. J Mol Med 1996;74:321-32.
118. Meyer M, Schillinger W, Pieske B, et al. Alterations of sarcoplasmic reticulum proteins in failing human dilated cardiomyopathy. Circulation 1995;92:778-84.
119. Hasenfuss G. Alterations of calcium-regulatory proteins in heart failure. Cardiovasc Res 1998;37:279-89.
120. de la Bastie D, Levitsky D, Rappaport L, et al. Function of the sarcoplasmic reticulum and expression of its Ca^{2+}-ATPase gene in pressure overload-induced cardiac hypertrophy in the rat. Circ Res 1990;66:554-64.
121. Movsesian MA. Calcium uptake by sarcoplasmic reticulum and its modulation by cAMP-dependent phosphorylation in normal and failing human myocardium. Basic Res Cardiol 1992;87:277-84.
122. Phillips RM, Narayan P, Gomez AM, et al. Sarcoplasmic reticulum in heart failure: central player or bystander? Cardiovasc Res 1998;37:346-51.
123. Lompre AM, Lambert F, Lakatta EG, Schwartz K. Expression of sarcoplasmic reticulum Ca^{2+}-ATPase and calsequestrin genes in rat heart during ontogenic development and aging. Circ Res 1991;69:1380-8.
124. Arai M, Otsu K, MacLennan DH, Alpert NR, Periasamy M. Effect of thyroid hormone on the expression of mRNA encoding sarcoplasmic reticulum proteins. Circ Res 1991;69:266-76.
125. Arai M, Alpert NR, MacLennan DH, Barton P, Periasamy M. Alterations in sarcoplasmic reticulum gene expression in human heart failure. A possible mechanism for alterations in systolic and diastolic properties of the failing myocardium. Circ Res 1993;72:463-9.
126. Movsesian MA, Karimi M, Green K, Jones LR. Ca^{2+}-transporting ATPase, phospholamban, and calsequestrin levels in nonfailing and failing human myocardium. Circulation 1994;90:653-7.

2. CORONARY ARTERY BYPASS FOR ADVANCED LEFT VENTRICULAR DYSFUNCTION

John A. Elefteriades, George Tellides, Habib Samady, Meher Yepremyan, Umer Darr, Franz J.Th. Wackers, and Barry Zaret

Introduction

Although courageous forays into the application of coronary artery bypass grafting (CABG) to the patient with advanced left ventricular dysfunction were made since the early days of open heart surgery, the opinion that the patient with advanced left ventricular dysfunction could not and should not be offered coronary artery bypass surgery prevailed well into the 1980's. The reluctance centered around three concerns: (1) that the risk of operation would be prohibitive, (2) that little symptomatic or longevity benefit would accrue from CABG, and (3) that CABG would merely punctuate an inevitable course of inexorable deterioration. Cardiologists were therefore reluctant to refer such patients for coronary revascularization and surgeons were reluctant to accept such patients. In terms of scientific evaluation, most large multicenter trials of coronary artery bypass grafting purposely excluded patients with advanced left ventricular dysfunction. (Ejection fraction was >35% in the Coronary Artery Surgery Study (CASS) and >50% for the European Coronary Surgery Study (ECSS)). [1, 2]

Despite the substantial dangers anticipated in the application of CABG to patients with advanced left ventricular dysfunction, the potential for recovery of function via grafting continued to add luster to the challenge. The very definition of "hibernating muscle", coined originally by Rahimtoola, embodies the concept that non-functioning, ischemic muscle can resume function upon provision of adequate blood supply.[3] The ultimate test of viability has always been, in fact, the restoration of function consequent upon revascularization.

The patient who poses the greatest potential for re-animation of hibernating muscle is the patient with coronary artery disease and advanced left ventricular dysfunction--the patient with so-called "advanced ischemic cardiomyopathy". It is not surprising that surgeons have attacked the problem of advanced ischemic cardiomyopathy, as the outlook with medical management alone is dismal. Figure 1, from Franciosa and Cohn, demonstrates vividly the desperate outlook for these patients. In their study, these authors examined the survival of patients with cardiomyopathy according to etiology. The poorest outlook by far was for patients with coronary artery disease as the cause of their myopathy, who manifested 80% mortality over 3 years. [4] While current

Roy Masters (editor), Surgical Options for the Treatment of Heart Failure, 15-31.

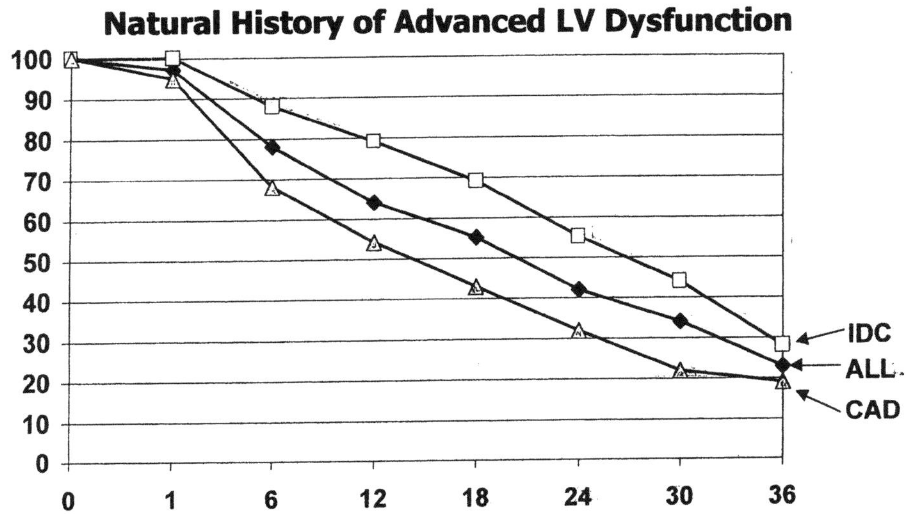

Figure 1. *Survival in heart failure. The center line indicates the overall survival for patients with left ventricular failure (ALL). The patients with idiopathic dilated cardiomyopathy cardiomyopathy (IDC), represented in the upper line, did somewhat better. The poorest outlook by far was had by the patients with coronary artery disease (CAD) as the cause of their myopathy, who manifested only 20% 3-year survival.*

From Reference 1, with permission.

therapy with ACE-inhibition and β-blockade may have rendered some improvement in outlook, most authorities agree that the impact has been small and that this continues to be a lethal disease.[5,6]

In the 1990's, a number of centers began to develop and publish organized clinical experience with coronary artery bypass grafting in advanced left ventricular dysfunction. These investigators and centers included Laks and colleagues at UCLA, Kron et al at the University of Virginia, Mickelborough at Toronto, Rose and colleagues at Columbia, Dreyfus in France, and our own group at Yale University, as well as others (Table 1).[7-19] The findings at these various centers with a concentrated interest in this subject are largely consonant. This chapter will review our own findings at Yale University in a relatively large group of patients undergoing CABG for advanced ischemic cardiomyopathy. Where there is discordance in findings or recommendations between our institution and the distinguished teams listed above, the data from the other centers will be emphasized specifically.

The questions to be addressed include:
--What is the mortality risk of CABG in advanced left ventricular dysfunction?
--What technical principles underlie the safe peri-operative management of low EF patient?
--What, if any, improvements in symptomatic state can be achieved, for angina or for congestive heart failure (CHF)?
--What, if any, improvement in EF can be documented objectively?
--What is the long-term survival after low-EF CABG?

Table 1. Secected studies of CABG in low EF from the present decade

Author (Date)	# of patients	EF (%) (range)	EF (%) (mean)	Hospital Mortality	Mean Followup	Post-Op EF (%)	Survival 1 yr	3 yr	5 yr	Comments
Louie (1991)	22	<30%	23%	13.6%	12	36%	72%	72%	–	Prefer EF > 20; LVEDD < 70mm
Christakis (1992)	487	≤20%	–	9.8%	–	–	–	–	–	
Lansman (1993)	42	≤ 20%	15.7%	4.8%		22.6%	88%	68%	57%	
Luciani (1993)	20	<30%	22%	20%	34	42%	80%	80%	80%	
Milano (1993)	118	≤ 25%		11%	–	27%	77%		57%	
Langenberg (1995)	96	≤ 25%	20%	8%	–	–	–	–		Poor distal targets are contraindication
Mickelborough (1995)	79	≤ 20%	18%	3.8%	44		94%	78%	68%	
Shapira (1995)	74	≤30%	23.5%	–	65	35.7%	96	91	86	Only hospital survivors tabulated
Kaul (1996)	210	≤ 20%		10%	43		82%	79%	73%	Many exclusion factors
Chan (1996)	57	≤ 35%	28%	1.7%	40	30%	86%	80%	73%	Thallium predicts EF improvement
Hausmann (1997)	514	≤ 30%	23.8%	7.1%	24	39%	?	?	?	Only patients with demonstrated ischemia operated
Radovanovic (1998)	120	≤20%	–	7%	36	–	83%	72%	58%	Extensive use of coronary enderterectomy
Elefteriades (1998)	188	≤ 30%	23.5%	5.3%	49	33.2%	86%	75%	60%	Late EF at 5Y: 31.7%

--What happens to EF long-term after CABG? Is it sustained or is there an inexorable decrement?

--What insights regarding pre-operative myocardial viability assessment can be drawn from the surgical experience?

--What are appropriate guidelines for patient selection?

The Yale Experience

At Yale University, we have taken an aggressive approach by widely applying myocardial revascularization for patients with advanced ischemic cardiomyopathy. Our group at Yale University has carefully studied a series of patients undergoing surgical revascularization for advanced left ventricular dysfunction operated by one surgeon (JAE). [4,5] We used 30% as our upper limit for EF in this series. Only patients who had a precise, objective, numerical determination of EF pre-operatively by ventriculography or equilibrium radionuclide angiocardiography (ERNA) were included. No "eyeball" estimates of EF were accepted, so as to allow precise comparison of pre- and post-operative ventricular function. Patients having concomitant valve replacement or left ventricular aneurysmectomy were purposely excluded in order to evaluate a homogeneous patient group.

There were 188 patients (156 M, 32 F) and the age ranged from 42 to 84 years, with a mean of 67. 75% of patients had angina and two-thirds had congestive heart failure, with one quarter manifesting frank pulmonary edema. One quarter had a prior history of significant ventricular arrhythmia. One quarter were already requiring ICU care at the time of CABG. EF ranged from 10 to 30%, with a mean of 23.3%. Two-thirds of the patients had EF at or below 25%. Follow-up ranged from 1 month to 12 years, with a mean of 40.4 months. Follow-up was 86.2% complete at 12 years.

Regarding the technical conduct of the operation, we followed the following principles and procedures.

--Despite concerns in the literature, we did utilize the internal mammary artery (IMA) routinely. The concerns that the initial mammary flow would be insufficient for these weak hearts, or that weak hearts would need inotropic support drugs which could cause mammary constriction, were simply not borne out. The IMA was utilized in 88% of all patients.

--The intra-aortic balloon pump (IABP) was used liberally for peri-operative support. Many of the patients were already on the balloon for therapeutic reasons, for angina or pump failure. We also utilized the IABP prophylactically on a selective basis to protect patients peri-operatively. The IABP is, of course, the only support measure that augments myocardial function without increasing oxygen demand. Evidence is mounting that such support is far more beneficial than "flogging" the heart with drugs to wean from bypass. [20-24] Our group believes strongly that much is lost if the IABP is placed only after such damaging unsuccessful attempts to wean from the heart-lung machine.

--We limited grafts to major vessels of adequate size to sustain long-term patency. The number of grafts ranged from 1 to 5, with a mean of 3. We did not "chase" small, diseased vessels unlikely to sustain patency, as these weak hearts do not tolerate unnecessary ischemia well.

--We did not use any special or complex cardioplegic measures. These procedures were done with cold, crystalloid cardioplegia given antegrade into the aortic root. Proximal anastomoses were done under side-biting control of the aorta after removal of the aortic cross-clamp.

--We pursued electrophysiologic studies vigorously when pre-operative or peri-operative arrhythmic events were observed or suspected. We believe that the implantable cardioverter-defibrillator (ICD) may play a very important role in sustaining life in the long-term future for such low EF coronary patients.

There were no peri-operative Q wave MI's. Many patients, of course, had pre-existing anterior or inferior Q-waves. The first 75 patients underwent CK-MB determinations post-operatively, and there were no subendocardial MI's. CK determinations were discontinued after that time for cost savings.

There were no deaths in the operating room and the operative mortality (30 day) was 10 of 188, or 5.3%. For patients not in ICU at the time of acceptance for CABG, mortality was 4 of 141, or 2.8%.

What symptomatic benefit was gleaned? Angina was essentially eliminated, going from class 3.2 pre-operatively to class 1.1 post-operatively. This was expected. We did not know what to expect in terms of CHF symptomatology. In fact, CHF improved dramatically, going from class 3.1 pre-operatively to class 1.4 post-operatively.

An important question has to do with how many of these patients went on to require transplantation. Only 2 of 188 patients, or 1.1%, required a heart transplant in long-term follow-up.

The EF improved dramatically, from a mean of 23.3% pre-operatively to 33.2% post-operatively (Figure 2.) This improvement represents an increase of 10 EF points

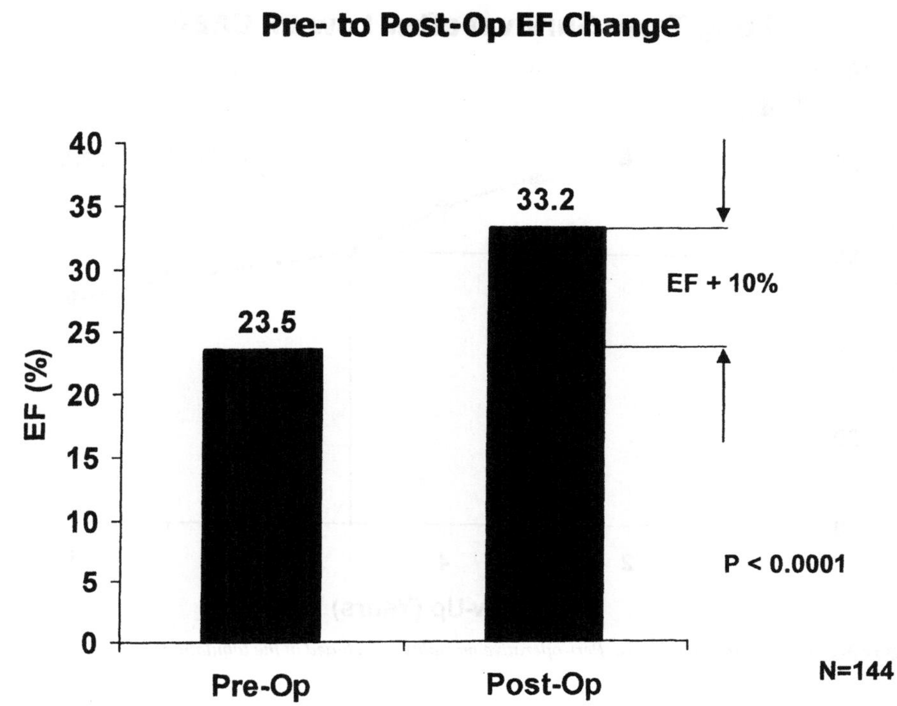

Figure 2. *Improvement in EF in the Yale series*

above the pre-op value--an improvement of 40% in function above the baseline level. This change is not only highly significant statistically--at the level of $p < 0.0001$--but also large enough to be of major physiologic importance.

The long-term survival is presented in Figure 3. The data is robust enough in number of patients and length of follow-up to yield reliable five-year data with small standard deviation. Five-year follow-up is essentially an "eternity" for these patients, in the context of their expected medical longevity. The survival for our low EF CABG patients at 3 years is 80%. At five years, the survival is 60%. These figures *include* the post-operative mortality. These survival rates far exceed the expected medical outlook. We will put these rates further into perspective at the end of this chapter.

We brought back as many patients as possible for late EF re-determination by ERNA. We are not aware of other experience that examines the course of EF over time after low-EF CABG. Our early EF determinations had been done usually at one week to one month post-operatively. For the patients having re-determination of EF late post-op, the mean interval between CABG and late EF re-determination was 64.8 months. We were pleased to find that EF was indeed fully preserved at the improved level. For this subset of patients having late EF re-determination, pre-op EF was 23.1%, early post-op EF improved to 30.8%, and the very late re-determined EF was slightly higher, at 31.7%. This finding suggests continued benefit in function over time from revascularization of viable muscle.

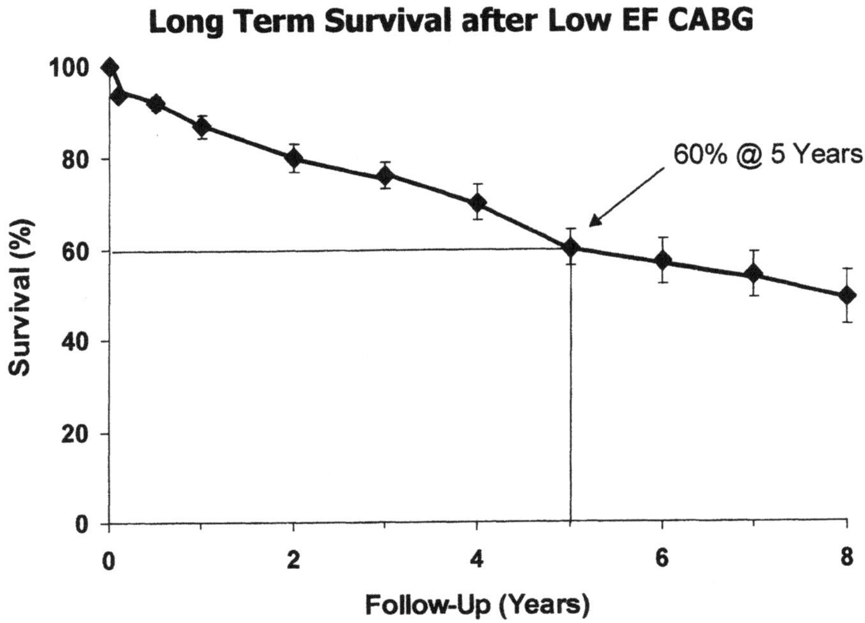

Figure 3. *Survival in the Yale series. Peri-operative mortality is included in the tabulations.*

The data from other interested centers is generally consonant with the Yale findings regarding many fundamental issues (Table 1). There is agreement that low EF patients can be operated relatively safely, that the measured ejection fraction generally improves, and that early to mid-term survival is adequate in the context of expectations for this category of patient. Our group's demonstration of good long-term survival and of maintenance of improved EF over the very long-term are additional findings encouraging aggressive application of CABG to the low EF patient.

Important questions in patient selection and management

We wish to analyze certain important questions in patient selection and management, emphasizing both the results from the literature as well as our own experience. Specifically, these questions are as follows:

Is clinical angina or objective evidence of ischemia essential for acceptance of the patient for operation? In careful studies, the UCLA, University of Virginia, the French group, and others have indeed demonstrated a beneficial impact of confirmed pre-operative ischemia, either in terms of clinical angina or documented ischemia by Thallium imaging, positron emission tomography, or echocardiography.[7,15,25-28] In particular, different groups have shown that patients who have evidence of ischemia do better in a number of ways: They have lower operative risk, they have better symptomatic improvement, they attain a larger EF improvement, and they achieve a better medium-term survival. Laks, Beller and colleagues at their insitutions have demonstrated the superiority of outcome of patients with evidence of viability convincingly and elegantly.

Nonetheless, our own group does not insist on angina or objective evidence of ischemia, for a number of reasons. We have found at our center no correlation between extent of ischemia on thallium imaging and EF improvement. (However, we have not pursued thallium imaging or positron emission tomography as fully or in as much detail in our patients as have Beller, Laks, and others.) Our series is unselected for angina or objective demonstrated evidence of viability, yet the overall results for operative risk, symptomatic improvement, EF improvement, and long-term survival are excellent. Furthermore, if the patient is not a transplant candidate, what else can be offered him other than revascularization? What else can be in his future besides further myocardial infarction from the uncorrected coronary blockages that got him to his condition of advanced ischemic cardiomyopathy? As revascularization can be offered at low operative risk, we feel it is indicated generally for patients with low EF and severe, proximal coronary artery disease, almost irrespective of clinical angina or objective manifestations of ischemia.

We offer two more points of evidence on this issue of a viability criterion. First, in our series, nearly all patients improved their EF, despite no application of a viability criterion. Figure 4 is a histogram of pre to post-op EF change. It can be seen that very few patients had any substantive decrease in EF post-operatively. Nearly all patients improved. Since restoration of function is the ultimate criterion for hibernation and viability, we take this to mean that nearly all patients have hibernating and viable infarct border zones, whether or not we can demonstrate them by viability imaging.

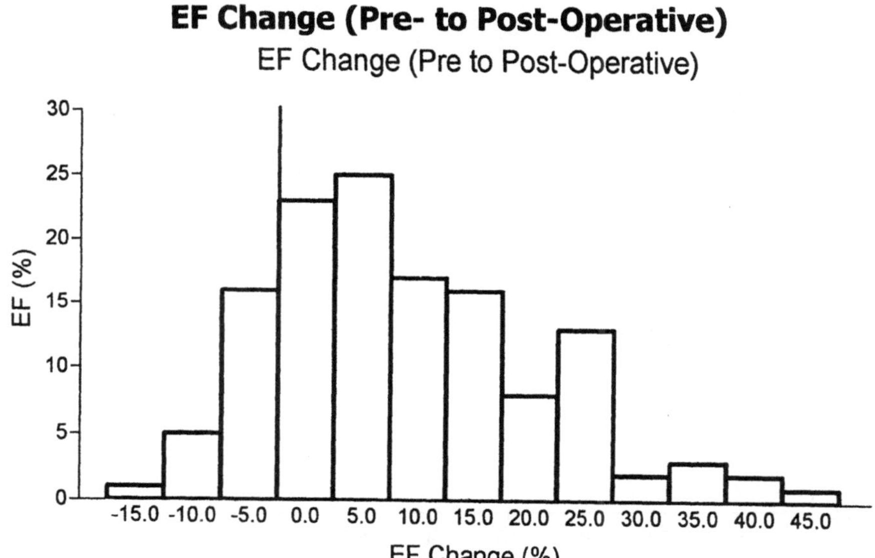

Figure 4. *Histogram of EF change. The number of patients is on the y-axis and the magnitude of EF changed on the x-axis. The line for zero EF change is indicated. It can be seen that very few patients had any substantive decrease in EF post-operatively.*

Further supporting an aggressive position (without insistence on demonstration of viability) is Figure 5, which compares survival curves for our patients who improved EF with those who did not. There was no significant difference in statistical comparison of these curves. This observation indicates that clinical benefit may accrue to these low EF patients after CABG even if "viability" was absent.

Is any ventricle too big, for low EF CABG? The UCLA group feels that operative candidates ideally should not exceed a left ventricular end-diastolic dimension (LVEDD) of 70 mm. At Yale, we do not feel that any ventricle is too big. We have accepted patients with ventricles up to 400 ml in size.

In fact, we divided our patients into two groups based on left ventricular size, "large" and "extra large". We used as our criterion a left ventricular end-systolic volume index (LVESVI) of 100 ml. The large group had LVESVI less than or equal to 100 and the extra large group exceeded 100. To give an idea of just how large these hearts are, an LVESVI of 100 in a patient with a BSA of 2 meters would give an LV end-systolic volume of 200 ml; if his EF is 30%, then his end-diastolic volume would be 300 ml. Thus our extra large group represents truly massive hearts. The extra large group had a lower EF than the large group, indicating more advanced ventricular dysfunction. However, even the extra large group did well with CABG surgery. Mortality was 4.1% and 4.3% respectively in the two groups. In fact, both the end-systolic and end-diastolic volumes came down with CABG, especially in the extra large group, indicating beneficial remodeling after revascularization.

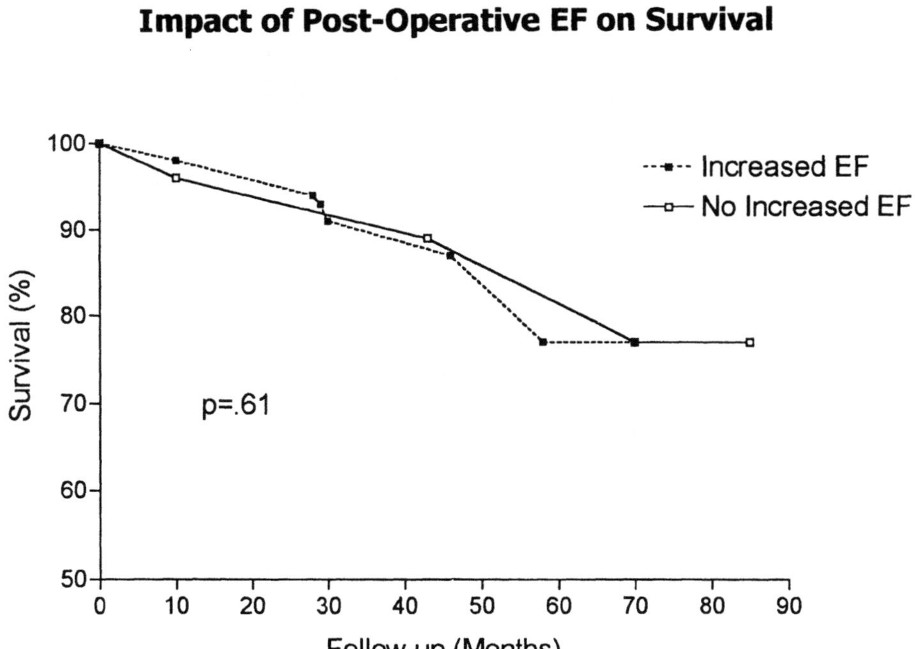

Figure 5. *Comparison of survival for patients who had increased and who did not have increased LV EF after low EF CABG. The two survival curves do not differ statistically. Only hospital survivors are tabulated.*

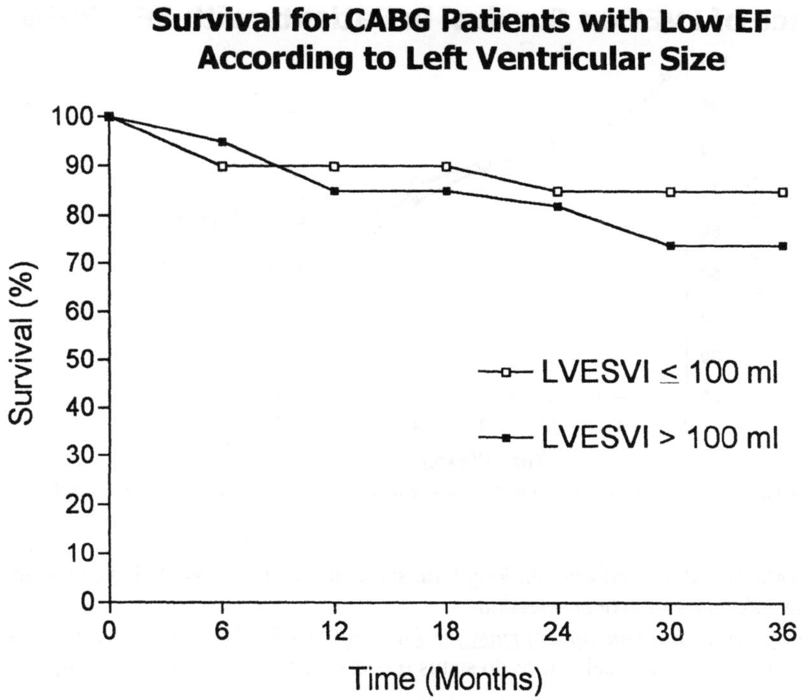

Figure 6. *Comparison of survival for patients with "large" (LVESVI ≤ 100 ml) and "extra large" (LVESVI > 100 ml) hearts. Only hospital survivors are tabulated.*

As Figure 6 indicates, even the "extra large" group had acceptable early and late survival, indistinguishable from that of the smaller group. For these reasons, we do not deny CABG based on ventricular size.

Is any EF too low? Our group, as well as the Kron group and the Mickelborough group, feel that no EF is too low.[13,29] The UCLA group prefers EF greater than 20%, which they have found to predict better outcome.[30]

Figure 7 compares survival in our patients with EF less than 20% to those with EF between 20 and 30%. There is no significant difference in long-term survival. This argues against denying surgery based on extreme depression of EF alone.

What other selection criteria may be important? We feel that right heart failure is an underappreciated and very important adverse risk factor. There is increasing emphasis in the general heart failure literature on right heart failure in patients with LV dysfunction. Associated right-sided failure has been found to be a powerful predicator of adverse outcome. Based on our own anecdotal impression of adverse outcome in the face of severe right heart failure, we undertook to investigate this factor specifically. We used RV EF on ERNA scan as our numerical indicator of right heart failure. We looked at early and late outcome after CABG in patients with RV EF > 40% and RV EF < 40%. Patients with right heart failure, manifest as RV EF less than 40%, had a markedly higher

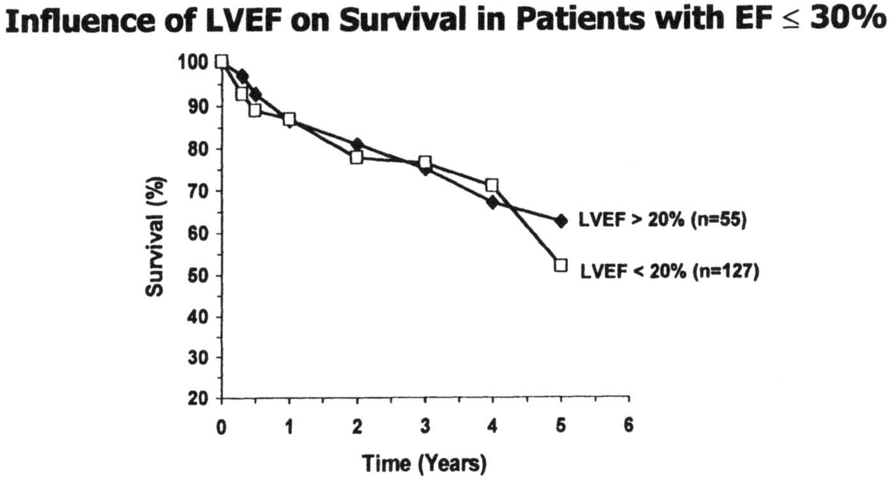

Figure 7. *Comparison of survival for patients with EF above and below 20%. Hospital mortality is included. There is no significant difference in survival.*

operative mortality and markedly poorer long-term survival (Figure 8). We believe that this an important risk factor in patient selection.

Are re-operative patients appropriate for low EF CABG? Both the University of Virginia group and our own feel that re-do status renders the low EF patient very high

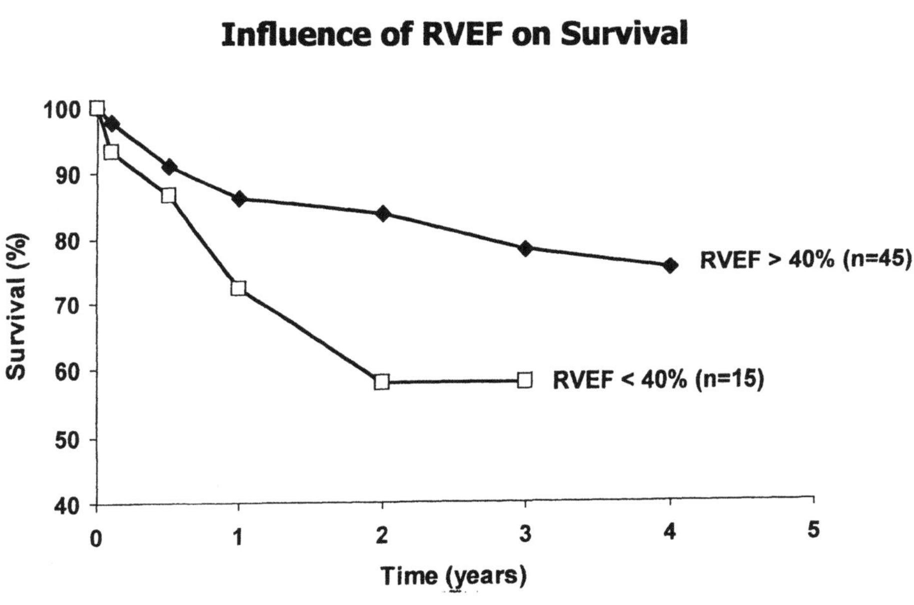

Figure 8. *Impact of right heart function on outcome after low EF CABG. Note higher early mortality and poorer long-term survival for the patients with right heart failure, manifested as RV EF < 40%. (The comparison of curves indicated a strong trend, but the number of patients with low RV EF was not large enough to achieve statistical significance.)*

risk for CABG.[31] Only 8% of our series represent re-do's. Many adverse events may accompany re-do CABG (despite experience and optimal technique), including graft atheroembolism. Unlike the patient with preserved function, the low EF patient does not have the margin to survive peri-operative myocardial infarction. In a precise statistical analysis, Kron and colleagues at University of Virginia found risk of peri-operative mortality to be a full 12% in their low EF re-do patients. We advise caution in accepting re-do patients for low EF CABG. Transplantation may be a better option.

Targets. There is general agreement among all centers on one additional selection criterion: In real estate, the important factor is "location, location, location". For low EF CABG, it is "targets, targets, targets". Without suitable distal sites at which to touch down, low EF CABG is not appropriate. The University of Virginia group have demonstrated this in a statistical analysis based on blinded re-reading of the pre-operative arteriograms.[12] Only Radovanovic, from Yugoslavia, encourages operation despite poor targets in low EF patients; he encourages extensive coronary endarterectomy for such patients.[32] Although his reported results are good, most authorities in this country shy away from this technique in advanced left ventricular dysfunction.

Presence of mitral regurgitation. We do not deny patients surgery on the basis of mild or moderate mitral insufficiency, which is quite common in these patients with advanced left ventricular dysfunction. Mitral insufficiency generally accompanies the process of left ventricular dilatation, which causes a shift in shape of the left ventricle from ovoid to spherical. We find that the severity of mitral insufficiency is often decreased by effective revascularization. The avoidance of direct surgery on the mitral valve in these patients is consistent with the approach of Carpentier, who has emphasized that a direct operative approach to the mitral valve in the low EF CABG patient adds to the extent of surgery and may remove a low-pressure left atrial decompression to which the weak left ventricle may have become accustomed. The excellent improvement in congestive heart failure realized in our Yale patients confirms that mitral regurgitation is not a problem in the long term after isolated coronary bypass in these patients. We do not address the mitral regurgitation surgically if it is ++ or +++, anticipating ameliorization after CABG, with its attendant beneficial effects on left ventricular *function* and, probably, *morphology* as well.

The ground-breaking work of Bolling is expanding the horizons of direct mitral valve surgery for the low EF patient.[33] His well-known series of low EF mitral valve repairs, however, excludes patients with concomitant CABG.

Clinical perspective: Low-EF CABG vs. Cardiac Transplantation

There is clearly overlap between the described series of low-EF patients undergoing CABG viv-a-vis those referred for cardiac transplantation for advanced ischemic cardiomyopathy. Kron eloquently discusses this issue in a key editorial.[34]

Several recent reports have addressed specifically the issue of conventional surgery as an alternative to heart transplantation. Sanchez, Louie, and Blakeman have each reported series of approximately 20 patients, referred initially for heart transplantation, who instead underwent "high-risk" conventional cardiac surgical procedures, mainly CABG.[35, 7, 36]

Reasonable functional status and survival were achieved. In an important study, Luciani and colleagues have attempted to compare outcomes for coronary revascularization with those for medical therapy and cardiac transplantation.[10] They identified 143 study patients with ischemic cardiomyopathy and an EF ≤ 30%. The medically treated patients fared the worst, with a 5-year survival of only 28%. The CABG patients had a relatively high operative mortality of 20% but achieved a 5-year survival of 80%. For transplantation, operative mortality was 11.6% and 5-year survival was 82%. Also, nineteen patients died waiting for transplantation. In terms of symptomatic state, the patients undergoing medical treatment deteriorated during treatment, the patients who underwent CABG improved somewhat, and the patients surviving heart transplantation achieved an excellent functional status. This report from Luciani and colleagues confirms the dismal survival with medical treatment alone and demonstrates that both CABG and transplantation can reasonably be considered for patients with advanced ischemic cardiomyopathy. Figure 9 presents the survival information from Luciani's series in graphic form. It must be borne in mind that despite the graphic representation, this was an observational study and not a randomized one.

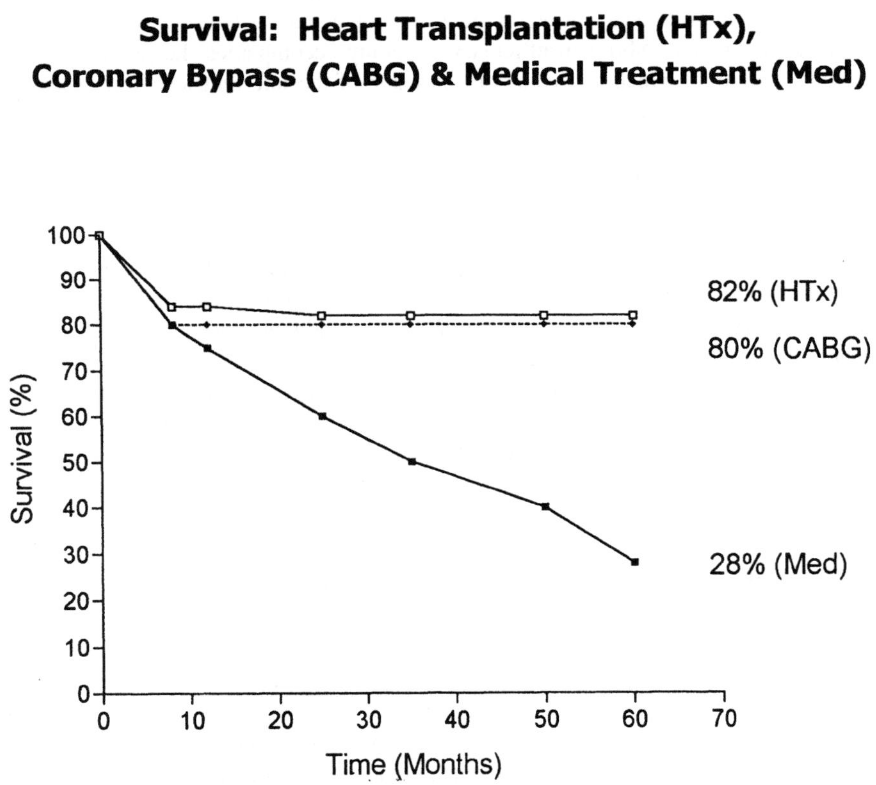

Figure 9. *Survival of patients with ischemic cardiomyopathy, treated by medications alone (dashed line, 72 patients), CABG (solid line, 20 patients), and transplantation (dotted line, 51 patients).*

From Reference 37, with permission.

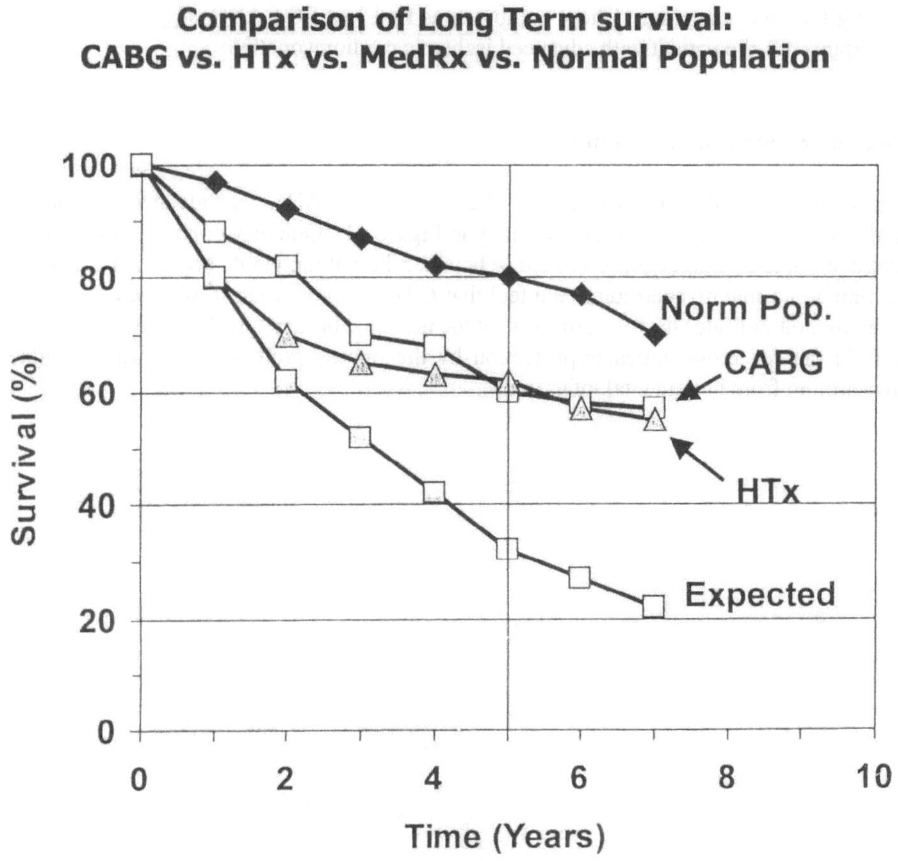

Figure 10. *Survival comparisons. The low EF CABG survival in the Yale series is compared to expected medical survival, survival after heart transplantation, and survival of an age and sex matched population. See text.*

Now, how do we put the long-term results in the low EF CABG patient discussed in this chapter further into clinical perspective? Figure 10 provides pertinent comparisons using long-term survival for our Yale low EF CABG patients. For comparison, the expected medical survival from Cohn's data is drawn. Also shown is the expected survival of an age and sex matched "normal" population. (A group of patients which is three-fourths male and sixty-seven years of age at onset dies at 4 to 5 percent per year normally.) Also drawn is the overall survival following heart transplantation in all patients from the International Heart Transplant Registry. One can see that the CABG survival far exceeds the expected medical survival. The survival curve after CABG is, in fact, lower than but essentially parallel to that of the normal population. Most importantly, the survival after low EF CABG is identical to that after transplantation--60% at 5 years. One must keep in mind also that the average transplant patient is much younger than our patients and that 15% of patients die waiting for transplantation. These comparisons find low EF CABG of great utility and importance for the patient with advanced ischemic cardiomyopathy.

Unifying Hypotheses and Summary

Our concept of the mechanisms of benefit from CABG in advanced ischemic cardiomyopathy is illustrated schematically in Figure 11. One may conceptualize (a) the central completed infarct zone, (b) the ischemic, hibernating, viable border zone, and (c) the remote normal myocardium. We feel that CABG is important in two ways: (1) the lightning bolt indicates the "reanimation" of the ischemic border zone by revascularization, and (2) the red cross indicates protection by the bypass grafts of the normal remote myocardium from incremental infarction.

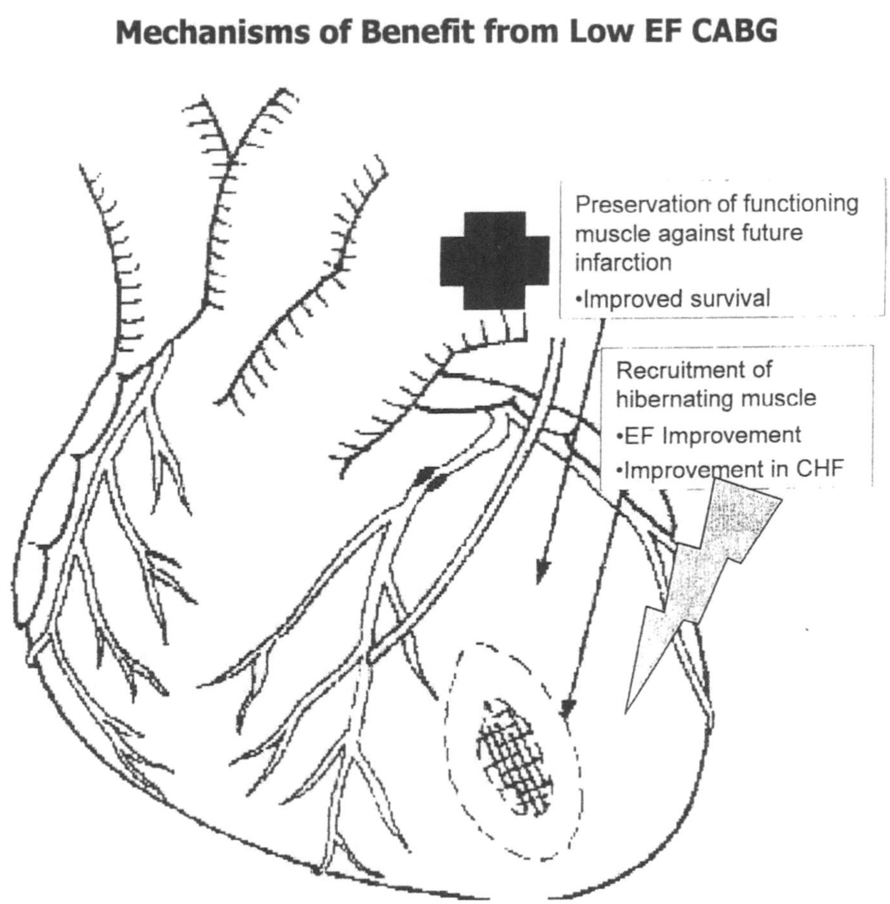

Figure 11. *Schematic presentation of proposed mechanisms of benefit from low EF CABG. See text.*

The unifying hypothesis is as follows. The recruitment of hibernating myocardium underlies the improvement in EF and improvement in symptomatic state consequent to CABG. The protection of viable myocardium from incremental infarction underlies the improvement in survival.

In summary, then, our experience (and that of others) with CABG in advanced ischemic cardiomyopathy has shown that:

--CABG can be performed safely. The overall mortality at our center was 5.3%. The figure of 2.8% mortality for our non-ICU patients more accurately represents the risk that should be considered in counseling the semi-elective patient being seen in one's office.

--Dramatic symptomatic improvement is realized, both in angina and in CHF status.

--Objective improvement in EF is powerfully demonstrated.

--The improvement in EF is durable over the very long-term.

--Excellent long-term survival is confirmed.

We feel that CABG should be applied aggressively to patients with severe, proximal coronary artery disease and severely depressed left ventricular function. We feel these patients need the operation much more than those with preserved EF, who can "take another myocardial hit" without mortal outcome.

We feel that CABG restores function to hibernating myocardial segments and represents a valuable alternative to heart transplantation in the patient with advanced ischemic cardiomyopathy.

References

1. CASS Principal Investigators. Coronary Artery Surgery Study (CASS): A randomized trial of coronary artery bypass surgery. Survival data. Circulation 1983;68:939-50.
2. European Coronary Surgery Study Group. Long-term results of prospective randomized study or coronary artery bypass surgery in stable angina pectoris. Lancet 1982;2:1173-80.
3. Rahimtoola SH. The hibernating myocardium. Am Heart J 1989; 117:211-3.
4. Franciosa JA, Wilen M, Ziesche S, et al. Survival in men with severe chronic left ventricular failure due to either coronary heart disease or idiopathic dilated cardiomyopathy. Am J Cardiol 1983;51:831-6.
5. Kannel WB. Epidemiological aspects of heart failure. Cardiol Clin 1989;7:1-9.
6. Guidelines for the evaluation and management of heart failure. Report of the American College of Cardiology/American Heart Association Task Force on Practice Guidelines. J Am Coll Cardiol 1995;26:1376-98.
7. Louie HW, Laks H, Milgalter E, et al. Ischemic cardiomyopathy: Criteria for coronary revascularization and cardiac transplantation. Circulation 1991;84[Suppl III]:III-290-III-295.
8. Christakis GT, Weisel RD, Fremes SE, et al. Coronary artery bypass grafting in patients with poor ventricular function. J Thoracic Cardiovasc Surg 1992;103:1083-92.
9. Lansman SL, Cohen M, Galla JD, et al. Coronary bypass with ejection fraction of 0.20 or less using centigrade cardioplegia: Long-term follow-up. Ann Thorac Surg 1993;56:480-6.
10. Luciani GB, Faggian G, Razzolini R, et al. Severe ischemic vantricular failure: Coronary operation or heart transplantation? Ann Thorac Surg 1993;55:719-23.
11. Milano CA, White WD, Smith LR, et al. Coronary artery bypass in patients with severely depressed ventricular function. Ann Thorac Surg 1993;56:487-93.
12. Langenberg SE, Buchanan SA, Blackbourne LH, et al. Predicting survival after coronary revascularization for ischemic cardiomyopathy. Ann Thorac Surg 1995;60:1193-7.
13. Mickelborough LL, Maruyama H, Takagi Y, et al. Results of revascularization in patients with severe left ventricular dysfunction. Circulation 1995;92[Suppl II]:II-73-II-79.
14. Kaul TK, Agnihotri A, Fields B, et al. Coronary artery bypass grafting in patients with an ejection fraction of twenty percent or less. J Thorac Cardiovasc Surg 1996;111:1001-12.
15. Chan RK, Raman J, Lee KJ, et al. Prediction of outcome after revascularization in patients with poor left ventricular function. Ann Thorac Surg 1996;61:1428-34.
16. Hausmann H, Topp H, Siniawski H, Holz S, Hetzer R. Decision-making in end-stage coronary artery disease: revascularization or heart transplantation? Ann Thorac Surg 1997;64:1296-302.
17. Shapira I, Isakov A, Yakirevich V, Topilsky M. Long-term results of coronary artery bypass surgery in patients with severely depressed left ventricular function. Chest 1995;108:1546-50.
18. Elefteriades JA, Morales DLS, Gradel C, et al. Results of coronary artery bypass grafting by a single surgeon in patients with left ventricular ejection fractions $\leq$ 30%. Am J Cardiol 1997;79:1573-8.
19. Elefteriades JA, Yepremyan M, Samady H, et al. Coronary Revascularization Outcomes. Plenary Sesion VII. 71st Annual Meeting of the American Heart Association, Dallas TX, November, 1998.
20. Elefteriades JA, Tolis G Jr, Levi E, et al. Coronary artery bypass grafting in severe left ventricular dysfunction: Excellent survival with improved ejection fraction and functional state. J Am Coll Cardiol 1993;22:1411-7
21. Dietl CA, Berkheimer MD, Woods EL, et al. Efficacy and cost-effectiveness of preoperative IABP in patients with ejection fraction of 0.25 or less. Ann Thorac Surg 1996;62:401-9.
22. Christenson JT, Badel P, Simonet F, Schmuziger M. Preoperative intraaortic balloon pump enhances cardiac performance and improves the outcome of redo CABG. Ann Thorac Surg1997;64:1237-44.
23. Christenson JT, Simonet F, Badel P, Schmuziger M. Evaluation of preoperative intra-aortic balloon pump support in high risk coronary patients. Eur J Cardiothorac Surg1997;11:1097-104.
24. Baumgartner FJ, Omari BO, Goldberg S, et al. Coronary artery bypass grafting in patients with profound ventricular dysfunction. Tex Heart Inst J 1998;25:125-9.
25. Beller GA. Assessing prognosis by means of radionuclide perfusion imaging: What technique and which variables should be used: J Am Coll Cardiol 1998;31:1286-90.
26. Di Carli MF, Asgarzadie F, Schelbert HR, et al. Quantitative relation between myocardial viability and improvement in heart failure symptoms after revascularization in patients with ischemic cardiomyopathy. Circulation 1995;92:3436-44.
27. Dreyfus G, Duboc D, Blasco A, et al. Cororary surgery can be an alternative to heart transplantation in selected patients with end-stage ischemic heart disease. Eur J Cardiothorac Surg 1993;7:482-8.
28. Maddahi J, Blitz A, Phelps M, Laks H. The use of positron emission tomography imaging in the management

of patients with ischemic cardiomyopathy. Adv Card Surg 1996;7:163-88.

29. Kern JA, Kron IL. High-Risk Myocardial Revascularization. In: Rose EA, Stevenson LW (eds). Management of End-Stage Heart Disease. Lippincott-Raven. Philadelphia. 1998.
30. Blitz A, Scholl F, Laks H. Surgery for Chronic Heart Failure. In: Poole-Wilson PA, Colucci WS, Massie BM, Chatterjee K, Coats AJS (eds). Heart Failure, Churchill Livingstone. New York. 1997.
31. Kron IL, Cope JT, Baker LD, Spotnitz HM. The risks of reoperative coronry artery bypass in chronic ischemic cardiomyopathy: Results of the CABG Patch trial. Circulation 1997;96[Suppl II]:II-21-II-25.
32. Radovanovic N, Jakovljevic D. Long-term follow-up after different open-heart surgical procedures. In: Radovanovic N and Jakovljevic, New Approach and Methods for Evaluation of Results in Cardiac Surgery–A Research Study. Institute of Cardiovascular Diseases. Novi Sad, Yugoslavia, 1998.
33. Pagani FD, Bolling SF. Valve surgery in patients with severe left ventricular dysfunction. In: Rose EA, Stephenson LW (eds.). Management of End-Stage Heart Disease. Lippincott-Raven, Philadelphia. 1998.
34. Kron IL. When does one replace the heart in ischemic cardiomyopathy? Ann Thorac Surg 1993;55:581-3.
35. Sanchez JA, Smith CR, Drusin RE, et al. High-risk reparative surgery: A neglected alternative to heart transplantation. Circulation 1990;82 [Suppl IV]:302-5.
36. Blakeman BM, Pifarre R, Sullivan H, et al. High-risk heart surgery in the heart transplant candidate. J Heart Transplant 1990;9:468-72.
37. Chan RK, Raman J, Lee KJ, et al. Prediction of outcome after revascularization in patients with poor left ventricular function. Ann Thor Surg 1996;61:1428-34.

3. VALVE SURGERY FOR REGURGITANT LESIONS OF THE AORTIC OR MITRAL VALVES IN ADVANCED LEFT VENTRICULAR DYSFUNCTION

Robert O. Bonow and Roy G. Masters

Introduction

Cardiologists and cardiac surgeons frequently must decide when it is appropriate to offer early surgical intervention to prevent compromise of left ventricular function from regurgitant lesions of the aortic or mitral valve. Both aortic and mitral regurgitation place a volume load on the left ventricle leading to dilatation and eventually impairment of left ventricular systolic function. This chapter however deals with the opposite issue: that of late surgical intervention after deterioration of left ventricular systolic function has occurred and reached advanced levels. Important questions to consider include (1) whether surgical intervention is contraindicated once advanced left ventricular dysfunction has become established (2) whether the risks of surgery are too high in this setting and (3) whether, even after successful surgery, improvements in left ventricular function, symptoms, or survival can realistically be anticipated.

A word should also be said about the medical management of regurgitant lesions with left ventricular dysfunction. Vasodilators and angiotensin converting enzyme (ACE) inhibitors have become popular in the treatment of left ventricular volume overload on the premise that afterload reduction is theoretically reasonable as a means to decrease regurgitant volume and improve forward stroke volume. These should result in reductions in left ventricular end-diastolic volume and wall stress and preservation of systolic function. Data indeed suggest a possible role for nifedipine in favorably influencing the long-term natural history of asymptomatic patients with normal left ventricular systolic function by resulting in a more gradual rate of development of symptoms or ventricular dysfunction.[1, 2] These data, however, do not pertain to patients with symptoms related to advanced left ventricular dysfunction. Further there are no long-term studies of the effect of ACE inhibition on natural history. Therefore although of prognostic benefit in ventricular dysfunction due to ischemic heart disease, vasodilators and ACE inhibitors have no demonstrated benefit in patients who have severe, symptomatic left ventricular dysfunction from aortic or mitral insufficiency. Such treatment might be reasonable as preparation for surgical intervention but should not be considered as an alternative to either valve

Roy Masters (editor), Surgical Options for the Treatment of Heart Failure, 33-47.

replacement or valve repair. The natural history of these patients indicates a poor outcome without surgery, and valve replacement or repair is the only means of preventing progressive ventricular damage from the hemodynamic valvular lesion.

Aortic insufficiency

The principle that the severity of left ventricular dysfunction has a marked influence on survival after aortic valve replacement for regurgitant lesions was first established during the 1970s (Figure 1).[3] Since that time numerous authors have supported the same conclusion that the long-term survival and functional results after valve replacement is worse in patients with impaired left ventricular function than those with preserved left ventricular function.[3-7] Despite this it is important to recognize that in many patients the impaired left ventricular systolic function is potentially reversible. Hence, ventricular function, and consequently prognosis, may improve after valve replacement in some patients.[8] In such patients, left ventricular dysfunction arises from the inability of left ventricular hypertrophy and chamber dilatation, which are adequate to preserve systolic function in mild-to-moderate regurgitation, to compensate for the progressive increases

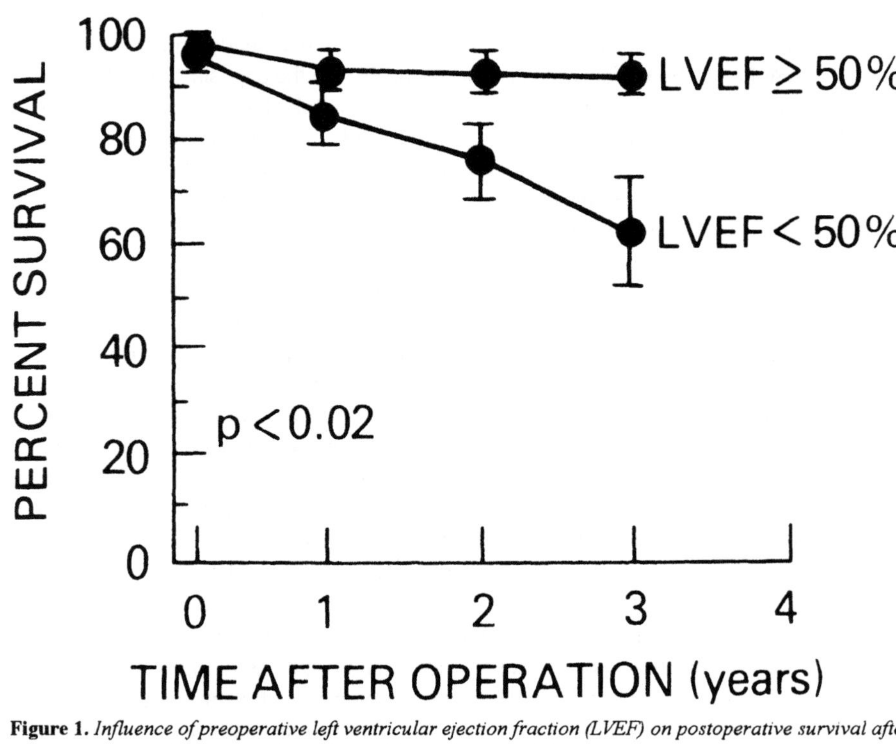

Figure 1. *Influence of preoperative left ventricular ejection fraction (LVEF) on postoperative survival after valve replacement in symptomatic patients with aortic regurgitation.*

(From Forman R, Firth BF, Barnard MS: Prognostic significance of preoperative left ventricular ejection fraction and valve lesion inpatients with aortic valve replacement. Am J Card 1980; 45:1120-1125. Page 122, Figure 1)

in afterload imposed by the regurgitant lesion. Depression of systolic function, owing predominantly to afterload mismatch, is a reversible process; prompt recognition and reversal of the volume overload by valve replacement can partially or completely restore ventricular volume and function to normal (Figure 2).[8-10]

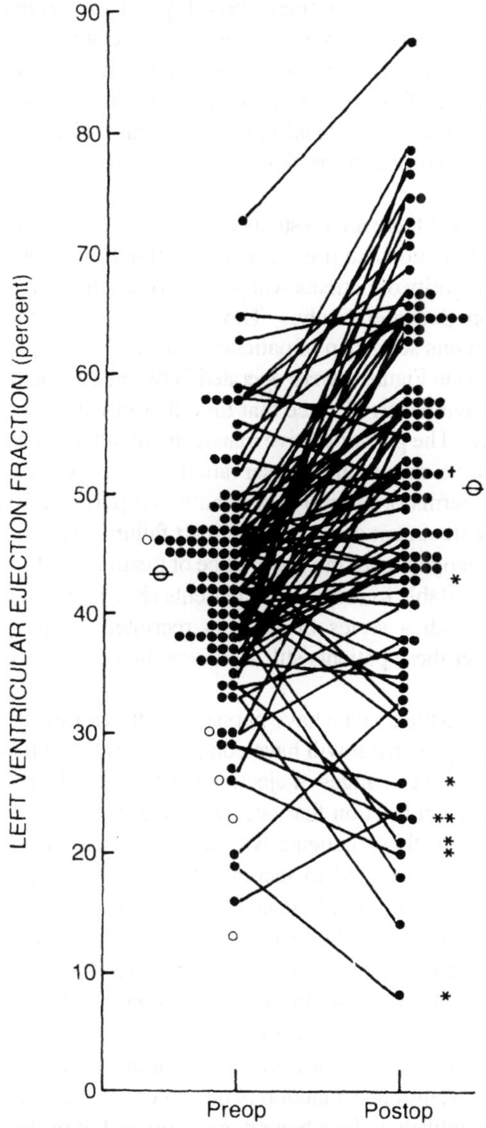

Figure 2. *Left ventricular ejection fraction at rest by radionuclide angiography before and after aortic valve replacement in 93 consecutive patients with chronic aortic regurgitation;* **open circles***: patients who died before their 6-month re-evaluation,* **asterisks***: patients who died from congestive heart failure after the 6-month study,* **cross***: one patient who died suddenly after the 6-month study.*

(From: Bonow RO: Radionuclide angiography in the management of aortic regurgitation. Circulation 1991;84(Suppl 1): I-296-302.Page I-297, Figure 1)

Although many patients in the current era undergo operation earlier in the natural history of their regurgitant lesions than previously, largely as a result of identification of appropriate noninvasive indicators of impending decompensation of the left ventricle, many patients still come to medical attention late, with advanced left ventricular dysfunction.[11-16] The concern with these patients is that some component, possibly a large component, of the left ventricular dysfunction at such a late stage may reflect an irreversible condition having made the transition to permanent myocardial disease which can no longer respond favorably to the correction in volume overload following surgery. By correcting the loading abnormality surgery may still have a beneficial clinical effect, but ventricular function may remain severely depressed with persistent heart failure and its adverse consequences on late survival (Figure 2).[8]

It is important to note that there are no studies which specifically focus on patients with severe left ventricular dysfunction and preoperative ejection fraction as low as 30%. It is clear, however, that the majority of patients with severe ventricular dysfunction show little improvement in function postoperatively. Those patients with the greatest risk of postoperative death are in this subgroup of patients (Figure 2).

The patients illustrated in Figure 2 were operated between 1978 and 1988.[8] A number of significant advances have occurred since that time that might alter the findings if this study were repeated today. The peri-operative management of these patients including the techniques of intraoperative myocardial preservation have improved. This may have beneficial effects both in terms of operative mortality and perioperative preservation of ventricular function. The treatment of congestive heart failure has improved dramatically as well, especially in the recognition of the importance of treatment with afterload reduction. This treatment was not available to many of the patients shown in Figure 2. Although the postoperative course of such a series of patients recruited in the present era could conceivably be much better these patients still represent the highest risk group of patients with aortic regurgitation.

It is also apparent that patients who have persistent left ventricular dysfunction 6 to 8 months after aortic valve replacement will have continued dysfunction during longer-term follow-up.[17] Late postoperative changes in ejection fraction are clearly influenced by the directional changes in ejection fraction that occurr during the first 6 months after valve replacement (Figure 3).[17] In those patients with an early increase in ejection fraction, ventricular systolic function continued to increase further with long-term follow-up. However those patients who manifested either no early improvement, or even an early decrement, in ventricular systolic function showed no improvement during the long-term follow-up period. Hence, late improvement in left ventricular function is rare in patients with persistent dysfunction at 6 to 8 months after operation, and this early postoperative assessment has important long-term prognostic implications in these individuals.

The identification of those patients with left ventricular dysfunction in whom substantial beneficial improvement in ventricular function is possible after valve replacement versus patients in whom there is unlikely to be a benefit is important but problematic. A number of factors influence both the survival and functional results after aortic valve replacement in patients with left ventricular dysfunction including (1) the severity of preoperative symptoms, (2) the severity of left ventricular dysfunction and (3) the duration of left ventricular dysfunction.[18,19] Pre-operative New York Heart Association functional class,

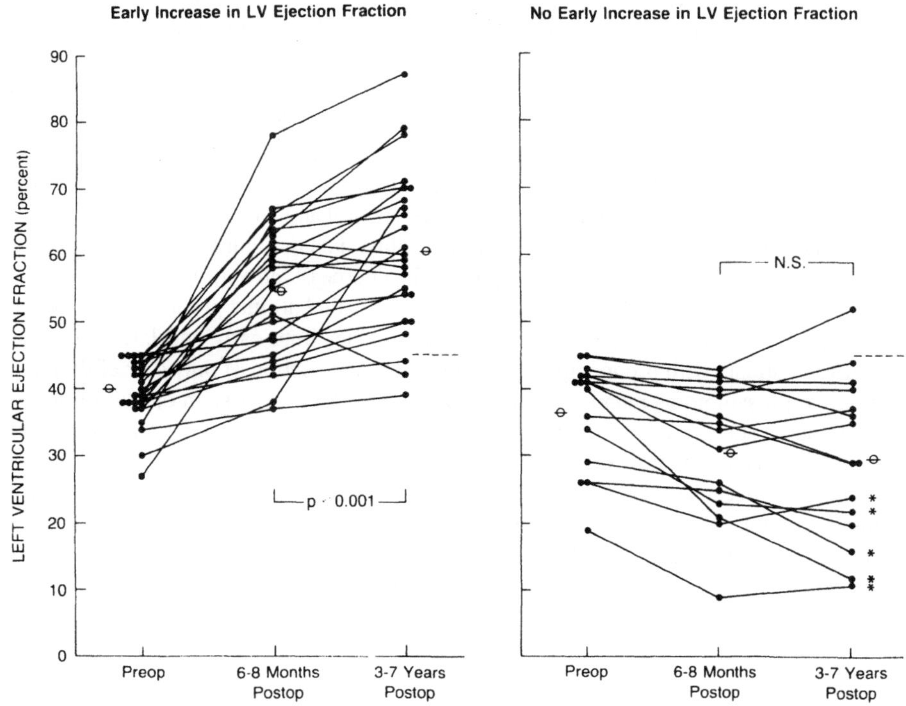

Figure 3. *Serial changes in left ventricular ejection in patients with decreased pre-operative ejection fractions before and after surgery.*

(From: Bonow RO, Dodd JT, Maron BJ, et al: Long-term serial changes in left ventricular function and reversal of ventricular dilatation after valve replacement for chronic aortic regurgitation. Circulation 1988; 78:1108-1120. Page 1113, Figure 3)

left ventricular end-systolic diameter and ejection have been shown to be significant determinants of long-term survival in multivariate analysis of 286 patients with aortic regurgitation.[18] Patients in New York Heart Association (NYHA) functional class III or IV have a worse outcome than patients with the same ejection fraction who is in functional class I or II. Similiarly the patient with an ejection fraction of 20% is probably at greater risk than the patient with an ejection fraction of 35%. By contrast a recent study of 175 patients with aortic regurgitation found that pre-operative ejection fraction but not diastolic dimension independently predicted late post-operative survival and post-operative ejection fraction.[19] These authors concluded that while extreme left ventricular dilation (≥80 mm) is frequently associated pre-operatively with a reduced ejection fraction it is not a marker of irreversible left ventricular dysfunction.[19] Finally the patient who is being followed carefully with noninvasive studies, which have previously shown preserved left ventricular function, who now demonstrates impaired systolic function and who is then operated on expeditiously is likely to show rebound in systolic function. One year of decreased function is an approximate time limit below which improvement in function can fairly be predicted.[20] In contrast, patients with aortic insufficiency and severe left ventricular dysfunction extending 18 months or longer likely have irreversible ventricular dysfunction. Further, the influence of these three factors, functional class, level of ventricular dysfunction and duration of dysfunction, is additive. For example, a patient with NYHA class IV symptoms who is operated on relatively early, when ejection fraction has fallen only to 35%, may still improve despite the advanced preoperative symptomatic state. The patients with severe symptoms, severe impairment of systolic function, and prolonged duration of dysfunction are at the greatest risk of having irreversible ventricular dysfunction and an inexorable process.

The influence of these three factors is further illustrated in Figure 4, which represents a continuum based on the severity of symptoms, the degree of left ventricular function and the duration of left ventricular dysfunction.[17] Patients with a normal preoperative ejection fraction have significantly higher ejection fraction values both early and late after their operation. Patients with preoperative left ventricular dysfunction of only a brief duration with only mild symptoms manifest a striking and significant increase in ejection fraction after operation, achieving levels that are identical to those achieved postoperatively in those patients who had a normal preoperative ejections fraction. Clearly this is a low-risk group, predominantly because they are identified early. Patients who have either more severe symptoms or left ventricular dysfunction of a longer duration are at greatest risk for persistent left ventricular dysfunction after valve replacement. In those patients improvements in post-operative ejection fraction cannot be predicted (Figure 4).[17]

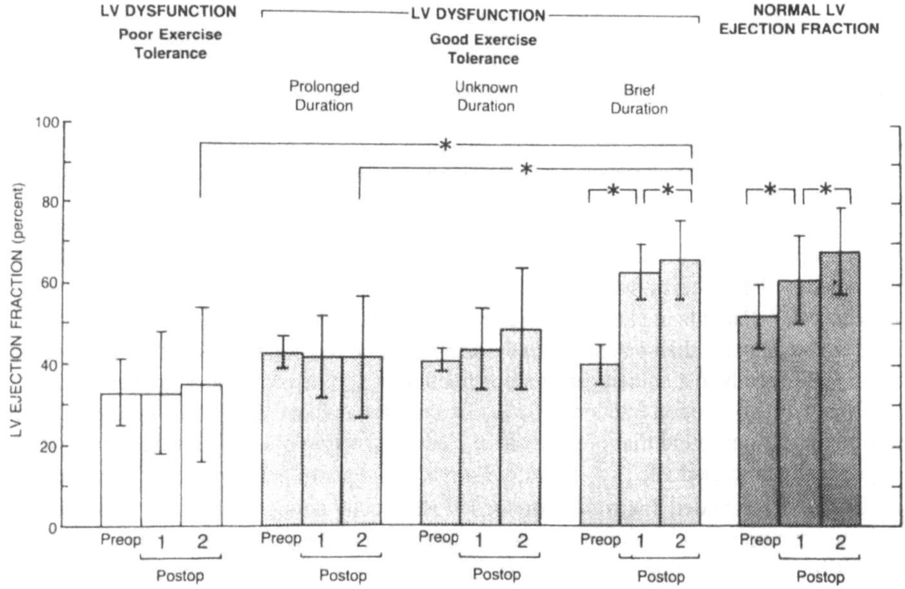

Figure 4. *Left ventricular ejection fraction at rest before and after aortic valve replacement in patients with normal pre-operative left ventricular ejection fraction and in patients with pre-operative left ventricular dysfunction who are subgrouped on the basis of symptom severity and duration of ventricular dysfunction.*

(From: Bonow RO, Dodd JT, Maron BJ, et al: Long-term serial changes in left ventricular function and reversal of ventricular dilatation after valve replacement for chronic aortic regurgitation. Circulation 1988; 78:1108-1120. Page 1116, Figure 6)

In the majority of patients, the increase in ejection fraction after valve replacement is parallelled by reduction in echocardiographic end-diastolic dimension (Figure 5).[17] With surgery, left ventricular end-diastolic dimension decreases markedly in the lower-risk patient groups; those with a normal pre-operative ejection fraction or with left ventricular dysfunction of only a brief duration with only mild symptoms. Left ventricular end-diastolic dimension is not reduced as favorably in the patients with left ventricular dysfunction who have either more severe symptoms or more prolonged duration of left ventricular dysfunction.[17]

Similar to post-operative ejection fraction, the post-operative end-diastolic dimension does not change appreciably from early to late postoperative determinations. There is rarely a gradual improvement in ventricular diastolic dimension; little change occurs after the 6-month determination.[17] In fact, the postoperative change in diastolic dimension occurs largely within the first 2 weeks of surgery; whatever diastolic dimension is achieved at 2 weeks is likely to be maintained for the next 5 or 6 years.[17] Therefore the early postoperative determinations are of important prognostic significance.

Thus, in patients with preoperative left ventricular dysfunction, survival and improved left ventricular function are strongly related to the severity of symptoms, the severity of ventricular dysfunction, and the duration of ventricular dysfunction. Patients with left ventricular dysfunction run a greater risk of irreversible dysfunction if surgery is delayed until more severe symptoms or more severe dysfunction develops. Consequently most investigators in the field would support the conclusion that even asymptomatic patients with aortic regurgitation and left ventricular dysfunction should undergo operation, before

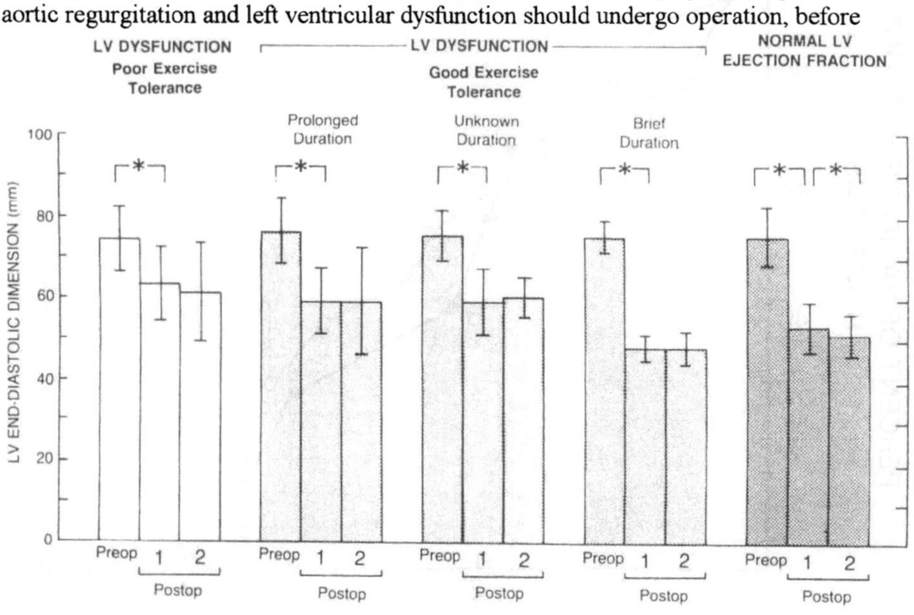

Figure 5. *Changes in left ventricular end-diastolic dimension by echocardiography in the same patients as in Figure 4.*

(From: Bonow RO, Dodd JT, Maron BJ, et al: Long-term serial changes in left ventricular function and reversal of ventricular dilatation after valve replacement for chronic aortic regurgitation. Circulation 1988; 78:1108-1120. Page 1117, Figure 7)

the onset of symptoms and limitation of exercise capacity. It is important to be aggressive in dealing with the patient who has evidence of left ventricular dysfunction from aortic insufficiency, and the most effective way to unload the left ventricle is with aortic valve replacement. This aggressive approach to operate on even asymptomatic patients with left ventricular dysfunction can be further justified by the available data that indicate that most patients with aortic regurgitation and left ventricular dysfunction develop symptoms within 2 to 3 years as indicated in Figure 6.[15, 18,19] There is not much gain in waiting and potentially much to lose, as the adverse prognostic factors of symptom severity and duration of dysfunction accumulate with time.

The other side of this issue is whether it is ever too late to operate. Are there patients with such severe left ventricular dysfunction from aortic insufficiency who, despite the presence of a surgically correctable valvular hemodynamic lesion, should not undergo operation because the likelihood of improvement is too low? This issue deserves careful analysis. The greater the left ventricular dysfunction and the greater the symptoms, the worse is the outcome. Without surgery, deterioration is even more inevitable, and the patient can be expected to have a poor outcome, with continued afterload mismatch, left ventricular dysfunction, and congestive heart failure. Despite overwhelming prospects of an adverse postoperative outcome based on preoperative prognostic risk factors, some

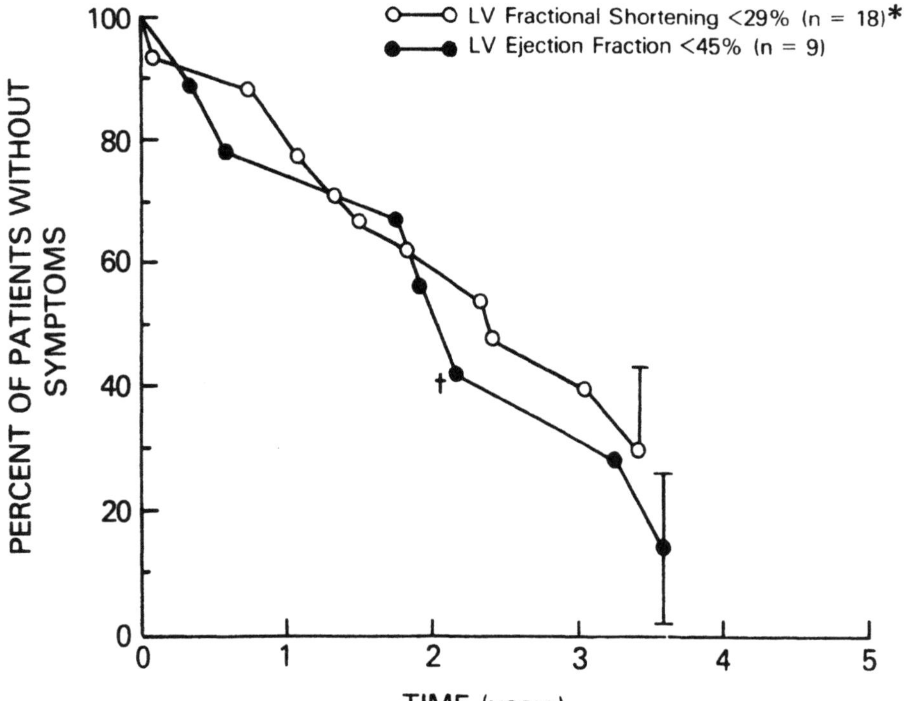

Figure 6. *Temporal relation in asymptomatic patients between left ventricular dysfunction and the onset of symptoms based on echocardiographic data* **(open circles)** *and radionuclide data* **(solid circles)**.

(From:Bonow RO: Radionuclide angiography in the management of aortic regurgitation. Circulation 1991; 84 (Suppl 1):I-296-302. Page I-299, Figure 3)

patients with severe left ventricular dysfunction do quite well, or at least better, with surgery. Aortic valve replacement decompresses the left ventricle and removes the afterload mismatch, improving the loading conditions that the ventricle will see in the future. A small minority of the patients in the high-risk group do better than anticipated, going on to a reasonable functional status and longevity. Age, other concomitant disease, and the wishes of the patient and family must be taken into account in these high-risk cases. Usually, in these advanced cases, one should operate. Although the lower the ejection fraction, the greater the risk, there is probably no definite threshold of ejection fraction below which it is definitely too late for valve replacement to be carried out. In the lowest ranges of ejection fraction, the issue does arise whether valve replacement should be the initial therapy or whether one should move to alternative therapies such as cardiac transplantation. In general, valve replacement should first be attempted. Valve replacement carries less of an economic and emotional burden for the patient. Although the operative mortality may be as high as 10% in this sub-group the patients usually do survive operation and can still undergo heart transplantation safely if heart failure continues or progresses.[6] The overall general recommendation is that it is never too late to make a trial of intervention with valve replacement in patients with left ventricular dysfunction arising from aortic insufficiency.[20]

Mitral insufficiency

The issues regarding the appropriate management of patients with mitral insufficiency and advanced left ventricular dysfunction are even more difficult than those associated with patients with aortic regurgitation. Left ventricular function is difficult to characterize in this setting because of the unloading effect of the regurgitation into the low-pressure left atrium. For the same degree of volume overload and increase in end-diastolic volume, patients with mitral regurgitation have reduced afterload compared with patients with aortic regurgitation.[21] Hence, virtually all measures of left ventricular systolic function tend to overestimate the true level of ventricular performance.

This problem is illustrated in the changes that occur in left ventricular ejection fraction in patients who undergo valve replacement for mitral insufficiency. In contrast to patients with aortic insufficiency, in whom ejection fraction generally improves after operation, with the exceptions noted previously, patients with mitral regurgitation generally show much higher ejection fractions before operation and a significant decline in ventricular function after operation (Figure 7), which can be striking in individual cases.[22-29]

Although ejection fraction overestimates true left ventricular systolic performance, it is important to emphasize that ejection fraction is one of the most important determinants of long-term survival after mitral valve surgery for mitral regurgitation.[18, 29, 30] Patients with normal preoperative ejection fraction have an excellent postoperative survival, whereas those with moderately to severely reduced ejection fraction are at considerable risk (Figure 8).[29]

The observation that conventional mitral valve replacement predisposes to deterioration of left ventricular systolic function in patients with normal preoperative

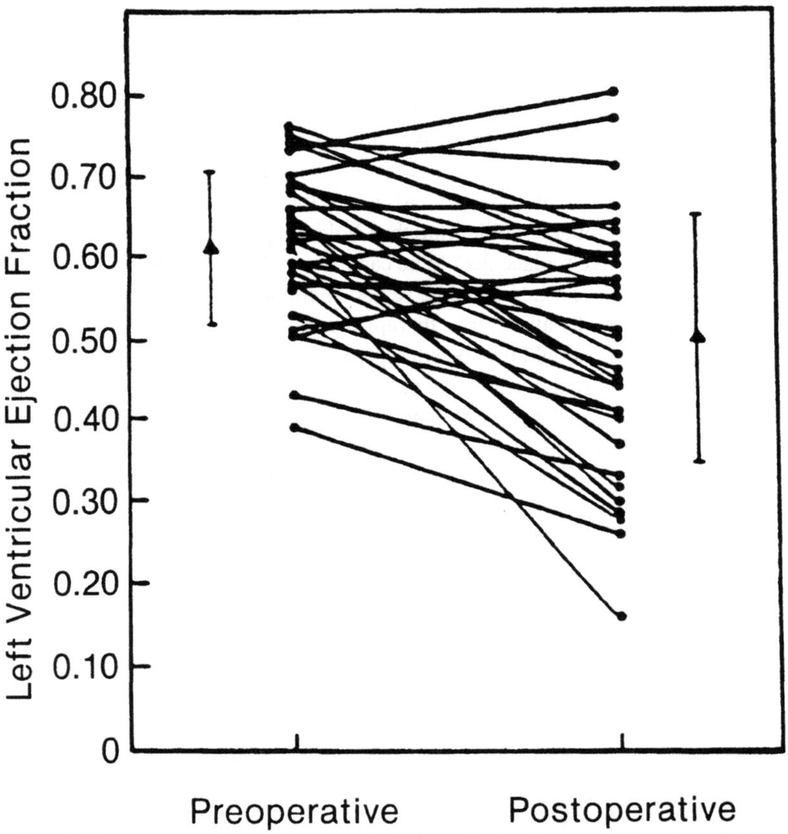

Figure 7. Individual pre-operative and post-operative left ventricular ejection fraction values in 34 patients who underwent multigated cardiac blood imaging 12 to 75 months after mitral valve replacement showing a mean decrease from .62±.009 to .50±.15 respectively.

(From: Phillips HR, Levine FH, Carter JE et al. Mitral valve replacement for isolated mitral regurgitation: Analysis of clinical course and late postoperative left ventricular ejection fraction. Am J Card 1981; 48:647-654. Page 651, Figure 3)

ejection fractions as well as those with low ejection fraction and dilated ventricles reflects complex physiologic and hemodynamic changes.[18, 22, 29] The exact mechanism of the postoperative depression of left ventricular performance still remains speculative despite the significant number of experimental and clinical studies.[31] The reduction of ejection fraction after mitral valve replacement develops in part from elimination of the low-pressure decompression of the left ventricle into the left atrium. Thus, valve replacement reduces preload and increases afterload, with resultant depression of ejection fraction.

Additional factors have come to light as appreciation has been gained for the importance of the mitral papillary apparatus in maintaining volume, geometry, and systolic performance of the left ventricle. This apparatus is disrupted in traditional mitral valve replacement with resection of the anterior and posterior leaflets. Lillehei and associates

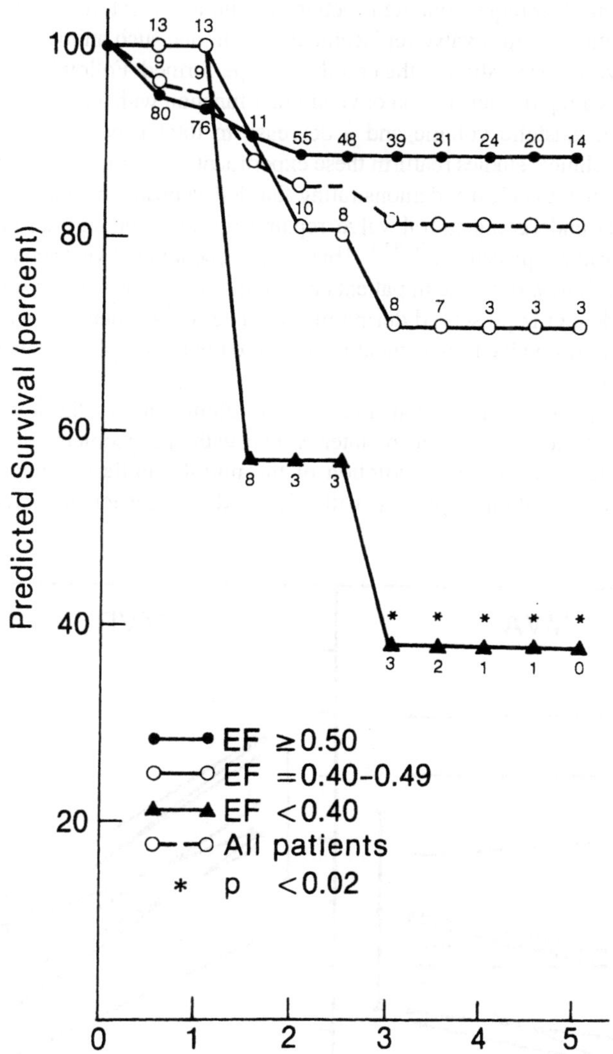

Figure 8. *Actuarial survival curves showing predicted survival following mitral valve replacement according to left ventricular fraction (EF).*

(From: Phillips HR, Levine FH, Carter JE et al. Mitral valve replacement for isolated mitral regurgitation: Analysis of clinical course and late postoperative left ventricular ejection fraction. Am J Card 1981; 48:647-654. Page 649, Figure 1)

first recognized the importance of preservation of the subvalvular apparatus.[32] Sarris and Miller supported the concept of the valvular-ventricular interaction and its importance in preserving systolic function postoperatively.[33] Experimentally within a few heartbeats of interruption of the papillary muscle apparatus there is an acute decrease in left ventricular function by approximately 30% with restoration to baseline when the chordae were reattached.[33] In keeping with these observations other experimental studies have confirmed that chordal-preserving techniques maintain better systolic and diastolic left ventricular function than conventional mitral valve replacement.[34-36] In one such animal study mitral valve replacement with preservation of the chordae was performed. Following division of the chordae there was a rapid deterioration of ventricular function with a decrease in stroke work, an increase in diastolic volume and a decrease in total generated mechan-ical energy.[34] Numerous clinical studies reaffirm these experimental findings of the importance of the subvalvular apparatus clearly demonstrating that left ventricular function is better preserved in patients undergoing mitral valve repair (Figure 9) or chordal-preserving techniques of mitral valve replacement.[26, 37-41] This improvement in left ventricular function translates into better clinical outcome in patients in whom mitral repair is performed or in whom the posterior leaflet is preserved during mitral valve replacement, versus those in whom conventional mitral valve replacement is performed with complete excision of the subvalvular apparatus.[39-45]

The issues of depression of ejection fraction from elimination of the low-pressure decompression into the left atrium and of interference with the geometry and systolic performance of the left ventricle by disruption of the mitral papillary apparatus enter strongly into the decision making in patients with advanced left ventricular dysfunction

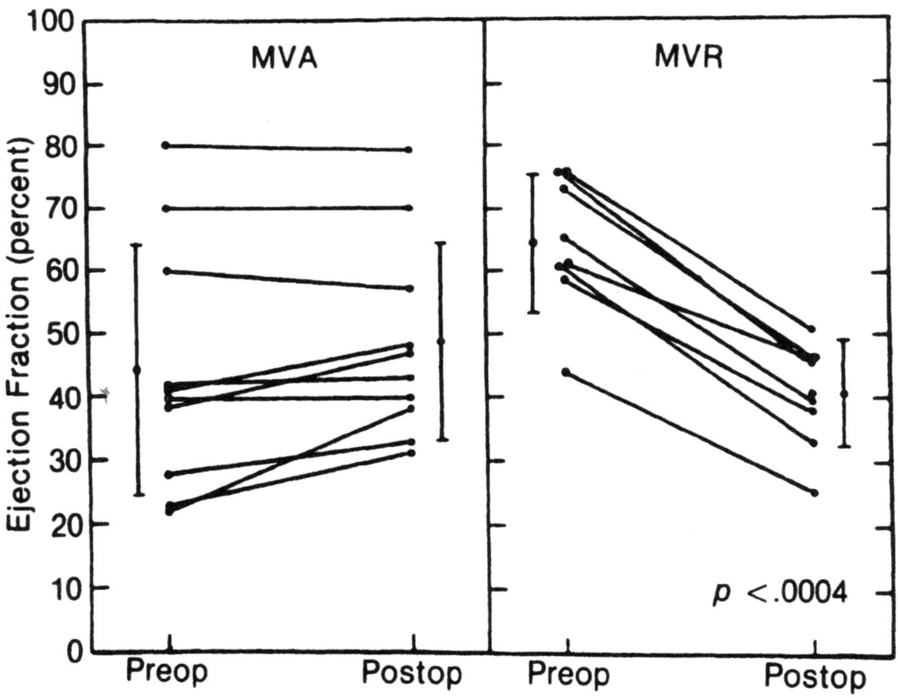

Figure 9. *Ventricular dysfunction following mitral valve repair (left) compared with mitral valve replacement (right).*

(From: Goldman ME, Mora F, Guarino T et al. Mitral valvuloplasty is superior to valve replacement for preservation of left ventricular function: An intraoperative two-dimensional echocardiographic study. J Am Coll Cardiol 1987: 10:568-575. Page 571, Figure 2)

and mitral regurgitation. Individual decisions depend in large part on which surgical procedure can be offered; preferably either valve repair or chordal-sparing valve replacement avoiding the disruption of the chordal apparatus.

The patient with moderate or severe impairment of contractile function may be at high risk for traditional valve replacement but do better over the long-term in terms of function and survival with a valve repair procedure or chordal-sparing replacement procedure. Among patients with severely depressed ventricular function, ventricular function does not appear to deteriorate further after valve repair (Figure 9).[38] However the data is limited on mitral valve surgery for patients with severe left ventricular dysfunction from chronic mitral regurgitation.

As with aortic regurgitation these considerations lead to the question of whether it is ever too late to operate for mitral valve regurgitation. In certain instances, the operative and postoperative risks may indeed be too great, particularly if the patient is not a candidate for a repair or chordal-sparing procedure - for specific anatomic or technical reasons. When the ejection fraction is below 25% or 30%, the risks may be truly prohibitive. Risk in this context refers not only to perioperative surgical mortality, but also to progressive long-term dysfunction and late mortality. If a repair or chordal-sparing procedure can technically be offered, a much lower threshold may be acceptable. The issue if often further complicated by the concomitant presence of coronary artery disease, in which case ischemia and hibernation may contribute to the left ventricular dysfunction. In such instances, revascularization in conjunction with valve surgery carries the potential for considerable improvement in left ventricular function from recruitment of dysfunctional ischemic muscle. Again, however, there are lower boundaries of function below which it may not be reasonable to operate as experience is small.

Summary

Patients with aortic regurgitation and severe left ventricular dysfunction remain candidates for aortic valve replacement, as long as the risks of late left ventricular dysfunction and congestive heart failure have been fully discussed with the patient, the patient's family, and the referring physician.

In contrast, patients with mitral regurgitation and severe systolic dysfunction are at considerable risk of more severe left ventricular dysfunction after operation, especially if mitral valve repair or chordal-sparing procedure cannot be performed. In patients who are candidates for such procedures that preserve the integrity of the subvalvular mitral apparatus, operation may be successful in selected patients despite moderate-to-severe depression of systolic function.

Prognosis is guarded to poor in patients with regurgitant valvular lesions and advanced left ventricular dysfunction, and the emerging alternative treatments discussed in other chapters in this book deserve consideration in these patients.

References

1. Bonow RO. Management of chronic aortic regurgitation. N Engl J Med 1994; 331:736-7.
2. Scognamiglio R, Rahimtoola S, Fasoli G et al. Nifedipine in asymptomatic patients with severe aortic regurgitation and normal left ventricular function. N Engl J Med 1994; 331:689-94.
3. Forman R, Firth BF, Barnard MS. Prognostic significance of pre-operative left ventriculaar ejection fraction and valve lesion in patients with aortic valve replacement. Am J Cardiol 1980; 45:1120-5.
4. Bonow RO, Picone AL, McIntosh CL et al. Survival and functional results after valve replacement for aortic regurgitation from 1976-1983: Impact of preoperative left ventricular function. Circulation 1985; 72:1244-56.
5. Cohn PF, Gorlin R, Cohn LH et al. Left ventricular ejection fraction as a prognostic guide in surgical treatment of coronary and valvular heart disease. Am J Cardiol 1974; 34:136-41.
6. Copeland JG, Griepp RB, Stinson EB et al. Long-term follow-up after isolated aortic valve replacement. J Thorac Cardiovasc Surg 1977; 74:875-89.
7. Greves J, Rahimtoola SH, McAnulty JH et al. Preoperative criteria predictive of late survival following valve replacement for severe aortic regurgitation. Am Heart J 1981; 101:300-8.
8. Bonow RO: Radionuclide angiography in the management of aortic regurgitation. Circulation 1991; 84 (Suppl 1):I-296-302.
9. Ross J Jr. Afterload mismatch in aortic and mitral valve disease: Implications for surgical therapy. J Am Coll Cardiol 1985; 5:811-26.
10. Ross J Jr. Afterload mismatch and preload reserve. A conceptual framework for the analysis of ventricular function. Prog Cardiovasc Dis 1976; 18:255-64.
11. Bonow RO, Lakatos E, Maron BJ et al. Serial long-term assessment of the natural history of asymptomatic patients with chronic aortic regurgitation and normal left ventricular systolic function. Circulation 1991; 84:1625-35.
12. Bonow RO, Rosing DR, Kent KM et al. Timing of operation for chronic aortic regurgitation. Am J Cardiol 1982; 50:325-36.
13. Daniel WG, Hood WP Jr, Siart A et al. Chronic aortic regurgitation: Reassessment of the prognostic value of preoperative left ventricular end-systolic dimension and fractional shortening. Circulation 1985; 71:669-80.
14. Fioretti P, Roelandt J, Bos RJ et al. Echocardiography in chronic aortic insufficiency: Is valve replacement too late when left ventricular end-systolic dimension reaches 55 mm? Circulation 1983; 67:216-21.
15. Gaasch WH, Andrias CW, Levine HJ. Chronic aortic regurgitation: The effect of aortic valve replacement on left ventricular volume, mass, and function. Circulation 1978; 58:825-36.
16. Gaasch WH, Carroll JD, Herbert HJ et al. Chronic aortic regurgitation: Prognostic value of left ventricular end-systolic dimension and end-diastolic radius/thickness ratio. J Am Coll Cardiol 1983; 1:775-82.
17. Bonow RO, Dodd JT, Maron BJ et al. Long-term serial changes in left ventricular function and reversal of ventricular dilatation after valve replacement for chronic aortic regurgitation. Circulation 1988; 78:1108-20.
18. Michel PL, Iung B, Jaoude SA et al. The effect of left ventricular systolic function on long term survival in mitral and aortic regurgitation. J Heart Valve Dis 1996; 4(Supp II):S160-169.
19. Klodas E, Enriquez-Sarano M, Tajik AJ et al. Aortic regurgitation complicated by extreme left ventricular dilation: long-term outcome after surgical correction. J Am Coll Cardiol 1996; 27:670-7.
20. Bonow RO, Nikas D, Elefteriades JA. Valve replacement for regurgitant lesions of theaortic or mitral valve in advanced left ventricular dycfunction. In: Cardiology Clinics 1995; Volume 13: WB Saunders, Toronto.
21. Wisenbaugh T, Spann JF, Carabello BA. Differences in myocardial performance and load between patients with similar amounts of chronic aortic versus chronic mitral regurgitation. J Am Coll Cardiol 1984; 3: 916-23.
22. Bonow RO. The value of radioisotope blood pool imaging for evaluation of valvular heart disease. In: Comparative Cardiac Imaging 1990; Aspen Publishers.
23. Gaasch WH, Zile MR. Left ventricular function after surgical correction of chronic mitral regurgitation. Eur Heart J 1991; 12(Suppl B):48-51.

24. Hansen DE, Cahill PD, DeCampli WM et al. Valvular-ventricular interaction: Importance of the mitral apparatus in canine left ventricular systolic performance. Circulation 1986; 73:1310-20.

25. Hilder FJ, Javier RP, Cohen LS. Myocardial dysfunction associated with valvar heart disease. Am J Cardiol 1972; 30:319-26.

26. Rozich JD, Carabello BA, Usher BW et al. Mitral valve replacement with and without chordal preservation in patients with chronic mitral regurgitation: Mechanisms for differences in postoperative ejection performance. Circulation 1992; 86:1718-26.

27. Schuler G, Peterson KL, Johnson A. Temporal response of left ventricular performance to mitral valve surgery. Circulation 1979; 59:1218-31.

28. Tyers G. Mitral valve replacement: What should be the standard technique? Ann Thorac Surg 1990; 49:861-2.

29. Phillips HR, Levine FH, Carter JE et al. Mitral valve replacement for isolated mitral regurgitation: Analysis of clinical course and late postoperative left ventricular ejection fraction. Am J Cardiol 1981; 48:647-54.

30. Enriquez-Sarano M, Tajik AJ, Schaff HV et al. Echocardiographic prediction of survival after surgical correction of organic mitral regurgitation. Circulation 1994; 90:830-7.

31. Yun KL, Rayhill SC, Niczyporuk MA et al. Mitral valve replacement in dilated canine hearts with chronic mitral regurgitation: Importance of the mitral subvalvular apparatus. Circulation 1991; 84 (Suppl 3): 112-24.

32. Lillehei CW, Levy MJ, Bonnabeau RC. Mitral valve replacement with preservation of papillary muscles and chordae tendineae. J Thorac Cardiovasc Surg 1964; 47:532-543.

33. Sarris GE, Cahill PD, Hansen DE et al. Restoration of left ventricular systolic performance after reattachment of the mitral chordae tendineae. J Thorac Cardiovasc Surg 1998; 95:969-79.

34. Moon MR, DeAnda A, Daughters GT, et al. Experimental evaluation of different chordal preservation methods during mitral valve replacement. Ann Thorac Surg 1994; 58:931-44.

35. Yun KL, Fann JI, Rayhill S et al. Importance of the mitral subvalvular apparatus for left ventricular segmental systolic mechanics. Circulation 1990; 82 (5 Suppl):IV89-104.

36. Yun KL, Niczyporuk MA, Sarris GE et al. Importance of mitral subvalvular apparatus in terms of cardiac energetics and systolic mechanics in the ejecting canine heart. J Clin Invest 1991; 87:247-51.

37. David TE, Uden DE, Strauss HD. The importance of the mitral apparatus in left ventricular function after correction of mitral regurgitation. Circulation 1983; 68 (Suppl II):1176-82.

38. Goldman ME, Mora F, Guarino T et al. Mitral valvuloplasty is superior to valve replacement for preservation of left ventricular function: An intraoperative two-dimensional echocardiographic study. J Am Coll Cardiol 1987: 10:568-75.

39. Hennein HA, Swain JA, McIntosh CL et al. Comparative assessment of chordal preservation versus chordal resection during mitral valve replacement. J Thorac Cardiovasc Surg 1980: 99:828-37.

40. Horstkotte D, Schulte HD, Bircks W et al. The effect of chordal preservation on late outcome after mitral valve replacement: A randomized study. J Heart Valve Dis 1993: 2:150-8.

41. Miki S, Kusuhara K, Ueda Y et al. Mitral valve replacement with preservation of chordae tendineae and papillary muscles. Ann Thorac Surg 1988: 45:28-34.

42. Carpentier A, Chauvaud S, Fabiani JN et al. Reconstructive surgery of mitral valve incompetence: Ten year appraisal. J Thorac Cardiovasc Surg 1980: 79:338-345.

43. Cosgrove DM, Stewart WJ: Mitral valvuloplasty. Curr Probl Cardiol 1989: 7:355-415.

44. Kaul TK, Ramsdale DR, Meek D et al. Mitral valve replacement in patients with severe mitral regurgitation and impaired left ventricular function. Int J Cardiol 1992: 35:169-79.

45. Yacoub M, Halim M, Radley-Smith R et al. Surgical treatment of mitral regurgitation caused by floppy valves: Repair versus replacement. Circulation 1981; 64(Suppl II):II-210-6.

4. LEFT VENTRICULAR ANEURYSM REPAIR FOR THE MANAGEMENT OF LEFT VENTRICULAR DYSFUNCTION

Lloyd C. Semelhago and Wilbert J. Keon

Historical Perspective

Although left ventricular aneurysms had previously been described by Hunter and others through their autopsy work it was not until the 1880s that aneurysms were proposed to occur as the result of coronary artery stenosis.[1] The relationship between myocardial infarction, fibrosis and aneurysm formation and coronary artery disease was first recognized at that time.[1] Likely Beck was the first to attempt the repair of a post-infarction left ventricular aneurysm when in 1944 he reinforced the ventricular wall with fascia lata.[2] Likoff and Bailey followed in 1955 by resecting an aneurysm without cardiopulmonary bypass using a specially designed side-biting left ventricular clamp that could be applied through a thoracotomy incision.[3] Subsequently, in 1958 Cooley reported the first successful open repair of a left ventricular aneurysm using cardioplumonary bypass and a buttressed linear closure.[4] The surgical repair of left ventricular aneurysms has since evolved to address such issues as left ventricular geometry and ventricular arrhythmias.[5-8]

Etiology

The majority of left ventricular aneurysms develop as a result of coronary artery disease with less than 5% being due to congenital, traumatic or infiltrative disorders.[9-11]

Although the incidence of aneurysms varies, up to 30% of patients surviving a major myocardial infarction develop a left ventricular aneurysm.[12] This appears no longer to be true and the prevalence of aneurysms appears to have lessened with the rapid access to the newer treatments for patients with acute myocardial infarction, in particular thrombolytics and angioplasty.[13] In patients treated early after infarction with thrombolytics the absence of aneurysm formation is associated with successful reperfusion.[14] Similiarly with postinfarction coronary angioplasty the frequency and size of left ventricular aneurysms has decreased.[15] The widespread use of both thrombolytic agents and postinfarction angioplasty result in greater preservation of the patency of the left anterior descending coronary artery (LAD).[14,15]

Roy Masters (editor), Surgical Options for the Treatment of Heart Failure, 49-59.

Prerequisite to the development of a left ventricular aneurysm is a transmural myocardial infarction particularly in those patients with poor intracoronary collateralization.[16] It has been speculated that a rich collateral blood supply to an area of infarction increases the number and size of the islands of viable myocytes in the area and decreases the probability that the necrosis is extensive enough to result in a thin-walled transmural scar.[13] Analyzing those who did not have successful reperfusion with thrombolysis the incidence of left ventricular aneurysm formation decreased from 58% to 10% if there was a rich network of collaterals.[16] In the setting of successful thrombolysis the incidence of aneurysm was only 4%.[16] Similiarly it has been demonstrated that total occlusion of the LAD coronary artery and poor collateral blood flow are significant determinants of aneurysm formation.[17] Conversely, multivessel coronary artery disease with either good collaterals or a patent left anterior descending coronary artery is uncommonly associated with a left ventricular aneurysm.[17]

Pathology

Either a true or a false left ventricular aneurysm may complicate an acute myocardial infarction.[18] True aneurysms occur after a transmural infarction as a consequence of myocardial destruction and localized remodeling. Early wall thinning due to myocyte stretching and wall weakness is followed by fibrous replacement of the infarct and further wall thinning. The aneurysm wall of a true aneurysm consists of full left ventricular thickness from endocardium to epicardium occassionally with dystrophic calcification.[18] Often the overlying pericardium is densely adherent to the epicardial surface of the aneurysm and in almost half of patients there is associated mural thrombus.[19] In contrast, false aneurysms, which are uncommon, occur as a sequela of transmural infarction and free wall rupture with containment of the rupture by adherent fibrous pericardium. The wall of these aneurysms is thin consisting of only the fibrous pericardium.

Approximately 85% of left ventricular aneurysms are located anterolaterally near the apex.[13] At the Ottawa Heart Institute of 95 patients having resection of a left ventricular aneurysm from 1983 to 1992, 15% were anterior, 37.6% were anterior-apical and 32.3% were apical.[18] Only 5-10% of aneurysms are posterior near the base of the heart and nearly one-half of these are false aneurysms.[13,18,20]

Natural History and Survival

The complexities of coronary artery disease and the difficulties with identifying patients with aneurysms in contrast to scar make analysis of the natural history and survival difficult. In a 1970s study of 590 patients, those with an akinetic area had a five-year survival of 69% whereas those with a left ventricular aneurysm had a five-year survival 54% and this decreased to 36% when the function of the remainder of the ventricle was reduced.[21] This study also reported differences in the mortality rates in aneurysm patients with single, double, and triple-vessel coronary artery disease.[21] The presence of symptoms and therfore likely the size of the aneurysm is also a risk factor for death in surgically untreated patients. In those patients without symptoms, and usually a small aneurysm, a ten-year survival of 90% has been reported whereas in patients with symptoms, and usually a large aneurysm, the ten-year survival was 46.3%.[22] The presence of dyskinesia in the aneurysm rather than akinesia also adversely affects survival.[23]

Left Ventricular Function

An aneurysm of the left ventricle places the left ventricle at a mechanical disadvantage and results in both diastolic and systolic dysfunction. Besides the localized geometric distortion an aneurysm results in global remodeling with generalized dilatation.[24] The thickness and curvature of the ventricular wall are determinants of afterload and as changes in these parameters occur significant changes in cardiac performance can be expected.[25] Also variations in the intrinsic properties of scar, muscle and bordering tissue add to the influence on both the systolic and diastolic function of the left ventricle.[26] In diastole the fibrotic aneurysm scar does not undergo normal distension and this failure to distend results in elevated left ventricular end-diastolic pressure (LVEDP). During systole the aneurysm moves paradoxically leading to reduced efficiency of the ventricle as a whole because systolic work is wasted on expansion of this segment.[27,28] This results in reduced cardiac output and ejection fraction . Finally, the increased ventricular size results in increased wall tension according to Laplace's Law. This increased tension results in higher oxygen consumption in the remaining myocardium and a decrease oxgen supply during diastole.

Because of the complexities of ventricular function in patients with left ventricular aneurysms assessment of myocardial function of the uninvolved segments has been difficult. Standard measurements of global function using ventriculography normally assume homogeneity and are thus unreliable in these patients. Wall thickening however, when assessed by echocardiography using multiple short-axis images, has been shown to be a more accurate measure of regional function in this setting.[25]

Indications for Repair

Although the absolute number of patients with left ventricular aneurysms has decreased the primary indications for surgical intervention have remained essentially unchanged and include (1) heart failure (2) angina pectoris (3) ventricular tachycardia and (4) thromboembolism.[29] By definition these classic indications apply to patients who are symptomatic. The indications for surgical intervention in asymptomatic patients however are much less clear. As noted previously, patients without symtoms and a small ventricular aneurysm enjoy a ten-year survival of almost 90%.[22] However the CASS study documented a substantially worse prognosis for patients with aneurysms associated with poor overall ventricular function and extensive coronary artery disease regardless of symptomalogy.[30,31] As well in a small prospective study the five-year survival was approximately 33% for patients with large aneurysms and approximately 70% for smaller ones.[32] On this basis if an aneurysm is truely small and the patient is indeed asymptomatic the decision to operate is guided on the basis of their coronary artery disease and left ventricular funcion. However the timing of surgery for asymptomatic patients with large left ventricular aneurysms poses a dilemma. While not all of these patients with large asymptomatic aneurysms develop global dysfunction it is unfortunately not possible to predict which ventricles will remain stable and which will deteriorate. The completely asyptomatic patient with a large ventricular aneurysm therefore should be followed very closely for signs and/or symptoms and if they develop it should be resected. Such signs include an increase in end-systole basilar diameter, a decrease in overall ejection fraction, worsening mitral regurgitation or progressive enlargement of the aneurysm.[29]

Occassionally true left ventricular aneurysms may develop early after acute myocardial infarction. Aneurysms that are at least three weeks old can be treated surgically with the same techniques that are used for the more chronic aneurysms.[29] Indeed in one series the hospital mortality was 5% for patients having surgery within eight weeks of infarction.[33]

Patients who survive cardiac rupture may develop a false aneurysm.[18] Because of the risk of rupture with hemorrhage, tamponade and death surgery is generally recommended without delay when a false aneurysm is identified.

Surgical Correction of Left Ventricular Aneurysm

Operative Preparation

The various types of contemporary aneurysm surgery are all performed via median sternotomy and cardiopulmonary bypass. For large aneurysms that extend to the septum or where there is a possibility of entering the right ventricle, bicaval cannulation is recommended. If a false aneurysm is suspected with extension anteriorly to the sternum cardiopulmnary bypass is established via the femoral artery and vein. Manipulation of the left ventricle to release adhesions in all cases is kept to a minimum while the heart is still ejecting to avoid embolization. Patients with recurrent ventricular arrhythmias undergo epicardial mapping at this time for cryoablation during resection of the aneurysmal wall and subendocardial scar. The use of cardioplegic arrest, however, is optional because some surgeons prefer to perform this surgery with either the heart beating or fibrillating.[29] Common to all methods of repair is the thorough evacuation of all thrombus.

Methods of Repair

Linear Repair (Figure 1)

The buttressed linear repair successfully performed by Cooley and his associates in 1958 is still commonly used today.[4] The aneurysm is opened by placing an incision parallel to and at least 2 cm lateral to the left anterior descending coronary artery. Care must be taken to avoid placing the incision too close to the LAD and entering the ventricular septum or too far away from the LAD and damaging the anterior papillary muscle.[29] Once an initial incision is made into the apex of the aneurysm the inside of the aneurysm

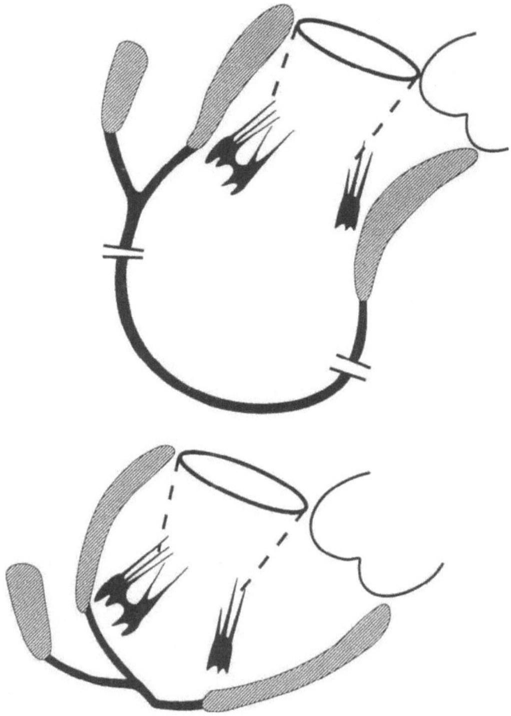

Figure 1. *Linear repair for repair of left ventricular aneurysm*

may be palpated or visualized to determine its extent and to guide the size of the ventriculotomy. Following exploration of the ventricular cavity for thrombus the incision is carried around the entire aneurysm leaving a thin rim of scar to facilitate closure. All thrombus is carefully evacuated. Classically the closure is linear using two parallel Teflon strips on the epicardial surface and a continuous horizontal mattress suture reinforced by a second row of over-and-over sutures. Two concerns of the linear closure technique are that it does not correct the portion of the distal septum that is involved in the aneurysm and it does not restore the original shape of the left ventricle.[29] To address the former, Mickelborough et al advocate a modified linear closure technique that incorporates patch exclusion of any aneurysmal septum.[34] To address the latter they advocate the placing of sutures further apart on the tissue than on the Teflon to plicate the length of the ventriculotomy and partially restore the shape of the ventricle.[34]

Endoventricular Repair of Jatene (Figure2)

In 1985 Jatene described his technique of aneurysm resection to restore both overall global ventricular geometry and myocardial fibre orientation to their original morphologic state.[35] This repair is based on the knowledge that in a large left ventricular aneurysm the directions of the normal muscle fibers are distorted and the belief that a closure by simply approximating the fibrous rim in a linear suture will result in an abnormally long and

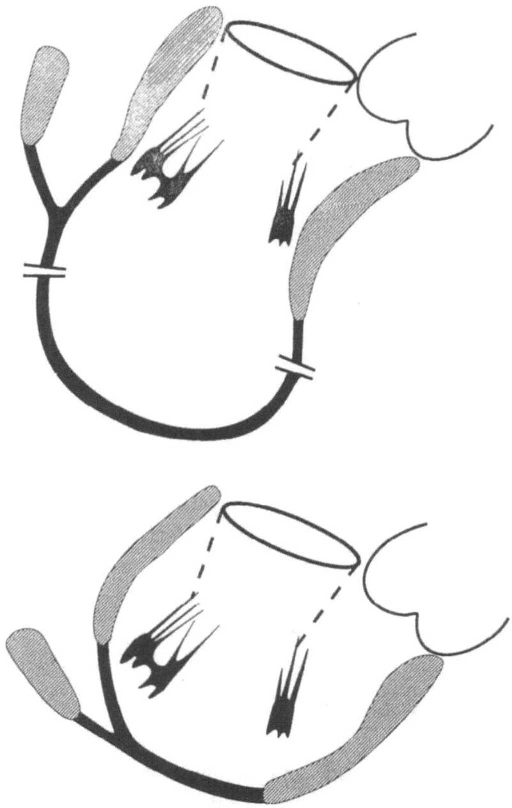

Figure 2. *Endoventricular aneurysm repair technique of Jatene*

narrow cavity. Further if the septum is involved, a paradoxical area will add to these problems.[35] Incorporating the concepts of Daggett et al, Jatene developed a technique to address these issues.[35, 36] Following resection of the aneurysm, leaving a rim of scar for suturing, the orifice of the aneurysm is reduced concentrically with U shaped stitches externally anchored on Teflon pledgets. An unstetchable Dacron patch whose shape duplicates that of the original infarcted area is fixed over the reduced orifice.[35] To determine the size and shape of the Dacron patch to be used one or two purse-string sutures are placed at the transition zone between normal and fibrous tissue and the purse-string sutures are carefully pulled to rebuild the left ventricular cavity. To address septal distension Jatene recommended the use of two or three mattress stitches with pledgets placed posterior to anterior to reduce elongation of the septal wall and prevent septal distension.[35]

Endoventricular Repair of Dor (Figure 3)

In 1984, almost simultaneous with the work of Jatene, Dor developed the technique of endoventricular circular patch plasty (EVCPP).[37,38] After opening the aneurysm through

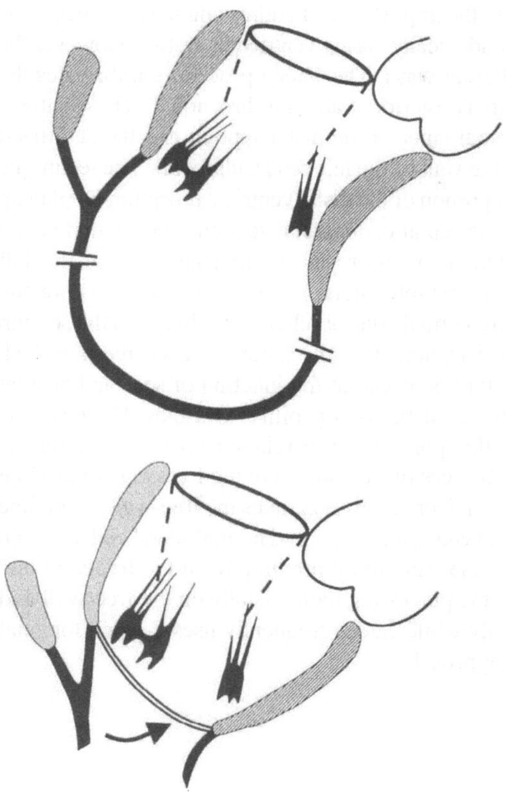

Figure 3. *Endoventricular circular patch plasty (EVCPP) of Dor*

the apex the junction between the endocardial scar and normal myocardioum is identified throughout the entire circumference of the aneurysm. A continuous 2-0 monofilament suture is placed around the entire circumference of the base of the aneurysm at the junction of scar and normal myocardium. The degree of tightening of this suture will determine the final size of the remaining opening in the ventricle and the size of the endocardial patch to be used. The patch is usually 2-3 cm in diameter and can be Dacron or pericardium. The patch is sutured at the level of the pursestring and glue is applied to the suture line to secure the closure. Finally the excluded sides of the ventricle beyond the endocardial patch can be resected or closed to one another. In the presence of large aneurysms, which is the usual case, the excluded edges should not be sutured together but rather should be tacked down to the edges of the patch. This prevents distortion of the right ventricle and ventricular septum.[38]

Comparison of the Techniques of Jatene and Dor

To clarify the similiarities and differences between these two approaches to the repair of left ventricular aneurysms Cox recently published a comparison of the two techniques.[39] Both the Dor and Jatene techniques emphasize the importance of addressing the dysfunctional distal septum which frequently moves paradoxically during ventricular systole. However the two techniques address this issue in different ways. The Jatene procedure imbricates the aneurysmal portion of the distal septum in a posterior to anterior direction.[40] These sutures stabilize the septum and restore the normal taper of the distal septum and the stabilized septum subsequently remains as part of the wall of the left ventricular wall. The technique of Dor however excludes the aneurysmal portion of the distal ventricular septum by placing the endocardial patch at the junction of the septal endocardial scar and the normal septal endocardium. Both techniques also attempt to restore the normal geomety of the left ventricular cavity to normal. Both use a circumferencial pursestring at the base of the aneurysm and tighten it to restore the more normal conical relationship between the septum and the free wall. In doing so the proper orientation of the myocardial fibers is reestablished. With both techniques the pursestring suture is placed at the junction of scar and normal endocardium but always distal to the bases of the two papillary muscles. However, as pointed out by Cox, the positioning of this pursestring in relationshp to the septum is different in the two techniques. Jatene advances the apical end of the free-wall suture line ono the distal septum at the apex (Figure 2). Dor simply continues the free-wall suture line onto the septum at the junction of the septal endocardial scar and normal septal endocardium (Figure 3). Whereas Jatene places the pursestring more proximally on the free-wall and more distally on the septum, Dor places the pursesting more distally on the free-wall and more proximally on the septum.[40] Finally while Jatene frequently uses a patch for final closure a patch is always used in Dor's approach.

Survival

Left ventricular aneurysm patients are not a homogenous group and this influences the interpretation of the surgical results.The hospital mortality after the repair of left ventricular aneurysm with and without coronary artery bypass is approximately 5%, although this varies greatly with the series.[29,40] Overall the long-term survival at one, three and five years is approximately 85%, 75% and 65% respectively.[29] Incremental risk factors for hospital death after surgery for left ventricular aneurysm include the pre-operative NYHA Class and myocardial score and having surgery before 1974.[29,41] In our own series 95 patients with 45% patients in Class 3 or 4 and 82% having bypass grafts the hospital survival was 91.6%.[18] For premature late death positive coefficients include the presence of right coronary stenosis ($\geq$ 75%) and the function of posterior basal left ventricle and negative coefficients include the presence of angina and the number of bypass grafts.[29,41]

Mickleborough et al using tailored scar excision and linear closure in 92 patients reported a 3% hospital mortality and a five-year actuarial survival of 80%.[34] Of the survivors in that study 89% were symptomatically improved and of a subset with both pre- and post-operative multiple gated aquisition scans left ventricular ejection fraction improved from 23% to 30%.[34] Jatene, in a series of 1381 patients with left ventricular aneurysms from 1977 to 1987, reported a surgical mortality of 5.8% and a late mortality of 4.5%.[40] To 1996 Dor et al had repaired aneurysms in 715 patients and a reported 30-day mortality rate was approximately 7% with a late improvement of ejection fraction of 0.10 post-operatively.[42] Risk factors for hospital mortality in their experience included refractory heart failure, ischemic ventricular septal defects, refractory ventricular tachycardia and the need for emergency surgery.[42]

References

1. Cohnheim J, Schulthess Rechberg AV. Uber die folgen der kranzarterien-verschliessung für das Hertz. Virchows Arch [A] 1881;85:503.
2. Beck CS. Operation for aneurysm of the heart. Ann Surg 1944;120:34-40.
3. Likoff W, Bailey CP. Ventriculoplasty: Excision of myocardial aneurysm, report of a successful case. JAMA 1955;158:915.
4. Cooley DA, Collins HA, Morris GC, Chapman DW. Ventricular aneurysm after myocardial infarction. Surgical excision with use of temporary cardiopulmonary bypass. JAMA 1958;167:557.
5. Daggett WM, Guyton RA, Mundth ED et al. Surgery for post-myocardial infarct ventricular septal defect. Ann Surg 1977;186:260-70.
6. Dor V, Saab M, Coste P, Kornaszewska M, Montiglio F. Left ventricular aneurysm: a new surgical approach. Thorac Cardiovasc Surg 1989;39:11-9.
7. Jatene AD. Left ventricular aneurysmectomy. Resection or reconstruction. J Thorac Cardiovasc Surg 1985;89:321-31.
8. Cooley DA. Ventricular endoaneurysmorrhaphy: a simplified repair for extensive postinfarction aneurysm. J Cardiac Surg 1989;4:200.
9. Grieco JG, Montoya A, Sullivan HJ, Bakhos M, Foy BK. Ventricular aneurysm due to blunt chest injury. Ann Thorac Surg 1989;47:322-9.
10. Davila JC, Enriquez F, Bergoglio S, et al. Congenital aneurysm of the left ventricle. Ann Thorac Surg 1965;1:697.
11. Valantine H, McKenna WJ, Nihoyannopoulos P, et al. Sarcoidosis: a pattern of clinical and morphological presentation. Br Heart J 1987;57:256.
12. Nagle RE, Williams DO. Natural history of ventricular aneurysm without surgical treatment. Br Heart J 1974;36:1037 (abst).
13. Kirklin JW and Barratt-Boyes BC. In: Cardiac Surgery, Second Edition, Churchill Livingstone, New York, 1992.
14. Kayden DS, Wackers FJ, Zaret BL. Left ventricular aneurysm formation after thrombolytic therapy for anterior infarction. TIMI phase I and open label 1985-86. Circulation 1987;76(Suppl IV):97.
15. Chen JS, Hwang CL, Lee DY, Chen YT. Regression of left ventricular aneurysm after delayed percutaneous transluminal coronary angioplasty (PTCA) in patients with acute myocardial infarction. Int J Cardiol 1995;48:39.
16. Hirai T, Fujita M, Nakajima H, et al. Importance of collateral circulation for prevention of left ventricular aneurysm formation in acute myocardial infarction. Circulation 1989;79:791-6.
17. Forman MB, Collins HW, Kopelman HA, et al. Determinants of left ventricular aneurym formation after anterior myocardial infarction: A clinical and angiographic study. J Am Coll Cardiol 1986;8:1256.
18. Veinot JP, Kos AI, Masters RG et al. Left ventricular aneurysms: clinicopathological review of 10 years experience. J Surg Path 1997; 2:107-14.
19. Dubnow MH, Burchell HB, Titus JL. Postinfarction ventricular aneurysm: A clinicopathologic and electrocardiographic study of 80 cases. Am Heart J 1965;70:753-8.
20. Buehler DL, Stinson EB, Oyer PE, Shumway NE. Surgical treatment of aneurysms of the inferior wall. J Thorac Cardiovasc Surg 1979;78:74-8.
21. Bruschke AVG, Proudfit WL, Sones FM Jr. Progress study of 590 consecutive nonsurgical cases of coronary disease followed 5-9 years. II. Ventriculographic and other correlations. Circulation 1973;47:1154-7.
22. Grondin P, Kretz JG, Bical O, et al. Natural history of saccular aneurysm of the left ventricle. J Thorac Cardiovasc Surg 1979;77:57-9.
23. Parmley WW, Chuck L, Kivowitz C et al. In vitro length-tension relations of human ventricular aneurysms: relation of stiffness to mechanical disadvantage. Am J Cardiol 1973;32:889-94.
24. Weisman H, Bush D, Mannisi, Bulkley B. Global cardiac remodeling after acute myocardial infarction. J Am Coll Cardiol 1985;5:1355-9.
25. Nicolosi AC, Spotnitz HM. Quantitative analysis of regional systolic function with left ventricular aneurysm. Circulation 1988;78:856-62.
26. Kitamura S, Kay JH, Krohn BG et al. Geometric and functional abnormalities of the left ventricle with a chronic localized noncontractile area. Am J Cardiol 1973;31:701-7.
27. Jan K. Distribution of myocardial stress and its influence on coronary blood flow. J Biochem 1985;18:815-8.
28. Streeter D, Vaishnav R, Pater D et al. Stress distribution in the canine left ventricle during diastole and systole. Biophys J 1970;10:345-8.
29. Cox JL. Left ventricular aneurysms: Pathologic observations and standard resection. Semi Thorac Cardiovasc

Surg 1997;9:113-22.

30. Faxon DP, Ryan TJ, David KB et al. Prognostic significance of angiographically documented left ventricular aneurysm from the coronary artery surgery (CASS)s study. Am j Cardiol 1982;50:157-64.
31. Faxon DP, Myers WO, McCabe CH et al. The influence of surgery on the natural history of angiographically documented left ventricular aneurysm. The coronary artery Surgery Study. Circulation 1986;74:110-8.
32. Mourdjinis A, Olsen E, Raphael MJ, Mounsey JPD. Clinical diagnosis and prognosis of ventricular aneurysm. Br Heart J 1968;30:497-513.
33. Walker WE, Stoney WS, Alford WC et al. Techniques and results of ventricular aneurysmectomy with emphasis on anteroseptal repair. J Thorac Cardiovasc Surg 1978;76:824-8.
34. Mickelborough LL, Maruyama H, Liu P, Mohamed S. Results of left ventricular aneurysmectomy with a tailored scar excision and primary closure technique. J Thorac Cardiovasc Surg 1994;107:690-8.
35. Jatene AD. Left ventricular aneurysmectomy. Resection or reconstruction. J Thorac Cardiovasc Surg 1985;89:321-31.
36. Daggett WM, Guyton RA, Mundth ED et al. Surgery for post-myocardial infarct ventricular septal defect. Ann Surg 1977;186:260-71.
37. Dor V, Saab M, Coste P et al. Left ventricular aneurysm: A new surgical approach. Thorac Cardiovasc Surg 1989;37:11-19.
38. Dor V. Left ventricular aneurysms: The endoventricular circular patch plasty. Sem Thorac Cardiovasc Surg 1997;9:123-30.
39. Surgical management of left ventricular aneurysms: A clarification of the similiarities and differences between the Jatene and Dor procedures. Sem Thorac Cardiovasc Surg 1997;9:131-8.
40. Jatene AD. Surgical management of left ventricular aneurysms. In: Buae AE, Geha AS, Hammond GL et al (eds): Gelnn's Thoracic and Cardiovascular Surgery. Appleton & Lange, Norwalk, 1991.
41. Barratt-Boyes BG, White HD, Agnew TM et al. The results of surgical treatment of left ventricular aneurysms: An assessment of risk factors affecting early and late mortality. J Thorac Cardiovasc Surg 1984;1:87-98.
42. Dor V, Sabatier M, DiDonato M et al. Late hemodynamic results after left ventricular patch repair associated with coronary grafting in patients with post- infarction akinetic or dyskinetic aneurysm of the left ventricle. J Thorac Cardiovasc Surg 1995;110:1291-301.

5. SELECTION AND MANAGEMENT OF THE POTENTIAL CANDIDATE FOR CARDIAC TRANSPLANTATION

Lynne Warner Stevenson

Introduction

The potential benefits of transplantation were already recognized in 1968, as reflected in the statement from the Bethesda conference chaired by Francis Moore: "Cardiac transplantation, still in an early stage of development, shows promise for the future treatment of many people with severe heart disease".[1] At that time there were 20 survivors of 50 heart transplant procedures. Since then, cardiac transplantation has evolved from an experimental to an accepted clinical procedure, endorsed by Medicare in 1986 as 'best therapy' for end-stage heart failure. The current survival rate is 80-85% at 1 year, 70% at 5 years and 40% at 10 years.[2] There have now been over 40,000 transplants performed in the world, involving over 250 heart transplant centres.

When transplantation was experimental, patients were selected from those facing imminent death. The indications were obvious, and the contraindications could be liberally defined by the investigators. Improving results led to consideration of candidates for whom the immediate need for transplant was less urgent, but the longer waiting times required earlier anticipation of that need. At the same time, continuing refinement of immunosuppression diminished the immediate negative impact of many conditions such as diabetes and older age, which were initially criteria for exclusion due to associated higher risks of post-transplant complications. These changes have widened the channels into an ever-expanding pool of potential candidates (Figure 1). It is currently estimated that up to 40,000 people each year in the United States would potentially benefit from cardiac transplantation, an estimate surprisingly consonant with the 10,000 - 40,000 estimated in 1968. The original estimate of potential donor heart availability at that time, however, was 45,000 yearly in the United States, compared to the 2,000-2,500 actually achieved yearly for the past 5 years. Interestingly, their original estimate of cost was U.S. $50,000 in 1968 dollars, which is only slightly lower than the absolute figure currently negotiated for some contracts in 1995 dollars.[1]

As cardiac transplantation has evolved, other medical and surgical alternatives to transplantation have also developed. Heart transplantation now represents only one facet of the therapies which should be offered by centres dedicated to the heart failure

Roy Masters (editor), Surgical Options for the Treatment of Heart Failure, 61-91.

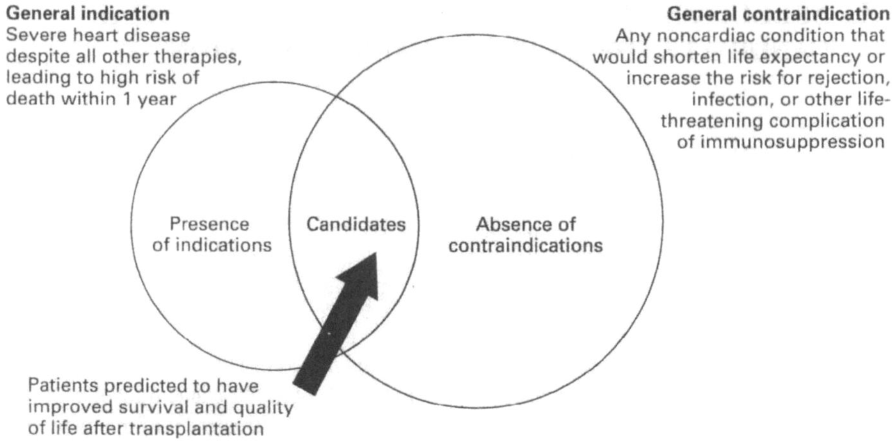

Figure 1. *Intersecting circles demonstrate the principle of selection for cardiac transplantation of candidates who demonstrate indications without serious contraindications. As the results of transplantation have improved the indications broaden and the contraindications become less strict.*

(From Stevenson, LW. Selection and management of a potential candidate for cardiac transplantation. In: Cooper DKC, Miller LW and Patterson GA (Eds) The transplantation and replacement of thoracic organs, 1996, Kluwer Academic Publishers: Figure 1, Page 161)

population. A left ventricular ejection fraction <25% no longer means that a new heart must be substituted in order for a patient to survive with a good quality of life. Surgery for reversible ischemia, distorted ventricular geometry, and valvular disease is successful in some patients despite poor left ventricular function and symptoms of heart failure.[3-5] Medical therapy has had a dramatic impact on the symptoms of heart failure, with less but still significant impact on survival, challenging previous assumptions of when left ventricular dysfunction becomes 'end-stage'.[6-8]

Approach to the Patient Referred for Cardiac Transplantation

The most common diagnosis in adults referred for transplantation is dilated heart failure, due in almost equal proportion to coronary artery disease and non-ischemic dilated cardiomyopathy. Primary restrictive cardiomyopathy, primary valvular disease, and congenital heart disease account for slightly fewer than 10% of all candidates, with rare cases of cardiac trauma or tumour.[2] The general approach to the identification of indications and contraindications is applicable regardless of etiology (Table 1), but most of the specific considerations below focus on advanced heart failure with low left ventricular ejection fraction.

Table 1. Approach to the potential candidate for heart transplantation

Address potentially reversible components of heart failure
Tailor medical therapy to relieve congestion
Evaluate functional capacity
Assess risks of deterioration or sudden death
Identify indications for transplant
Exclude contraindications to transplantation
Determine candidacy for transplantation: now, when needed, or conditional
Maintain and re-evaluate

(From Stevenson, LW. Selection and management of a potential candidate for cardiac transplantation. In: Cooper DKC, Miller LW and Patterson GA (Eds) The transplantation and replacement of thoracic organs, 1996, Kluwer Academic Publishers: Table 1, Page 162)

Factors Which are Potentially Reversible

All patients should undergo extensive investigation to identify the primary cause and any potentially reversible factors contributing to decompensation (Table 2). Occasionally a systemic cause of disease is identified which will preclude cardiac transplantation due to expected effects on other organs after transplantation. A low left ventricular ejection fraction may in some cases reflect major areas of hibernating or stunned myocardium, which may demonstrate improved function after revascularization with coronary artery bypass grafting or catheter-based interventional procedures.[4, 5] Angina is frequently absent, and thallium redistribution after reinjection or prolonged delay is not always

Table 2. Potentially reversible factors in heart transplantation

Intrinsic factors
Recent-onset cardiomyopathy
Extensive myocardial ischemia with potential for revascularization
Secondary viral infection superimposed on primary disease
Major alcohol consumption
Tachycardias
Metabolic factors: thyroid disease, electrolyte distrubances, obesity
Anemia or other high-output state
Factors of therapy
Ineffective drug regimen:
ineffective doses or combinations of vasodilators
inadequate diuresis
Non-compliance:
with drug regimen
with salt and fluid restriction
Concomitant drug therapy causing:
increased fluid retention
depressed contractility

(From Stevenson, LW. Selection and management of a potential candidate for cardiac transplantation. In: Cooper DKC, Miller LW and Patterson GA (Eds) The transplantation and replacement of thoracic organs, 1996, Kluwer Academic Publishers: Table 2, Page 162)

present. Areas of glucose uptake in regions with decreased flow may identify viability otherwise not evident. A history of multiple reoperations or chronic diabetes mellitus may predict worse outcome. The quality of distal vessels appears critical for success, particularly in this population.

Recent practice surveys from metropolitan transplant centres suggest that no more than 3 - 10% of potential transplant candidates with coronary artery disease may be appropriate revascularization candidates. [9] There is even less information available regarding valve replacement in patients with severely reduced ejection fractions, although it is generally considered indicated in any patient with significant aortic stenosis, and recent experience suggests that mitral valve reconstruction may be feasible and helpful in some patients.[3] Vigorous searching for surgically reversible conditions is warranted, however, due to the implications both for the patient whose own heart may improve without transplantation and for another patient who may receive the donor heart which is spared. Considering the limitation of donor hearts, an operative risk for an alternative procedure which is higher than for the same procedure in a patient with good ventricular function is not itself an indication for cardiac transplantation. Those who survive often demonstrate gradual improvement after 'salvage surgery', or at least stabilize sufficiently to undergo elective transplantation after discharge. Reliance upon 'transplant back-up' for post-cardiotomy shock, however, may be dangerous, as outcomes are uncertain for such patients. Patients requiring mechanical assistance to bridge from post-cardiotomy shock have been reported to have poorer outcome than patients receiving a primary bridge, although those surviving to transplantation have subsequent survival comparable to elective transplantation.[10,11]

Recent cardiomyopathy, defined as less than 6 months of symptoms in the absence of major coronary artery or primary valvular disease, may improve spontaneously in up to 50% of patients, whether or not associated with a recent viral infection or with myocarditis on endomyocardial biopsy. When the clinical severity of symptoms leads to referral for transplantation, major improvement defined as > 0.15% increase in left ventricular ejection fraction occurred in 27% of patients in one series, most often in those with the least elevation in filling pressure and the least mitral regurgitation at the time of referral.[12] For patients with this defined improvement, subsequent prognosis is excellent, although exercise capacity may remain somewhat impaired by diastolic dysfunction.[13] Recent-onset cardiomyopathy which does not improve, however, confers worse short-term prognosis than for patients with more chronic disease (Figure 2), particularly in patients under 33 years.[12] Occasionally, young patients present with a fulminant picture of acute cardiac and other organ failure, usually in association with a viral syndrome, from which the chance of complete recovery may exceed 50%, although high-dose catecholamine support, and occasionally mechanical ventricular support, may be necessary for 5 - 10 days. The incidence of this syndrome varies from year to year and is usually highest in the winter months.

Cardiomyopathy presenting within the last trimester of pregnancy or initial post-partem months has a higher chance of improvement than cardiomyopathy of other etiologies.[14] Symptoms often improve remarkably after assisted diuresis post-partum of the excess volume of water accumulated during pregnancy. Heart failure presenting earlier in pregnancy often reflects exacerbation of previous conditions.

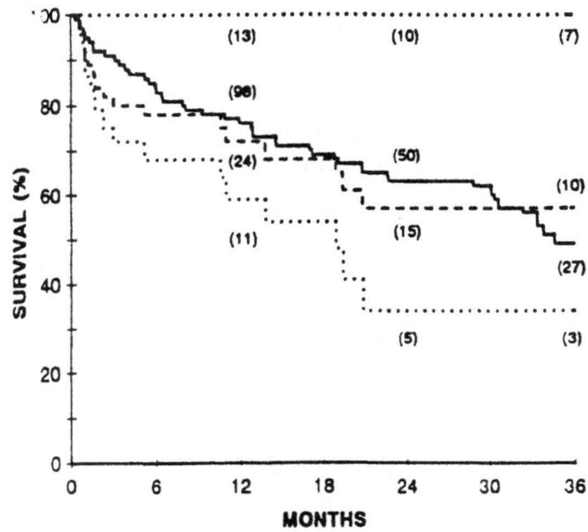

Figure 2. *Survival for 297 patients with primary dilated cardiomyopathy referred for cardiac transplantation. The survival with chronic cardiomyopathy was not different from the total survival of all patients with recent-onset cardiomyopathy, but this recent-onset group could be divided into: (a) those with > 15% ejection fraction improvement to > 30% and (b) those with no improvement for whom survival was significantly worse (p=0.0009).*[12]

(From Stevenson, LW. Selection and management of a potential candidate for cardiac transplantation. In: Cooper DKC, Miller LW and Patterson GA (Eds) The transplantation and replacement of thoracic organs, 1996, Kluwer Academic Publishers: Figure 2, Page 163)

Patients with known heart failure due to cardiomyopathy or coronary artery disease often demonstrate prolonged deterioration after respiratory and viral syndromes, perhaps as a result of the negative inotropic effects of cytokines, the accompanying tachycardia, or increased metabolic demands. Many patients are first referred for transplantation within weeks after such an episode. Restoration of fluid balance and adjustment of vasodilator therapy frequently allows recovery to previous levels of compensation within the next few months.

Approximately 10% of cardiomyopathy in the United States has been attributed to heavy alcohol consumption, although the incidence may be underestimated.[15] Consumption of two drinks daily, which is common in the general population, may be sufficient to worsen heart failure of other primary causes. Occasionally dramatic improvement in the left ventricular ejection fractions of patients with old myocardial infarctions is sometimes explained later by the patient's retrospective admission of heavy alcohol consumption prior to referral. Complete abstinence from alcohol should be mandated for at least 3 - 6 months prior to transplantation candidacy, both to demonstrate the irreversibility of decompensation and to ensure the patient's ability to avoid excessive alcohol consumption after transplantation, although modest consumption is then acceptable. Tachycardia is increasingly recognized as a primary cause of cardiomyopathy in both adults and children.[16] Supraventricular tachycardia and relatively slow ventricular tachycardia may not be initially recognized. Atrial fibrillation, present in approximately 20% of patients referred for cardiac transplantation, is frequently associated with excessive ventricular rates during exertion. Conversion to sinus rhythm usually leads to clinical improvement, but has also frequently been associated with major improvements in the left ventricular ejection fraction.[17] Amiodarone is the safest and most effective antiarrhythmic agent in this population, of whom more than half may still be in sinus rhythm a year after cardioversion on amiodarone.[18] Atrioventricular node ablation and pacemaker implantation may be considered when atrial fibrillation is refractory and the rate cannot be well controlled.

Obesity has been implicated as a primary cause of cardiomyopathy. Weight loss is achievable and frequently easier during heart failure, even though activity is curtailed. Weight loss itself allows more effective distribution of limited cardiac output but, in addition, is frequently associated with significant improvement in left ventricular function, such that cardiac transplantation need not be considered.[19] This should be emphasized to all potential transplant candidates. A pattern of weight maintenance is also critical to avoid morbid weight gain after transplantation, which limits rehabilitation, contributes to osteoporotic complications, and has been associated with transplant vasculopathy.

Tailored Therapy Prior to Transplantation

At the time of serious consideration for transplantation, most patients have a left ventricular ejection fraction < 25% (Table 3) (although this is not necessary for acceptance, see below) and symptoms of heart failure which limit daily life. These symptoms are dominated by elevated intracardiac filling pressures which on the left side cause orthopnea, paroxysmal nocturnal dyspnea (PND), and immediate dyspnea on light exertion (IDLE). (In contrast,

Table 3. Profile of 265 patients discharged after referral with Class IV symptoms and ejection fraction ≤ 25%

Ejection fraction (%)		18 ± 5
CHF duration (months)		33 ± 34
Left ventricular end-diastolic dimension (mm)		75 ± 10
Mitral regurgitation (0-3)		2.0 ± 0.8
Tricuspid regurgitation (0-3)		1.7 ± 0.9
Seerum sodium (mEq/l)		134 ± 5
Hemodynamics	*Initial*	*On revised therapy*
Right atrial pressure	13 ± 7	7 ± 4
Systolic blood pressure	106 ± 14	96 ± 13
Pulmonary wedge pressure	27 ± 9	17 ± 16
Systemic arterial pressure	85 ± 11	76 ± 10
Cardiac index (1 min^{-1} m^{-2})	1.9 ± 0.6	2.5 ± 0.5
Heart rate (beats / min)	94 ± 17	91 ± 15

(From Stevenson, LW. Selection and management of a potential candidate for cardiac transplantation. In: Cooper DKC, Miller LW and Patterson GA (Eds) The transplantation and replacement of thoracic organs, 1996, Kluwer Academic Publishers: Table 3, Page 163)

dyspnea occurring only after several minutes of moderate exertion is more often due to the failure to increase cardiac output to levels adequate for aerobic metabolism during increased demand.) Elevated right-sided cardiac filling pressures cause the symptoms of systemic venous congestion, which can be manifest as gastrointestinal discomfort, anorexia, early satiety, ascites, and peripheral edema. Most patients have a history of recent hospitalizations during which intravenous diuretics, often in conjunction with a brief course of an intravenous inotropic agent, such as dobutamine or milrinone, have caused only a temporary clinical improvement, following which the congestion rapidly recurs.

The majority of patients at the time of referral are already receiving a standard 'triple therapy' which includes digoxin, diuretics, and angiotensin-converting-enzyme (ACE) inhibitors, which have in some cases been reduced or stopped due to hypotension. Although effective doses of vasodilators have been established in trials of mild to moderate heart failure, the use of different doses or different combinations frequently improves clinical status in patients with more severe heart failure. [6 - 8, 20] For all potential candidates, transplant evaluation provides a vital opportunity to redesign the medical regimen, which is of central concern regardless of whether or not the patient is ultimately found to be a candidate for transplantation.

Therapy for severely symptomatic patients is dominated by the need to reduce congestive symptoms and thus the filling pressures which cause those symptoms. The first challenge is to recognize the excess volume present in most of these patients.[21] Although many patients have 3 to 5 litres of excess fluid at the time of evaluation, the lungs are usually clear of rales in chronic heart failure and peripheral edema and / or ascites occur in fewer than 30% of these patients. Orthopnea and jugular venous distension are the most reliable clinical indicators of volume overload, and almost always indicate the need for further therapy.

Previous therapy to relieve congestion has often been hampered by concern that therapy to decrease volume status will further depress cardiac output. This misconception is often strengthened by small rises in creatinine and blood urea nitrogen during diuresis, which is more often a direct result of reflex responses to decreased atrial distension than an indication of falling cardiac output. The majority of patients with chronically dilated heart failure will achieve their highest cardiac outputs with pulmonary capillary wedge pressures in the range of 12 to 15 mmHg. [22] Forward stroke volume often increase by 30-50%, due largely to forward redistribution of mitral regurgitant flow. [23]

Resting hemodynamic compensation is maintained on standard doses of diuretics and vasodilators despite low left ventricular ejection fractions in most patients with left ventricular dysfunction, who have not been shown to benefit from hemodynamic monitoring to achieve more precise goals when already clinically compensated. Cardiac transplantation is rarely indicated in such patients except for other indications such as refractory angina or arrhythmias. Adjustment of vasodilators or diuretics can be guided by clinical assessment in some patients with mild hemodynamic abnormalities. When severe symptoms persist after empiric therapy, however, further intervention can frequently still restore compensation (Table 4). [20]

In the Bethesda conference on cardiac transplantation, the summary of general recommendations specifies that functional status should not be assessed until patients have

Table 4. Suggested indications for invasive monitoring of hemodynamics during therapy of congestion

Congestion with concomitant hypoperfusion suggested by: Mental obtundation Pulse pressure < 25% Cool extremities Declining renal function Hemodynamic intolerance to ACEI (likely when systolic blood pressure < 90 mmHg or serum sodium < 133 mEq/l)
Congestion in the presence of: Active ischemia Symptomatic ventricular arrhythmias Suspected active pulmonary disease Impaired baseline renal function
Congestion persisting or recurring despite all of: ACEI as tolerated Combination high-dose diuretics Sodium and water restriction
Serious consideration of heart transplantation for symptoms of heart failure

ACEI – antiotensin-converting-enzyme inhibitors

(From Stevenson, LW. Selection and management of a potential candidate for cardiac transplantation. In: Cooper DKC, Miller LW and Patterson GA (Eds) The transplantation and replacement of thoracic organs, 1996, Kluwer Academic Publishers: Table 4, Page 164)

undergone aggressive therapy with combinations of vasodilator and diuretic therapies. [24] "Therapy should be adjusted until clinical congestion has been resolved or until further therapy has been repeatedly limited by severe hypotension (generally systolic blood pressure < 80 mmHg) or marked azotemia. Patients should not be considered to have refractory hemodynamic decompensation until therapy with intravenous followed by oral vasodilators and diuretic agents has been pursued using continuous hemodynamic monitoring to approach hemodynamic goals". [24]

Hemodynamic monitoring allows the coupled optimization of both volume status and vascular resistances using simultaneous diuretic and vasodilator therapy, which can rarely otherwise be achieved safely and completely once decompensation is severe (Table 5). Hemodynamic status is often easiest to optimize initially during titration of intravenous vasodilators, such as nitroprusside. Intravenous inotropic agents such as dobutamine have also been used but are less predictive of ultimately successful maintenance on oral regimens because the inotropic component cannot currently be duplicated with available oral drugs. Use of longer-acting inotropic agents is occasionally necessary for prolonged intravenous support, but the long half-life complicates monitored weaning onto oral agents. In addition to restoring clinical stability, reduction of left ventricular filling pressures over several days often demonstrates reversibility of pulmonary hypertension which during acute therapy appeared fixed.

The oral regimens established by tailored therapy often consist of relatively high doses of angiotensin-converting-enzyme inhibitors. Some data suggest that the best survival may be obtained in this population when angiotensin-converting-enzyme inhibitors are combined

Table 5. Tailored therapy for advanced heart failure

1. Steady diuresis to diminish large fluid reservoirs such as major ascites or ansarca
2. Measurement of baseline hemodynamics
3. Intravenous nitroprusside and diuretics tailored to hemodynamic goals
   - PCW $\leq$ 15 mmHg
   - SVR $\leq$ 1200 dynes cm^{-5}
   - RA $\leq$ 8 mmHg
   - SBP $\geq$ 80 mmHg
4. Definition of optimal hymodynamics by 24-48 hours
5. Titration of high-dose oral vasodilators as nitroprusside is weaned
   - Combinations of: captopril, isosorbide dinitrate, hydralazine as needed as alternative or additional therapy
6. Monitored ambulation and diuretic adjustment for 24-48 hours
7. Maintain digoxin levels 1.0-2.0 ng/dl, if no contraindication
8. Detailed patient education
9. Flexible outpatient diuretic regimen including PRN metolazone
10. Progressive walking program
11. Vigilant follow-up

with oral nitrates. [8] Patients with the most severe decompensation, as indicated by very low serum sodium and / or the inability to tolerate sufficient doses of ACE inhibitors to optimize loading conditions, often derive sustained benefit from the combination of hydralazine and oral nitrate therapy.[8]

Tailoring of therapy for hemodynamic goals in class IV heart failure often leads to dramatic improvement in hemodynamics and clinical status (Table 3). Prolonged maintenance of hemodynamic goals has also been associated with measured reductions in atrial size, reduction in the severity of mitral and tricuspid regurgitation and with improvement in peak oxygen consumption (Table 6). [25-27] In combination with patient

Table 6. Outcome of tailored therapy in patients referred for cardiac transplantation

	Pre-referral	*Post-referral*
NYHA Class	3.3	2.4*
Orthopnea (0-4 scale)	3	0.2*
Jugular venuous distension (0-4 scale)	3	0.5*
Edema (0-4 scale)	1	0.1*
Atrial overload		
Left atrial overload (cc)	100	65*
Right atrial volume (cc)	85	52*
Mitral regurgitant units	33	13*
Tricuspid regurgitant units	36	18*
Peak $\dot{V}O_2$ (ml kg^{-1} min^{-1})	11	15*
Hospital / 6 months	2.0	0.2*

* $p < 0.05$ compared to baseline

(From Stevenson, LW. Selection and management of a potential candidate for cardiac transplantation. In: Cooper DKC, Miller LW and Patterson GA (Eds) The transplantation and replacement of thoracic organs, 1996, Kluwer Academic Publishers: Table 6, Page 165)

Table 7. Outpatient therapies for advanced heart failure

Routine Use	*Selected Use*	*Detrimental*	*Under Clinical Investigation*
ACE inhibitors Digoxin Diuretics Nitrates Potassium Replacement Exercise For CAD patients: ASA HMG CoA enzyme inhibitors	β Blockers Amiodarone A II receptor Antagonists Spironolactone Anticoagulation Hydralazine Magnesium AICD Nocturnal oxygen CPAP Ultrafiltration	Amrinone, milrinone Ibopamine Vesnarinone Home prostacyclin Infusion Type 1 anti-arrhythmics Mebefradil Diltiazem Nifedipine Mebefradil Nonsteroidal anti-inflammatory agents	Carvedilol Amlodipine NEP inhibitors Moxonidine Endothelin antagonists Home inotropic infusion Intermittent inotropic Infusion Ubiquitin (Coenzyme Q10) L-Carnitine CPAP

education, progressive exercise and meticulous ongoing care by an experienced heart failure team, this approach has been shown to reduce the rehospitalization rate by over 75%.[27] The impact of this care extends not only to the patient who can postpone transplantation but also to the patient who can await transplantation in greater comfort and in a more favourable condition for surgery and perhaps most importantly to the larger majority of patients for whom transplantation is not an option.

Adjunctive Outpatient Therapies for Heart Failure

On the foundation of tailored therapy, other therapies may offer additional benefit in selected patients (Table 7). The use of adrenergic blocking agents has been shown to improve ejection fraction and clinical status in some patients with heart failure, but their benefit in decompensated heart failure has not been demonstrated.[28, 29] The limited experience in advanced heart failure involves patients who were free of apparent volume overload or congestive symptoms when the drug was cautiously initiated in very low doses.[30] While patients frequently experience some fatigue during initiation of these drugs, administration should usually be stopped if accompanied by fluid retention unresponsive to diuretics or by evidence of hypoperfusion. Although it is controversial, withdrawal should be considered in patients presenting with severe decompensation such that intravenous inotropic therapy is initiated. Amiodarone has been associated with similar increases in ejection fraction, possibly related to similar decreases in heart rate.[31] Unlike other antiarrhythmic agents studied in heart failure, amiodarone does not appear to increase mortality. In fact, several lines of evidence suggest that amiodarone may actually improve survival in advanced heart failure.[32, 33] This effect appears to be independent of the degree of baseline arrhythmia and to result in decreased heart failure endpoints, as well as sudden death.[32]

Multiple non-glycosidic oral inotropic agents have been investigated in heart failure populations, all of which have increased mortality. Intermittent or continuous ambulatory infusion of dobutamine or milrinone are given occasionally even routinely by some programs in some patients, but sustained benefit has not been proven, and concern remains that they may hasten death.

Indications for Cardiac Transplantation

The goal of cardiac transplantation is to maximize the benefit derived from each donor heart transplanted (Figure 3). Benefit is a function of both quality and length of life, with different relative values assigned by different patients. If the goal were instead to maximize overall survival after transplantation, the optimal recipient would be a healthy young athlete, who would himself derive negative benefit from the procedure. For the patient who remains critical in an intensive care unit despite consideration of all other medical and surgical options, the expected benefit of transplantation for both function and survival is obvious. For the patient who remains unstable, in or out of the hospital, with recurrent symptoms of congestion, the benefit is also obvious.

A major challenge of selection is the identification of the ambulatory patient at home who has sufficient clinical limitation or sufficient risk of deterioration and death to warrant the risks and limitations of cardiac transplantation. Many of the adverse prognostic factors validated in large heart failure trials are consistently present in the patients considered for cardiac transplantation. Factors proposed more specifically in severe heart failure relate to cardiac and hemodynamic parameters, the substrate for arrhythmias, and the systemic cardiovascular and neuroendocrine integration.[34 - 40]

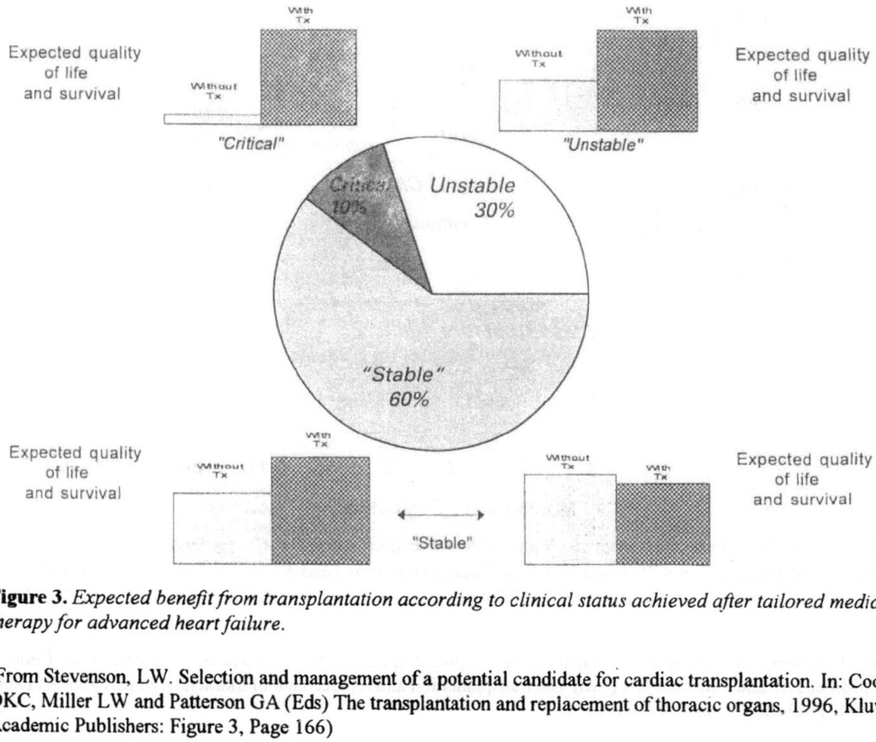

Figure 3. *Expected benefit from transplantation according to clinical status achieved after tailored medical therapy for advanced heart failure.*

(From Stevenson, LW. Selection and management of a potential candidate for cardiac transplantation. In: Cooper DKC, Miller LW and Patterson GA (Eds) The transplantation and replacement of thoracic organs, 1996, Kluwer Academic Publishers: Figure 3, Page 166)

Symptions of Heart Failure

The presence of class IV symptoms of heart failure was originally considered to indicate 'end-stage' heart failure and thus represented the major indication for transplantation. Since the early days of transplantation, however, medical therapy has evolved such that even patients with class IV symptoms can often improve to regain good quality of life. Although survival remains limited, it has improved (Figure 4). While the extended prognosis of advanced heart failure remains worse than that of transplantation, the limitations both of donor supply and of lifespan after transplantation require that the indications for transplantation be based on the expected increment in 1-2-year prognosis, with frequent reassessment. Considering the 70-80% 2-year survival after transplantation at major centres, it has been suggested that cardiac transplant candidates should have a predicted 2-year survival of < 50% without transplant.[41]

Left Ventricular Ejection Fraction

Left ventricular ejection fraction below 20-25% has also been suggested to confer an unacceptable risk of mortality.[42] While this is certainly true when a population covering the spectrum from mild to severe disease is included, the prognostic value of left ventricular ejection fraction once it is below 25-30% is less clear. If only those patients with class III or IV symptoms are considered, the left ventricular ejection fraction is not very helpful once

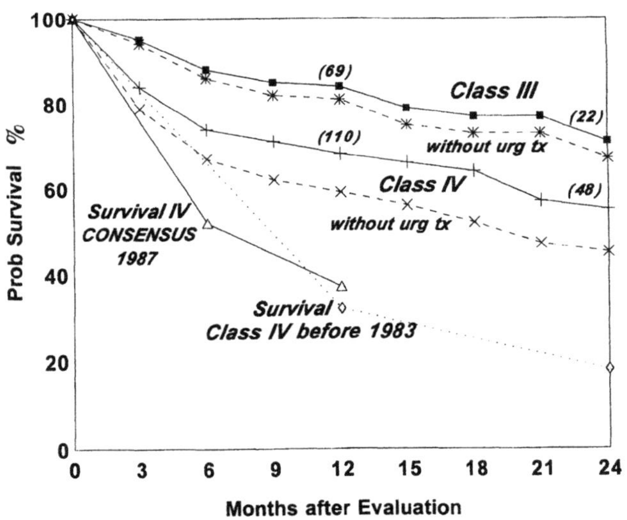

Figure 4. *Overall survival and survival without urgent transplantation for 404 patients presenting with left ventricular ejection fraction ≤25% and New York Heart Association class III (n=265). Recent survival of class IV patients is compared to those described by Wilson et al in 1983 and the CONSENSUS trial in 1987.*[34, 86]

(From Stevenson, LW. Selection and management of a potential candidate for cardiac transplantation. In: Cooper DKC, Miller LW and Patterson GA (Eds) The transplantation and replacement of thoracic organs, 1996, Kluwer Academic Publishers: Figure 4, Page 167)

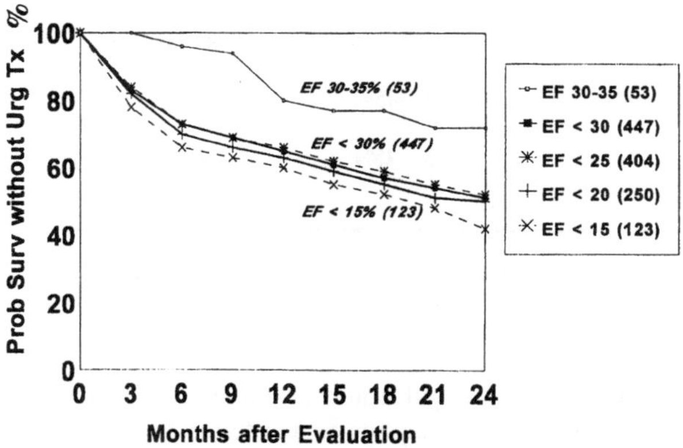

Figure 5. *Relationship of left ventricular ejection fraction to actuarial survival without urgent transplantation in 500 patients presenting with New York Heart Association class III or IV symptoms from 1988-1993 in one center. Ejection fraction >30% was associated with better survival but once below 30% progressively lower ejection fraction did not portend worse survival.*

(From Stevenson, LW. Selection and management of a potential candidate for cardiac transplantation. In: Cooper DKC, Miller LW and Patterson GA (Eds) The transplantation and replacement of thoracic organs, 1996, Kluwer Academic Publishers: Figure 5, Page 167)

it is lower (Figure 5)[43]. Interestingly, potential transplant candidates with massive left ventricular dilatation have a significantly worse prognosis than those with moderate dilatation, even when etiology of disease and degree of hemodynamic compromise are comparable.[44] Even for presentation with class IV symptoms and left ventricular ejection fraction < 20%, prognosis after discharge on tailored medical therapy is not uniformly dismal: 45% survival without urgent transplant.[43] (When comparing the outcome of other therapies to transplantation, it is important to consider the patients who are saved by 'urgent' transplantation as failures of alternative medical therapy, who would presumably have died had they not been hospitalized and supported until transplantation).

Peak Oxygen Consumption

Measurement of peak oxygen consumption during exercise provides an index of overall cardiovascular reserve that is useful both to quantitate functional limitation and to estimate prognosis (Table 8). In the Veterans Administration Heart Failure trials of mild to moderate heart failure a peak oxygen consumption < 14.5 ml kg^{-1} min^{-1} predicted worse survival whether left ventricular ejection fraction was above or below 28%.[45] The experiences of Szlachic and Likoff in other populations confirmed the measurement of peak

Table 8. Peak oxygen consumption and expected benefit from transplantation.

Peak VO_2 with heart failure	*Expected after transplant*	*Estimated 1-year survival with heart failure*	*Estimated 1-year survival after transplant*	*Decision regarding transplant*
< 10	< 14–18	< 50–60%	≤ 80–90%	Transplant (if eligible)
10–14	14–18	60–75%	80–90%	Toward transplant
14–18	14–18	70–85%	80–90%	Away from transplant
> 18	> 14–18	80–95%	≥ 80–90%	No transplant (unless other indications)

(From Stevenson, LW. Selection and management of a potential candidate for cardiac transplantation. In: Cooper DKC, Miller LW and Patterson GA (Eds) The transplantation and replacement of thoracic organs, 1996, Kluwer Academic Publishers: Table 8, Page 166)

oxygen as an independent prognostic guide in heart failure.[46-47] Mancini et al provided the initial validation of peak oxygen consumption as a criterion for transplant candidacy from their analysis of 114 potential transplant candidates, suggesting a critical value of 14 ml kg^{-1} min^{-1}.[48] Other experience has identified values between 10 and 14 ml kg^{-1} min^{-1} (Figure 6A).[49-50]

Some differences between programs may reflect varying practices of excluding patients with obvious resting symptoms. In addition, bicycle exercise yields peak oxygen consumption values slightly lower than treadmill exercise. Synthesis of the currently available information suggests that patients who are unable to perform exercise or who can achieve peak oxygen consumption of < 10-12 ml kg^{-1} min^{-1} have the worst prognosis. The importance of indexing to predicted values remains controversial (Figure 6B). Patients with peak oxygen consumption over 16-18 ml kg^{-1} min^{-1} have 2-year survival rates similar to that of cardiac transplantation, in the absence of other confounding factors such as active ischemia or rapid deterioration (Table 8).

Many patients are unwilling to accept the burdens and risks of immunosuppression unless a major improvement in functional capacity is anticipated in addition to the survival benefit. For some patients with stable heart failure by clinical criteria quality of life may not be significantly improved after transplantation.[51 - 53] Despite a left ventricular ejection fraction usually within normal limits, exercise capacity after transplantation is limited by multiple cardiac and systemic factors. Peak oxygen consumption and other measures of exercise capacity such as the 6-minute walk distance are often similar between patients with stable heart failure and cardiac transplant recipients, in the range of 50-70% of values predicted on the basis of age, size, and gender.[52] The perception of prolonged fatigue after exertion is less easy to quantify, but appears less common after transplantation.

The current guidelines for cardiac transplantation focus on peak oxygen consumption as the basis for predicting improvements in survival and functional capacity after transplantation (Table 9).[24] While considerable debate surrounds the issue of whether to adjust for age- and gender-predicted maximal values, the threshold of peak oxygen

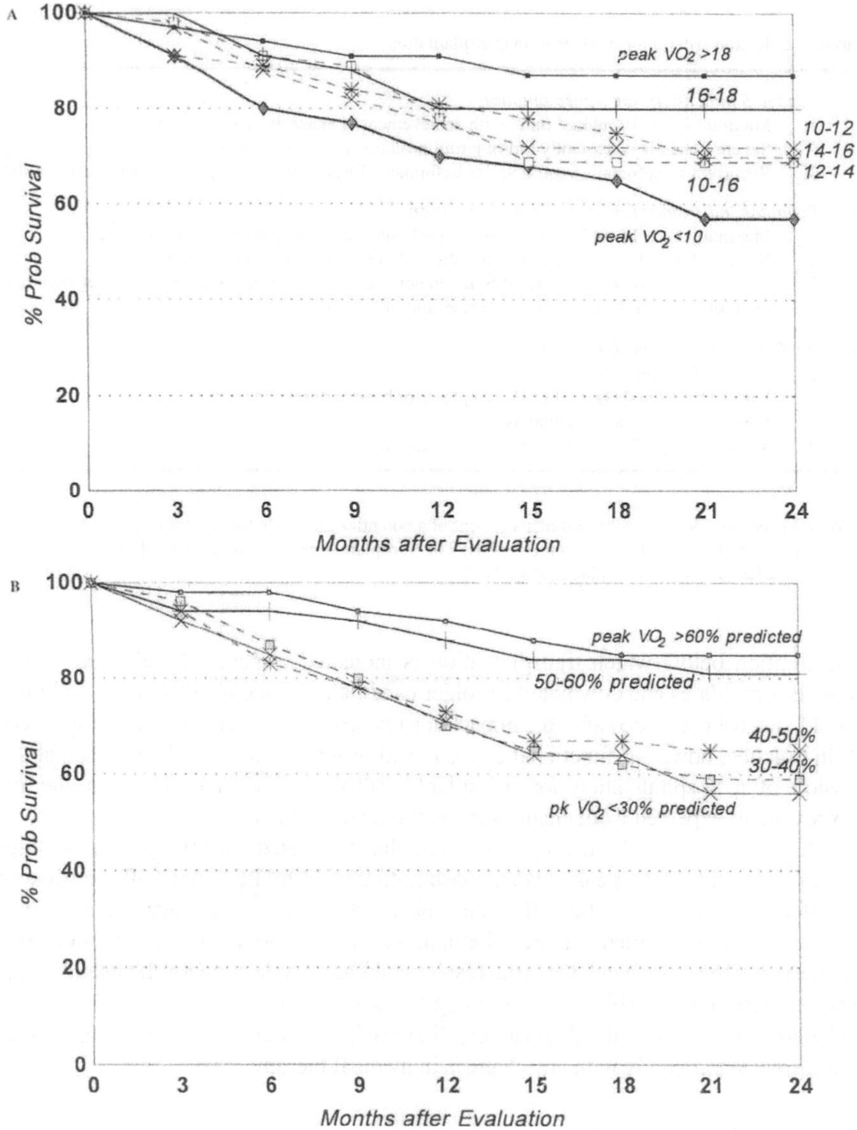

Figure 6. *Actuarial survival without hospitalization for urgent transplantation analyzed for 320 patients undergoing cardiopulmonary exercise testing during the initial evaluation. Top: Analysis according to peak oxygen consumption (ml kg^{-1} min^{-1}) achieved <10 (n=73), 10-12 (n=67), 12-14 (n=62), 14-16 (n=46), 16-18 (n=37) and >18 (n=35). Bottom: Analysis according to percentage of predicted peak oxygen consumption which was actually achieved, demonstrating a threshold value of 50% with additional discrimination.*[87]

(From Stevenson, LW. Selection and management of a potential candidate for cardiac transplantation. In: Cooper DKC, Miller LW and Patterson GA (Eds) The transplantation and replacement of thoracic organs, 1996, Kluwer Academic Publishers: Figure 6, Page 168)

Table 9. Selection criteria for benefits from transplantation.

I.	*Accepted indications for transplantation*	
	1.	Maximal $\dot{V}O_2 < 10$ ml kg^{-1} min^{-1} with achievement of anaerobic metabolism
	2.	Severe ischemia consistently limiting routine activity not amenable to bypass surgery or angioplasty
	3.	Recurrent symptomatic ventricular arrhythmias refractory to all accepted therapeutic modalities
II.	*Probable indications for cardiac transplantation*	
	1.	Maximal $\dot{V}O_2 < 14$ ml kg^{-1} min^{-1} and major limitation of the patient's daily activities
	2.	Recurrent unstable ischemia not amenable to bypass surgery or angioplasty
	3.	Instability of fluid balance / renal function not due to patient non-compliance with regimen of weight monitoring, flexible use of diuretic drugs and salt restriction
III.	*Inadequate indications for transplantation*	
	1.	Ejection fraction ≤ 20%
	2.	History functional class III or IV symptoms of heart failure
	3.	Previous ventricular arrhythmias
	4.	Maximal $\dot{V}O_2 > 15$ ml kg^{-1} min^{-1} without other indications

(From Stevenson, LW. Selection and management of a potential candidate for cardiac transplantation. In: Cooper DKC, Miller LW and Patterson GA (Eds) The transplantation and replacement of thoracic organs, 1996, Kluwer Academic Publishers: Table 9, Page 169)

consumption below which transplantation is indicated is generally adjusted upward for younger candidates and downward for older candidates. Functional capacity and prognosis should ideally be assessed after the impact of a revised medical regimen can be appreciated.[51, 52] In practice, however, functional capacity and prognosis are usually assessed at the conclusion of a hospitalization for transplant evaluation, and interpreted in the light of improvement expected from changes in the medical regimen.

A patient referred, for example, after months of repeated hospitalizations for congestive symptoms might have a peak oxygen consumption of 11 ml kg^{-1} min^{-1} after evaluation, but the effective diuresis of 10 kg of fluid and enhanced vasodilator regimen might allow further symptomatic improvement and peripheral muscle reconditioning due to relief of exertional dyspnea. On the other hand, the same result would be an indication for the listing of a patient who is referred on a stable regimen of angiotensin-converting-enzyme inhibitors, diuretics and digoxin with an initial pulmonary capillary wedge pressure of 14 mmHg, who is unlikely to improve significantly with any changes in medical therapy.

Restrictive Cardiomyopathy

A severely reduced left ventricular ejection fraction is neither necessary nor sufficient indication for transplantation (Table 9). Although the majority of patients referred have an ejection fraction below 25%, patients may also have severe symptoms of congestion due to restrictive disease in which the ventricle is minimally dilated and the ejection fraction is 30-45%. Such patients may have severe difficulty maintaining their fluid balance even with meticulous salt and fluid restriction. Amyloidosis needs to be excluded in such patients, even in the absence of a characteristic echocardiographic appearance. When restrictive disease has progressed slowly over many years liver function should be carefully assessed because these patients may be among the few to develop true irreversible 'cardiac cirrhosis'.

Hypertrophic Cardiomyopathy
Cardiac transplantation is rarely indicated for hypertrophic cardiomyopathy when still in the hypercontractile stage. Diuretics and agents that decrease contractility can generally control congestive symptoms. Dual chamber pacing, myomectomy and mitral valve replacement should be considered. In the minority of patients who progress to 'burned-out' cardiomyopathy, congestive symptoms and exercise intolerance may become severe with only modest reduction of contractility to ejection fractions in the range of 30-40% due to concomitant impairment in compliance. The natural history of these patients has not been well established, but their clinical limitation suggests that quality of life and outcome may be sufficiently compromised to warrant cardiac transplantation.

Other Indications
Transplantation is occasionally indicated for reasons other than heart failure. Intractable angina may be an indication when multiple revascularization procedures have failed and no further attempts at surgical or catheter-based intervention are feasible. The left ventricular ejection fraction is usually below 30% in such patients, because those with better left ventricular function are generally candidates for some form of revascularization procedure. Transplantation is occasionally performed in patients disabled by recurrent discharges from automatic implantable defibrillators despite all attempts at catheter ablation and chemical control. Unusual trauma or isolated intracardiac tumours are rare indications for transplantation.

Contraindications to Cardiac Transplantation

Evaluation for transplantation includes a careful search for any non-cardiac condition that limits life expectancy or increases the risk of complications from the procedure, particularly from immunosuppression (Table 10). [24,54] Although this component of evaluation might logically take place after a patient has demonstrated indications for transplantation, in practice it is often more efficient to perform it simultaneously. Furthermore, in patients who initially appear too well for transplantation, but may deteriorate, transplantation can be performed more expeditiously when eligibility has already been established.

The appropriate candidate for cardiac transplantation is sick enough to need a new heart, but sufficiently well in terms of overall condition and non-cardiac organ function to expect a good result. Age limits are controversial and usually expressed in relative rather than absolute terms. Highly selected older patients have good 1-year survival, but large series demonstrate decreased longer survival in order patients. [55 - 57] The older candidates are usually evaluated very carefully for evidence of diseases which commonly cause co-morbidity in this age group.

Table 10. Contraindications to cardiac transplantation.

General eligibility
Absence of any non-cardiac condition that would itself shorten life expectancy or increase the risk of death from rejection or from complications of immunosuppression, particularly infection
Specific contraindications
Approximate age limit of 60–65 years (various programs)
Active infection
Active ulcer disease
Severe diabetes mellitus with end-organ damage
Severe peripheral vascular disease
Pulmonary function (FEV_1, FVC) < 60%* or history of chronic bronchitis
Creatinine clearance < 40–50 ml/min*
Bilirubin > 2.5 mg/dl, transaminases > 2 x normal*
Pulmonary artery systolic pressure > 60 mmHg*
Mean transpulmonary gradient > 15 mmHg*
High risk of life-threatening non-compliance
- Inability to make strong commitment to transplantation
- Cognitive impairment severe enough to limit comprehension of medical regimen
- Psychiatric instability severe enough to jeopardize incentive for adherence to medical regimen
- History of recurring alcohol or drug abuse
- Failure of establish stable address or telephone number
- Previous demonstration of repeated non-compliance with medication or follow-up

(From Stevenson, LW. Selection and management of a potential candidate for cardiac transplantation. In: Cooper DKC, Miller LW and Patterson GA (Eds) The transplantation and replacement of thoracic organs, 1996, Kluwer Academic Publishers: Table 10, Page 170)

Active Systemic Disease

Considerations regarding the etiology of disease are important to exclude patients with active systemic disease such as lupus erythematosus, rheumatoid arthritis or scleroderma which could cause disease after transplantation. In most programs amyloidosis is a contraindication due to the tendency for systemic progression and recurrence in the allograft.[58] Chagas' disease may reactivate after cardiac transplantation, but is a common disease in South America, where immunosuppressive therapy has been successfully used after transplantation.[59]

Considerable emotional debate may develop regarding patients with chronic conditions with the potential to deteriorate after transplantation, as some patients at high risk will nonetheless do well after transplantation. The severe shortage of donor hearts curtails the systematic validation of each apparent contraindication. As described by Copeland, selection must therefore reflect 'a combination of empirically derived contraindications with limited natural history and considerable common sense'.[60]

Diabetes mellitus is no longer an absolute contraindication for transplantation, although, severity of disease in terms of duration and insulin doses renders candidacy less likely. Initiation and augmentation of immunosuppression render glucose control very difficult and hyperglycemia predisposes to infection. Patients with diabetes are evaluated carefully for evidence of other organ damage such as proteinuria and nephropathy, peripheral neuropathy, retinopathy and small-vessel peripheral vascular disease which are generally considered grounds for exclusion. Adult survivors of juvenile-onset diabetes are generally excluded for one or more of the above conditions.

Psychosocial Factors

Failure to adhere to a rigorous regimen of medications, biopsies, and clinic visits remains a major factor in rejection and mortality for all organ transplant recipients.[61,62] The heavy psychological and financial burdens of chronic heart failure followed by transplantation, combined with labile mood changes during glucocorticoid augmentation, can precipitate lethal episodes of overt suicidal behaviour or more commonly passive attempts to commit suicide through withdrawal of immunosuppression. Considerable debate surrounds the importance of various psychiatric and psychological conditions. Similarly, the importance of family support varies from patient to patient. Relative weaknesses in one area may be compensated by other strengths. The multiple factors relating to the patients and their support systems may best be combined into a profile from which the chances for longterm compliance can be assessed (Table 10). One of the many reasons that effective transplantation programs include integrated heart failure programs is the opportunity for reassessment of patients with non-compliance history, who might later demonstrate sufficient compliance on complicated medical therapy to warrant acceptance.[63]

Previous Malignant Disease

The incidence of malignancy is increased in organ transplant recipients and other patients on chronic immunosuppression, presumably due to impaired policing of potentially oncogenic viruses and malignant clones, particularly of lymphomas, which may occur up to 40 times more frequently in transplant recipients.[64] Transplantation is generally not performed within 3-5 years of neoplasms other than superficial skin lesions. A history of tumours with a predilection for recurrence, such as breast cancer and renal cell cancer, requires vigorous screening for recurrent disease. There is a growing population, however, of patients with successful transplantation late after successful chemotherapy with adriamycin-containing regimens for lymphoma, particularly Hodgkin's lymphoma.

Irreversible Pulmonary Hypertension

Multiple criteria for selection of recipients are profoundly affected by hemodynamic compromise, which may need to be addressed before candidacy can be confirmed (Table 10). Demonstration of sufficiently low pulmonary vascular resistance may require several days of vigorous reduction of left-sided filling pressures with vasodilators and diuretics, occasionally requiring support with inotrope-dilators also. Early pulmonary hypertension presents a heavy burden to the donor right ventricle, even if pulmonary pressures later decrease. Acute right heart failure continues to be a major factor in early postoperative morbidity.

Pulmonary hypertension is generally evaluated not by one number alone, but by a combination of calculations, including pulmonary vascular resistance, which should generally be reducible to below 240-300 dynes-cm^{-5}, pulmonary artery systolic pressure which should be reducible to levels below 50-60 mmHg and transpulmonary gradient. The transpulmonary gradient, calculated as the mean pulmonary artery pressure minus the pulmonary capillary wedge pressure, usually shows the least change during pharmacologic therapy and should be below 12-15 mmHg.[65] Although evaluation in some centres includes acute titration of intravenous nitroprusside to systemic blood pressure tolerance, reversibility of pulmonary hypertension in patients with pulmonary capillary wedge pressures chronically above 25 mmHg may be easier to demonstrate after sustained reductions in filling pressures over several days.[66] The average patient with symptoms at rest, or with minimal exertion, has chronically elevated ventricular filling pressures and some reversible elevation in pulmonary pressures (Table 11). A brief trial of prostaglandin E1 may occasionally help to demonstrate reversibility after other modalities and assist in planning of postoperative hemodynamic management. Nitric oxide appears to be a potent pulmonary vasodilator, but its use should be tempered with caution, as it frequently leads to elevation in left-sided filling pressures, most likely due to increased right-sided cardiac output to the failing left ventricle. Heterotopic transplantation ('piggy-back' of the new heart on the old) has at times been employed for irreversible pulmonary hypertension, but this procedure has been associated with a 1-month mortality of 25% compared to 10% for othotopic transplantation, and it is now rarely performed.[67,68]

Impaired Pulmonary Function

Pulmonary function testing should be postponed until after hemodynamic optimization in patients with obvious resting congestion. Both obstructive and restrictive patterns may be observed with pulmonary congestion.[69] Maintained reduction of filling pressures and volume status, often for several days, allows optimal performance. General thresholds for

Table 11. Pre-operative reversibility of pulmonary hypertension during tailored therapy prior to transplantation in 100 patients later receiving transplanation.

	Initial PVR > 240 dyne-s-cm^{-5}	*Initial PAS > 50 mmHg*	*Initial TPG > 15 mmHg*
No	59% (9%) †	35% (6%) †	86% (7%) †
Yes	41% (5%)	65% (8%)	14% (7%)
If yes, reversible *	25% (11%)	41% (3%)	8% (17%)
Not reversible	16% (0%)	24% (10%)	6% (0%)

Numbers in parentheses indicate 30-day mortality after transplantation. †

PAS = pulmonary artery systolic pressure; PVR = pulmonary vascular resistance; TPG = transpulmonary gradient) (mean pulmonary artery pressure minus pulmonary capilliary wedge pressure)

*** Reversibility determined after 72 h of therapy tailored to reduce pulmonary capillary wedge to 15 mmHg, followed occasionally by a trial of prostaglandin E_1, if necessary.**

† Reproducibility of this post-transplant survival may depend in part on the vigor with which pulmonary congestion is prevented preoperatively, the preservation and age of the donor heart, and early postoperative hemodynamic management.

(From Stevenson, LW. Selection and management of a potential candidate for cardiac transplantation. In: Cooper DKC, Miller LW and Patterson GA (Eds) The transplantation and replacement of thoracic organs, 1996, Kluwer Academic Publishers: Table 11, Page 171)

acceptability have been 50-70% of predicted forced vital capacity and forced expired volume. Cessation of smoking is generally required by most programs for at least 3 months, both to reduce perioperative pulmonary complications and to decrease the chance of postoperative smoking, which may increase the risk of early graft coronary artery disease.[70] Compliance with smoking cessation may be assessed with unscheduled urinary nicotine levels. Regardless of pulmonary function test results, a history of chronic sputum production and a 'smoker's cough' is sometimes considered a contraindication due to risks of pulmonary infection during immunosuppresion. No organized data have been collected on post-transplant outcome for patients with mild intrinsic asthma, which has generally not been considered a complication unless it has required intensive chronic therapy or multiple hospitalizations.

Hepatic Dysfunction

Hepatic function is also optimized by vigorous diuresis and vasodilator therapy to reduce right-sided filling pressures and tricuspid regurgitation. This is important not only to establish transplant candidacy, but to minimize coagulopathy which may become profound after cardiopulmonary during transplantation. All patterns of abnormal liver function have been observed with 'passive congestion'. Depressed cardiac output is much less important for hepatic function, except when circulatory collapse leads to 'shock liver', when elevation of transaminases into the thousands may occur. This pattern should be allowed to recover during support with either circulatory support devices or drugs prior to transplantation to avoid postoperative hepatic failure.

Renal Dysfunction

Unlike pulmonary and hepatic function, renal function is more dependent on adequate cardiac output. In fact, even when cardiac output is adequate, renal function may decline temporarily after brisk diuresis of chronically congested patients, perhaps due to sudden decompensation of distended atria and resultant reflex increase in renal vasoconstriction, and perhaps compounded by decreased atrial natriuretic peptide secretion.[71, 72]. Several days of inotropic infusions may be required to optimize renal function in some cases. Creatinine clearance of at least 50 ml/min is preferred, but lower rates may occasionally be accepted if clearly the result of acute decompensation, with normal renal size on ultrasound and absence of proteinuria. Disproportionate elevation of blood urea nitrogen is common. Patients with creatinine over 2 mg/ml, blood urea nitrogen over 50 mg/dl or preoperative dependence on inotropic infusions, are at particularly high risk for early postoperative renal dysfunction, which may in some cases be decreased by the use of antithymocyte globulins rather than cyclosporin in the immediate postoperative period.

The Critically Ill Patient

Evaluation presents a particular challenge when performed in a candidate seen first in critical condition. When the patient's major organ and cerebral function are acutely compromised, decisions regarding medical risk and patient commitment are based on experienced guesswork and emotional bias. Peripheral vascular disease is often underappreciated while renal and hepatic dysfunction believed (or hoped) to be reversible may become major impediments to postoperative recovery. A common ordeal is the decision regarding a young patient with a previous history of non-compliance or substance abuse for whom there is no time to confirm a commitment to reform. Some patients in critical condition must be refused transplantation, with the cost of immediate disappointment preventing the tragedy of protracted postoperative misery prior to death, and the tragedy of the premature end of a donor heart. Transplantation for otherwise doomed patients, however, is often the most rewarding, with the infinite relative increment in both quality and length of life (Figure 3). Increasing availability of mechanical circulatory support may allow many such patients to achieve stabilization and rehabilitation before transplant, following which the chance of favourable post-transplant outcome may be highest.

Documented Risk Factors
Collaboration between transplant programs is now yielding increasing information regarding the likelihood of good post-transplant outcomes. Of the two major multicenter experiences, the International Society for Heart and Lung Transplantation (ISHLT) Registry has established older age, left ventricular ejection fraction <11%, mechanical support while waiting, and female gender as risk factors for death after transplantation.[2] It should be noted, however, that some risk factors for post-transplant death also identify high risk without transplantation. The Cardiac Transplant Research Database provided the first multivariate analysis of death, demonstrating older age, elevated serum creatinine, low cardiac output and mechanical ventilation prior to transplantation to be associated with worse survival, while female gender was associated with more rejection but equivalent survival.[73] A separate study of program attributes found the most important program factor in patient survival to be the previous experience of the transplant cardiologist, with strong contribution from the transplant nurse coordinator.[74]

Candidates on the Waiting List: Management and Re-Evaluation

The average waiting period for candidates has increased from 6 weeks for all candidates in 1984 to over 6 months on average. Patients waiting at home frequently do not undergo cardiac transplantation for over a year after listing, particularly if they have blood group O. During the prolonged waiting time, outpatients require careful management and re-evaluation for both deterioration and improvement. As recommended by the Consensus Conference on Transplantation, waiting candidates should be seen at least monthly by the heart failure/transplant cardiologist at the centre where the transplant will be performed.[9] Assessment of clinical stability by history, particularly for evidence of congestion, examination of postural vital signs and jugular venous pressure and laboratory monitoring of electrolytes, renal and hepatic function and anticoagulation are critical to ensure that the candidates are in optimal condition for transplantation. More frequent visits with the primary physician are often necessary.

Medical management for transplant candidates is dominated by the same principles developed to decrease the need for transplantation and provide alternative hope to ineligible patients. Maintenance of low filling pressures not only serves to minimize congestive pulmonary and abdominal symptoms and improve nutrition, but also reduces the risk of postoperative pulmonary hypertension, prolonged intubation, coagulopathy and hepatic dysfunction during the postoperative course. Patients should be compliant with a regimen which includes, in most cases, restriction to <2 g of sodium and <2 L of fluid daily and always a daily weight diary which guides patient adjustment of diuretic dosage. The spectrum of medications in this population is shown in Table 7.

Anticoagulation

The issue of anticoagulation for patients with low left ventricular ejection fractions and dilated ventricles remains controversial. It is accepted that patients with an additional risk factor such as atrial fibrillation, history of previous embolic event or pedunculated thrombus need anticoagulation, with the strongest risk factor being atrial fibrillation with its yearly embolism risk as high as 18% in the presence of heart failure.[75] In 120 transplant candidates without any of these risk factors, the incidence of embolic events during a mean follow-up of 300 days without anticoagulation was 4%.[76] The official National Practice Guidelines for Heart Failure do not at this time recommend routine anticoagulation for heart failure patients without other risk factors.[77] The decision reflects the estimated balance of risks of embolic events, which can lead to tragic strokes and death, and the risks of hemorrhage, which can rarely lead to intracranial hemorrhage or other life-threatening events. The risks of bleeding are low when anticoagulation is monitored closely and doses decreased for amiodarone and impaired hepatic function. Perioperative bleeding is often greater after coumadin therapy despite administration of vitamin K prior to the transplant.

Ventricular Dysrhythmia

Non-sustained ventricular tachycardia occurs in 50-80% of patients with heart failure severe enough to warrant evaluation for transplantation.[40] Although sudden death occurs in 15-30% of these patients its relationship to previous non-sustained ventricular tachycardia remains controversial. The risk of sudden death is increased in heart failure patients with a history of syncope, which is an indication for admission and evaluation.

Therapy for asymptomatic non-sustained ventricular tachycardia has generally not been undertaken unless the runs are long and rapid. Type 1 antiarrhythmic agents appear to increase the risk of sudden death in heart failure patients, and are rarely used except occasionally to decrease the frequency of discharges from an implantable cardioverter-defibrillator. Therapy with amiodarone does not worsen and may improve survival in severe heart failure, with benefits for ventricular function and heart failure endpoints as well as sudden death.[32] The GESICA trial studied patients with an overall mortality of 55% at 2 years, similar to that of ambulatory transplant candidates with class IV history, and found a 28% decrease of mortality with amiodarone[32] The differences between this trial and the Veterans Administration trial may reflect in part the different disease severity.[33] Perioperative pulmonary and hemodynamic problems attributed to prolonged amiodarone use have been described in other surgical populations, but have rarely occurred after transplantation.[78]

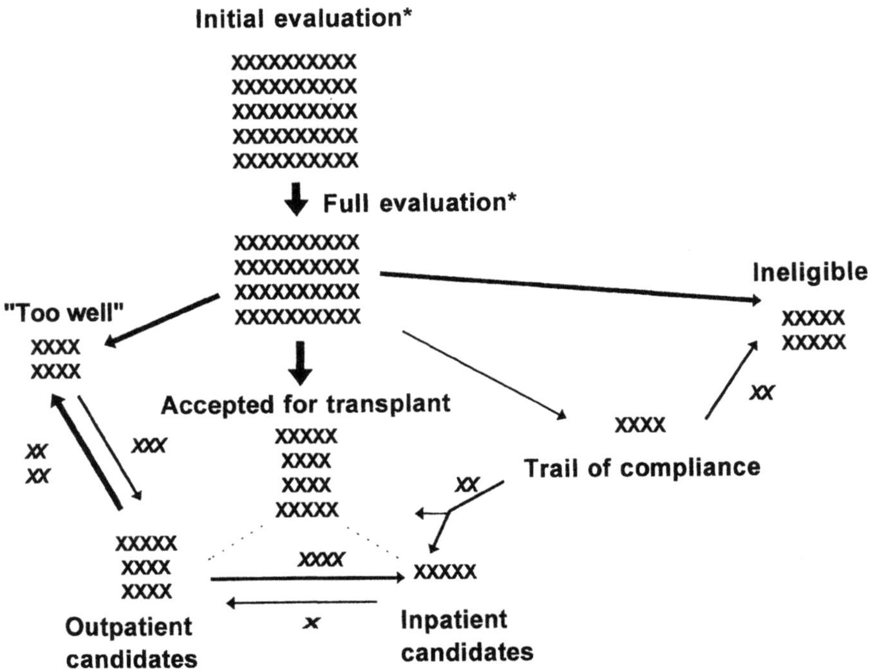

Figure 7. *Progress through evaluation and continual re-evaluation for cardiac transplantation demonstrating the dynamic nature of candidacy.*

(From Stevensön, LW. Selection and management of a potential candidate for cardiac transplantation. In: Cooper DKC, Miller LW and Patterson GA (Eds) The transplantation and replacement of thoracic organs, 1996, Kluwer Academic Publishers: Figure 7, Page 173)

Hospitalization

Candidacy is a dynamic state from which movement is possible, particularly during the lengthening waiting periods (Figure 7). Deterioration to require hospitalization has in the past occurred in up to 30% of candidates during the first 6 months and may become more frequent with growing adherence to more defined criteria of disease severity before listing.[79] The pre-transplant database of 1340 patients listed at 11 major US institutions described the pre-transplant mortality of 23% in patients listed as urgent (Status 1) and 17% mortality if listed originally as Status II.[80] Hospitalization may be indicated to prevent imminent death or to prevent serious organ system deterioration which could compromise the outcome of transplantation (Table 12). Progressive right heart failure and worsening renal or hepatic dysfunction could be indications for hospitalization even if the candidate finds them compatible with life at home. Escalating fluid retention can increase perioperative pulmonary hypertension, prolong intubation requirements, and worsen coagulopathy but also seem to be associated anecdotally with an increased risk of unexpected death at home, which may in part be related to the difficulties of controlling potassium, both high and low, during fluctuating diuresis and electrolyte replacement.

Table 12. Frequent indications for hospital admission of waiting candidates.

General considerations
To prevent death at home
To prevent conditions which jeopardize perioperative outcome

Specific considerations
Unstable angina
Syncope
Frequent Implantable cardioventer defibrillator discharges
Suspected embolic event
Congestion refractory despite good compliance to increased diuretics, which:
  a) renders patients bedridden
  b) causes marked hepatic congestion
  c) may worsen borderline pulmonary hypertension
Systolic blood pressure persistently < 70–75 mmHg
Pulse pressure < 12 mmHg, particularly with cool extremities
Creatinine > 2.0 and rising

(From Stevenson, LW. Selection and management of a potential candidate for cardiac transplantation. In: Cooper DKC, Miller LW and Patterson GA (Eds) The transplantation and replacement of thoracic organs, 1996, Kluwer Academic Publishers: Table 12, Page 174)

Although patients with the most severe compromise can expect the greatest improvement from transplantation, perioperative condition is a critical determinant of postoperative outcome and should be optimized.

Mechanical Circulatory Support

The indications for mechanical circulatory support continue to evolve. The hemodynamic criteria often suggested for heart failure were actually originally proposed for the very different setting of post-cardiotomy shock needing intra-aortic balloon counterpulsation.[81] These criteria include cardiac index <2.0 $l\ min^{-1}\ m^{-2}$, pulmonary capillary wedge pressure >20 mmHg, systolic blood pressure <90 mmHg and systemic vascular resistance >2100 dynes-cm^{-5}, which are typical of many heart failure patients who can be not only stabilized but also discharged after adjustment of medical therapy. The clinical impact of hemodynamic parameters varies greatly, particularly in relation to the duration of compromise, but at the most severe end of the spectrum, mechanical support would generally be indicated for continued inability to maintain a systolic blood pressure >75 mmHg, cardiac index >1.5 $l\ min^{-1}\ m^{-2}$, and pulmonary venous saturation >50% on maximal pharmacologic support. (Severely elevated filling pressures, on the other hand, generally indicate the potential for improvement from further adjustment of medical therapy). More subtle trends of declining cardiac index and renal function on maximal therapy are difficult to interpret, but are at least as important as the absolute measured numbers.[82]

Patients who require mechanical support in the absence of coronary artery disease may be considered for direct placement of left ventricular assist devices without intervening therapy with an intra-aortic balloon, from which the benefit is controversial in this population.

Patients with coronary disease who demonstrate continued dependence on intra-aortic balloon counterpulsation may eventually also be considered for placement of a left ventricular assist device, which allows ambulation and rehabilitation prior to transplantation. Over 300 left ventricular assist devices, both the HeartMate and Novacor models, have been implanted in the United States.[83] Complications include infection, usually through the drive line, bleeding, and thromboemboli from the heart and from the device itself, which appear to be less common with the HeartMate due to the endothelialization of the blood-contacting surface.

Recent experience with left ventricular assistance as bridging to transplantation has shown approximately 70% survival to transplantation. The clear benefit of bridging devices for improving pre-transplant rehabilitation and post-transplant recovery has led to consideration of devices for 'destination as well as bridging' therapy.[84]

Re-evaluation

The long waiting periods also allow demonstration of improvement in some patients able to wait at home. The highest period of risk for outpatients may be the first few months, after which some of the factors which led to deterioration and referral may resolve spontaneously, and the benefits of optimal medical therapy may be realized. The Bethesda Conference and the Consensus Conference on Selection both emphasize the important of periodic re-evaluation of waiting candidates.[9, 24] Suggested criteria for re-evaluation include an assessment of clinical stability and demonstration of improved exercise capacity measured by peak oxygen consumption (Table 13). Up to 30% of ambulatory patients initially listed with initial average peak oxygen consumption <14 ml kg^{-1} min^{-1} (average 11) demonstrated sufficient improvement to leave the list, with a subsequent 2-year survival of 92%.[51]

Table 13. Assessment of clinical stability for re-evaluation of waiting candidates.

Clinical criteria

1. Stable fluid balance without orthopnea, elevated jugular venous pressures, or other evidence of congestion on the flexible diuretic regimen
2. Stable blood pressure with systolic at least 80 mmHg
3. Stable serum sodium (usually > 133 mEq/l)
4. Stable renal function (blood urea nitrogen usually < 60 mg/dl)
5. Absence of symptomatic ventricular arrhythmias
6. Absence of frequent angina
7. Absence of severe drug side-effects
8. Stable or improving activity level without syspnea during self-care or 1 block exertion

Exercise criteria (if initial peak oxygen consumption < 14 ml kg^{-1} min^{-1})

1. Improvement in peak oxygen consumption ≥ 2 ml kg^{-1} min^{-1}
2. Peak oxygen consumption of ≥ 12 ml kg^{-1} min^{-1}

(From Stevenson, LW. Selection and management of a potential candidate for cardiac transplantation. In: Cooper DKC, Miller LW and Patterson GA (Eds) The transplantation and replacement of thoracic organs, 1996, Kluwer Academic Publishers: Table 13, Page 174)

Comment

The personal dedication of the early heart transplantation teams combined with the advances in surgical techniques and immunosuppression have established this as the best current therapy for patients with truly end-stage heart failure. Once patients are referred for transplantation with New York Heart Association class IV symptoms and an ejection fraction <25%, even if they can be maintained out of the hospital, their survival without urgent transplant is less than 50% at 2 years. [43] This compared to a 60% chance of surviving to 6 years and a 35% chance of surviving 10 years after transplantation with current protocols.[2, 43] Most recipients achieve a good to excellent quality of life, although less than 50% return to full-time employment.[85]

As originally projected at the time of the first Bethesda conference on transplantation over 25 years ago, however, the promise of transplantation has not been fulfilled.[1] Despite arduous efforts the donor heart supply is limited to 2000-2500 per year in the United States, compared to the 40,000-45,000 originally projected in 1968. Over 70% of these hearts are being used for patients waiting in hospitals. It has been said that heart transplantation is currently to heart failure what the lottery is to poverty (attributed to Arnold Katz and others).

Left ventricular assist devices currently offer hope for those hospitalized patients who might otherwise not survive until transplantation. Although now employed only as 'bridges' to transplantation, increasing refinement and experience suggest that permanent ambulatory devises may extend a highway even to patient ineligible for transplantation. At the other end of the spectrum of heart failure, there is now increasing evidence that early intervention can reduce the development of heart failure. [86, 87] Even after the symptoms of heart failure have appeared, new approaches to both medical and surgical therapy may prolong the period of cardiac and clinical compensation. [3-5, 20] In particular, recognition of the contributions of mitral regurgitation and left ventricular distortion to be progression of heart failure has stimulated the development of new surgical approaches to cardiac remodelling.

A beneficial side-effect of cardiac transplantation has been the increased medical and public focus on the problem of heart failure, which affects over 3 million patients in the United States, almost 1 million of whom have class III-IV symptoms. The magnitude of the miseries and costs of this problem warrant increasing focus on innovation and collaboration at all levels of research and clinical care.

References

1. Moore FD. Fifth Bethesda Conference Report: Cardiac and other organ transplantation. Am J Cardiol 1968;22:896.
2. Hosenpud JD, Bennet CE, Keek BRN, Fiel B, Novick RJ. The Registry of the International Society for Heart and Lung Transplantation: Fourteenth official report, 1997. J Heart Lung Transplant 1997;13:691.
3. Bach DS, Bolling SF. Early improvement in congestive heart failure after correction of secondary mitral regurgitation in end-stage cardiomyopathy. Am Heart J 1995;129:1165.
4. Louie HW, Laks H, Milgalter E, et al. Ischemic cardiomyopathy: criteria for coronary revascularization and cardiac transplantation. Circulation 1991 (Suppl.III):290.
5. Elefteriades JA, Tolis G, Levi E, Mills LK, Zaret BL. Coronary artery bypass grafting in severe left ventricular dysfunction: excellent survival with improved ejection fraction and functional state. J Am Coll Cardiol 1993;22:1411.
6. Cohn JN, Johnson G, Ziesche S, et al. A comparison of enalapril with hydralazine-isosorbide dinitrate in the treatment of chronic congestive heart failure. N Engl J Med 1991;325:303.
7. The SOLVD Investigators: effect of enalapril on mortality and the development of heart failure in asymptomatic patients with reduced left ventricular ejection fractions. N Engl J Med 1992;327:685.
8. Fonarow GC, Chelimsky-Fallick C, Stevenson LW, et al. Effect of direct vasodilation with hydralazine versus angiotensin-converting enzyme inhibition with captopril on mortality in advanced heart failure: the Hy-C trial. J Am Coll Cardiol 1992;19:842.
9. Miller LW, Kubo SH, Young JB, et al. report of the consensus conference on candidate selection for cardiac transplantation. J Heart Lung Transplant 1995;14:562.
10. Votapka TV, Pennington DG. Circulatory assist devices in congestive heart failure. Cardiol Clin 1994;12:143.
11. Frazier OH, Rose EA, Macmanus Q, et al. Multicenter clinical evaluation of the HeartMate 1000IP left ventricular assist device. Ann Thorac Surg 1992;53:1080.
12. Steimle AE, Stevenson LW, Fonarow GC, Hamilton MA, Moriguchi JD. Prediction of improvement in recent onset cardiomyopathy after referral for heart transplantation. J Am Coll Cardiol 1994;23:553.
13. Semigran MJ, Thaik CM, Fifer MA, et al. Exercise capacity and systolic and diastolic ventricular function after recovery from acute dilated cardiomyopathy. J Am Coll Cardiol 1994;24:462.
14. O'Connell JB, Constanzo-Nordin MR, Bubramanian R, et al. Peripartum cardiomyopathy: clinical, hemodynamic, histologic, and prognostic characteristics. J Am Coll Cardiol 1986;8:52.
15. Regan TJ. Alcohol and the cardiovascular system: a review. J Am Med Assoc 1991;264: 377.
16. Packer DL, Bardy GH, Worley SJ, et al. Tachycardia-induced cardiomyopathy: a reversible form of left ventricular dysfunction. Am J Cardiol 1986;54:563.
17. Grogan M, Smith HC, Gersh BJ, Wood DW. Left ventricular dysfunction due to atrial fibrillation in patients initially believed to have idiopathic dilated cardiomyopathy. Am J Cardiol 1992;69:1570.
18. Middlekauff HR, Weiner I, Stevenson WG, Saxon LA, Stevenson LW. Low dose amiodarone for atrial fibrillation in advanced heart failure restores sinus rhythm and improves functional capacity. Circulation 1992;86:I-808.
19. Alexander JK. The cardiomyopathy of obesity. Prog Cardiovasc Dis 1985;27:325.
20. Stevenson LW. Tailored therapy before transplantation for treatment of advanced heart failure: effective use of vasodilators and diuretics. J Heart Lung Transplant. 1991;10:468.
21. Stevenson LW, Perloff JK. The limited reliability of physical signs for the estimation of hemodynamics in chronic heart failure. J Am Med Assoc 1989;261:884.
22. Stevenson LW, Tillisch JH. Maintenance of cardiac output with normal filling pressures in dilated heart failure. Circulation 1986;74:1303.
23. Stevenson LW, Brunken RC, Belil D, et al. Afterload reduction with vasodilators and diuretics decreases mitral valve regurgitation during upright exercise in advanced heart failure. J Am Coll Cardio 1990;15:174.
24. Mudge GH, Goldstein S, Addonizio LJ, et al. Task force 3: recipient guidelines/prioritization. J Am Coll Cardiol 1993;22:21.
25. Steimle AE, Stevenson LW, Chelimsky-Fallick C, Fonarow GA, Tillisch JH. Prolonged maintenance of cardiac output with normal filling pressures during chronic therapy for advanced heart failure. Circulation 1993;88:I-59A.
26. Steimle AE, Stevenson LW, Chelimsky-Fallick C, et al. Sustained hemodynamic efficacy of therapy tailored to reduce filling pressures in survivors with advanced heart failure. Circulation 1997;96:1165.
27. Fonarow GC, Stevenson LW, Walden JA, et al. Impact of a comprehensive management program on the hospitalization rate for patients with advanced heart failure. J Am Coll Cardiol 1997;30:725.

28. Waagstein F, Caidahl K, Wallentin I, Bergh C-H, Hjalmarson A. Long-term beta-blockade in congestive cardiomyopathy: effects of short and long-term metoprolol treatment followed by withdrawal and readmission of metoprolol. Circulation 1989; 80:551.
29. Waagstein F, Bristow MR, Swedberg K, et al. Beneficial effects of metoprolol in idiopathic dilated cardiomyopathy. Lancet 1993;342:1442.
30. Erlebacher JA, Bhardway M, Suresh A, Leber GB, Goldweit RS. Beta-blocker treatment of idiopathic and ischemic dilated cardiomyopathy in patients with ejection fractions < 20%. Am J Coll Cardiol 1993;71:1467.
31. Hamer AWF, Arkles LB, Johns JA. Beneficial effects of low dose amiodarone in patients with congestive heart failure: a placebo-controlled trial. J Am Coll Cardiol 1989;14:1768.
32. Doval HC, Nul DR, Grancello et al. Randomized trial of low-dose amiodarone in severe congestive heart failure. Lancet 1994;344:493.
33. Singh SN, Fletcher RD, Fisehr SG, et al. Amiodarone in patients with congestive heart failure and asymptomatic ventricular arrhythmia. N Engl J Med 1995;333:77.
34. Wilson JR, Schwartz JS, St. John Sutton M et al. Prognosis in severe heart failure: relating to hemodynamic measurements and ventricular ectopic activity. J Am Coll Cardiol 1983;2:403.
35. DiSalvo TG, Mathier M, Semigran MJ, Dec GW. Preserved right ventricular ejection fraction predicts exercise capacity and survival in advanced heart failure. J Am Coll Cardiol 1995;25:1143.
36. Lee WH, Packer M. Prognostic importance of serum sodium concentration and its modification by converting enzyme inhibition in patients with severe chronic heart failure. Circulation 1986;73:257.
37. Cohn JN, Levine TB, Olivari MT, et al. Plasma norepinephrine as a guide to prognosis in patients with chronic congestive heart failure. N Engl J Med 1984;311:819.
38. Steimle AE, Stevenson LW, Hamilton MA, Fonarow GA. Prediction of spontaneous improvement in recent onset cardiomyopathy after referral for transplantation. Circulation 1993;88:I-93A.
39. Stevenson LW, Fonarow G, Hamilton M, Tillisch JH. Why cardiac output is not a good hemodynamic target for therapy in advanced heart failure. Circulation 1994;90:I-611.
40. Stevenson WG, Stevenson LW, Middlekauff HR, Saxon LA. Sudden death prevention in patient with advanced left ventricular dysfunction. Circulation 1993;88:2953.
41. O'Connell JB, Gunnar RM, Evans RW, Fricker FJ, et al. Task force 1: organization of heart transplantation in the U.S. J Am Coll Cardiol 1993;22:8.
42. Keogh AM, Freund J, Baron DW, Hickie JB. Timing of transplantation in idiopathic dilated cardiomyopathy. Am J Cardiol 1988;61:418.
43. Stevenson LW, Couper G, Natterson BJ, et al. Target heart failure population for new therapies. Circulation 1995 (In press).
44. Lee TH, Hamilton MA, Stevenson LW, et al. Impact of left ventricular cavity size on survival in advanced heart failure. Am J Cardiol 1993;72:672.
45. Cohn J, Johnson G, Shabetai R, et al. Ejection fraction, peak exercise oxygen consumption, cardiothoracic ratio, ventricular arrhythmias, and plasma norepinephrine as determinants of prognosis in heart failure. Circulation 1993;87(Suppl.VI):V15.
46. Szlachic J, Massie B, Kramer B, Topic N, Tubau J. Correlates and prognostic implication of exercise capacity in chronic congestive heart failure. Am J Cardiol 1985;55:1037.
47. Likoff M, Chandler S, Kay H. Clinical determinants of mortality in chronic congestive heart failure secondary to idiopathic dilated or ischemic cardiomyopathy. Am J Cardiol 1987;59:634.
48. Mancini DM, Eisen H, Kussmaul W, et al. Value of peak exercise oxygen consumption for optimal timing of cardiac transplantation in ambulatory patients with heart failure. Circulation 1991;83:778.
49. Haywood GA, Rickenbacher PR, Trindade PT, et al. Deaths in patients awaiting heart transplantation: the need to identify high risk category to patients. Circulation 1994;90:I-360.
50. Stevenson LW, Steimle AE, Chelimsky-Fallick C, et al. Outcomes predicted by peak oxygen consumption during evaluation of 333 patients with advanced heart failure. Circulation 1993;88:I-94A.
51. Stevenson LW, Steimle AE, Fonarow G, et al. Improvement in exercise capacity of candidates awaiting heart transplantation. J Am Coll Cardiol 1995;25:163.
52. Stevenson LW, Sietsema K, Tillisch JH, et al. Exercise capacity for survivors of cardiac transplantation or sustained medical therapy for stable heart failure. Circulation 1990; 81:78.
53. Walden JA, Stevenson LW, Dracup K, et al. Extended comparison of quality of life between stable heart failure patient and heart transplant recipients. J Heart Lung Transplant 1994;13:1109.
54. Stevenson LW, Miller L. Cardiac transplantation as therapy for heart failure. Curr Prob Cardiol 1991;16:219.
55. Olivari MT, Antolick A, Kaye MP, Jamieson SW, Ring WS. Heart transplantation in elderly patients. J Heart Transplant 1988;7:258.

56. Grattan MT, Moreno-Cabral CE, Starnes VA, et al. Eight year results of cyclosporin-treated patient with cardiac transplants. J Thorac Cardiovasc Surg 1990;99:500.
57. Kave MP. The Registry of the International Society for Heart and Lung Transplantation: Tenth Official report - 1993. J Heart Lung Transplant 1993;12:541.
58. Hosenpud JD, DeMarco T, Frazier H, et al. Progression of systemic disease and reduced long-term survival in patients with cardiac amyloidosis undergoing heart transplantation. Circulation 1991;84:III-338.
59. Stolf NAG, Higushi L, Bocchi E, et al. Heart transplantation in patients with Chagas' disease cardiomyopathy. J Heart Transplant 1987;5:307.
60. Copeland JG, Emery RW, Levinson MM, et al. Selection of patients for cardiac transplantation. Circulation 1987;75:2.
61. Olbrisch ME, Levenson JL. Psychological evaluation of heart transplantation candidates: an international survey of process, criteria and outcomes. J Heart Lung Transplant 1991;10:948.
62. Rodriguez MD, Colon A, Santiago-Delphin EA. Psychosocial profile of noncompliant patients. Transplant Proc 1991;23:1807.
63. Herrick CM, Mealey PC, Tischner LL, Holland DS. Combined heart failure-transplant program: advantages in assessing medical compliance. J Heart Transplant 1987;6:141.
64. Penn I. Cancers after cyclosporin therapy. Transplant Proc 1988;20:276.
65. Erickson KW, Costanzo-Nordin MR, O'Sullivan EJ, et al. Influence of preoperative transpulmonary gradient on late mortality after orthotopic heart transplantation. J Heart Transplant 1990;9:526.
66. Costard-Jackle A, Fowler MB. Influence of preoperative pulmonary artery pressure on mortality after heart transplantation: testing of potential reversibility of pulmonary hypertension with nitroprusside is useful in defining a high risk group. J Am Coll Cardiol 1992:19:48.
67. Kaye MP. The Registry of the International Society for Heart and Lung Transplantation: Ninth official report. J Heart Lung Transplant 1992;599:11.
68. Desruennes M, Muneretto C, Grandjbakhch I, et al. Heterotopic heart transplantation: current status in 1988. J Heart Transplant 1989;8:475.
69. Wright RS, Levine MS, Bellamy EP, et al. Ventilatory and diffusion abnormalities in potential heart-transplant recipients. Chest 1990;98:816.
70. Radovancevic B, Poindexter S, Birovljev S, et al. Risk factors for development of accelerated coronary artery disease in cardiac transplant recipients. Eur J Cardiothorac Surg 1990;4:309.
71. Myers BD, Peterson C, Molina C, et al. Role of cardiac atria in the human renal response to changing plasma volume. Am J Physiol 1988;254:F562.
72. Wei CM, Kao PC, Lin JT, Heublein DM, Schaff HV, Burnett JC Jr. Circulating b-atrial natriuretic factor in congestive heart failure. Circulation 1993;88:1016.
73. Bourge RC, Naftal DC, Costanzo M, et al. Risk factors for death after cardiac transplantation: a multi-institutional study. J Heart Lung Transplant 1993;12:549.
74. Laffel GL, Barnett AI, Finkelstein S, et al. The relation between experience and outcome in heart transplantation. N Engl J Med 1992;327:1220.
75. Flaker GC, Blackshear JL, McBride R, et al. Antiarrhythmic drug therapy and cardiac mortality in atrial fibrillation. The Stroke Prevention in Atrial Fibrillation Investigators. J Am Coll Cardiol 1992;20:527.
76. Natterson PD, Stevenson WG, Saxon LA, Middlekauff HR, Stevenson LW. Risk of arterial embolization in 224 patients awaiting cardiac transplantation. Am Heart J 1995;129:564.
77. Konstram MA, Dracup K, Baker DW, et al. Heart failure: evaluation and care of patient with left-ventricular systolic dysfunction. Rockville, MD: US Dept. of Health and Human Services; 1994.
78. Chelimsky-Fallick C, Middlekauff HR, Stevenson WG, et al. Amiodarone therapy does not compromise subsequent heart transplantation. J Am Coll Cardiol 1992;20:1556.
79. Stevenson LW, Warner SL, Steimle AE, et al. The impending crisis awaiting cardiac transplantation: modelling a solution based on selection. Circulation 1994;89:450.
80. Stevenson LW, Bourge RC, Naftel DC, et al. Deterioration and death on the current waiting list: a multicenter study of patients awaiting heart transplantation. Circulation 1995;92:I-124.
81. Norman JC, Colley DA, Igo SR, et al. Prognostic indices for survival during postcardiotomy intra-aortic balloon pumping. J Thorac Cardiovasc Surg 1977;74:709.
82. Loisance DY, Deleuze PH, Houel R, et al. Pharmacologic bridge to cardiac transplantation: current limitations. Ann Thorac Surg 1993;55:310.
83. McCarthy PM, Sabik JF. Implantable circulatory support devices as a bridge to heart transplantation. Sem Thorac Cardiovasc Surg 1994;6:174.
84. Rose EA, Stevenson LW (Eds). Management of End-Stage Heart Disease, Lippincott-Raven, Philadelphia, 1998.
85. Evans RW. Executive Summary: The National Cooperative Transplantation Study. Report BHARC-100-

91-020. Seattle: Battelle Seattle Research Center, June 1991.
86. Pfeffer MA, Braunwald E, Moye LA, et al. (on behalf of the SAVE investigators). Effect of captopril on mortality and morbidity in patients with left ventricular dysfunction after myocardial infarction: results of the survival and ventricular enlargement trial. N Engl J Med 1992;327:669.
87. The SOLVD Investigators: Effect of enalapril on survival in patients with reduced left ventricular ejection fractions and congestive heart failure. N Engl J Med 1991;325:293.
88. CONSENSUS trial study group. Effects of enalapril on mortality in severe congestive heart failure: results of the Cooperative New Scandinavian Enalapril Survival Study. N Engl J Med 1987;316:1429.
89. Stevenson LW. Role of exercise in the evaluation of candidates for cardiac transplantation: In: Wasserman K, editor. Exercise gas exchange in heart disease. New York: Futura;1996;27

6. THE REGISTRY OF THE INTERNATIONAL SOCIETY FOR HEART AND LUNG TRANSPLANTATION: FIFTEENTH OFFICIAL REPORT — 1998

Jeffrey D. Hosenpud, Leah E. Bennett, Berkeley M. Keck, Bennie Fiol, Mark M. Boucek, Richard J. Novick

Over the past 12 months, The Registry of the International Society for Heart and Lung Transplantation added 20 new transplantation programs and a total of 7073 additional thoracic organ recipients. All of the national and multinational registries are now fully integrated into our registry, and electronic data submission via the Internet will be instituted by mid 1998 for those centers not participating in larger registries. For the first time, the entire data set was used to calculate multivariate risks rather than the U.S. data set alone, and we have continued to extend the time frame for both univariate and multivariate analyses. For this report, risk factors for 5-year outcome and morbidity at 3 years are presented.

Data Set and Statistical Methodology

This report represents data on 45,993 heart transplantations reported from 301 heart transplantation programs, 2428 heart-lung transplantations reported from 122 programs, and 4777 single lung and 3278 double lung transplantations reported from a total of 150 lung transplantation programs. For purposes of analysis, the data set was closed as of March 1, 1998. Survival was calculated actuarially (Harris and Albert, Survivorship analysis for clinical studies, New York, Marcel Decker, 1991, pp 12-5), and actuarial survival curves were contrasted by use of the Wilcoxon and log-rank tests. Logistic regression methods (Hosmer and Lemeshow, Applied logistic regression, New York, John Wiley & Sons, 1989, pp 1-134) were used to determine which variables were associated with survival after transplantation. A multivariate logistic regression analysis was then applied to the entire data set, but limited to those patients who had all of the model variables available in their records to determine the independent predictors of survival. Furthermore, the odds ratio of each variable was expressed as a comparison of survival between groups, with a value of 1.0 indicating no survival benefit, less than 1.0 indicating increased survival, and greater than 1.0 increased mortality rates after transplantation.

Roy Masters (editor), Surgical Options for the Treatment of Heart Failure, 93-115.

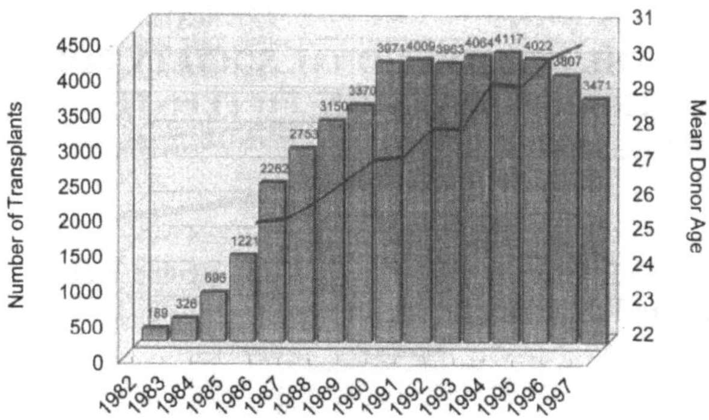

Figure 1. *Heart transplantation volumes and donor age by year.*

Heart Transplantation

Figure 1 shows the number of heart transplantations reported to the Registry from the years 1982 to 1997 in the bars, with donor age as a line graph (Y2 axis). As in last year's report, the heart transplantation volume has reached a plateau and may in fact be declining slightly, in spite of the practice of using older donors to "expand" the donor pool. The age distribution for patients receiving heart transplants is shown in Figure 2, with clustering between the ages of 35 and 64 years. Pediatric heart transplantations likewise have reached a plateau (Figure 3). Figure 4 demonstrates the indications for adult heart transplantation, with coronary artery disease and cardiomyopathy representing approximately equal numbers and both together representing the vast majority of cases. The percentage of cases for each of these two diagnoses has varied from year to year, with cardiomyopathy being the majority of cases in the early 1980s, supplanted by coronary artery disease in the late 1980s and early 1990s at a time when the age criteria for heart transplantation was being liberalized. During the past 5 years there is relatively equal representation from both patients with

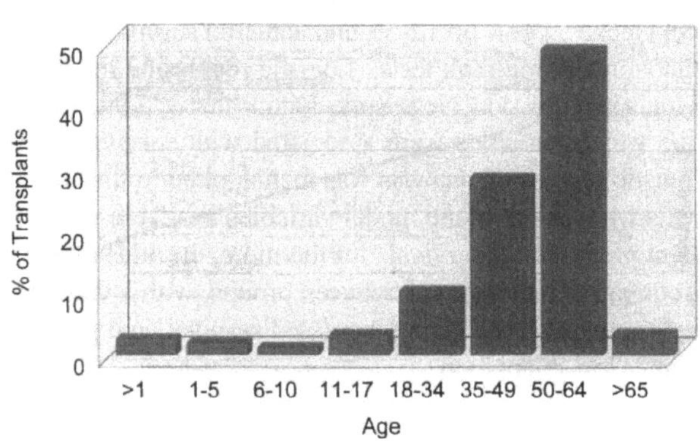

Figure 2. *Age distribution of heart transplant recipients.*

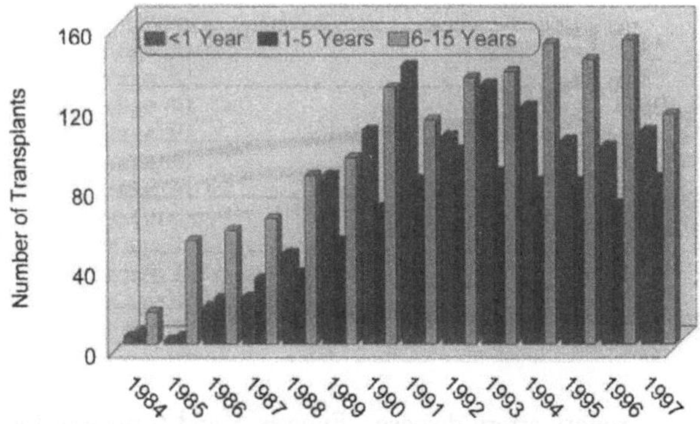

Figure 3. *Pediatric heart transplantation volumes by age.*

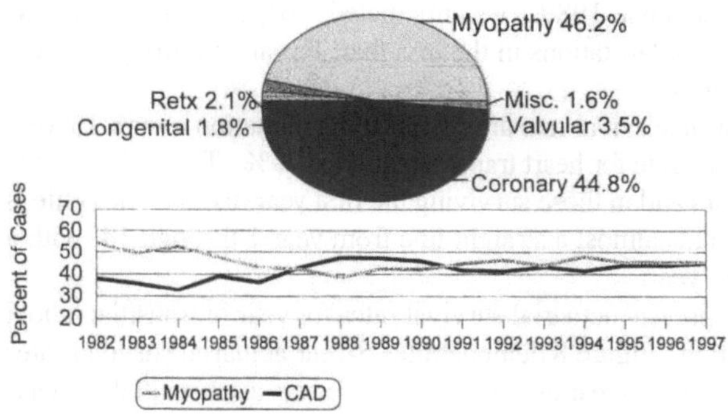

Figure 4. *Adult heart transplantation indications.* **Retx** = *retransplantation,* **CAD** = *coronary artery disease*

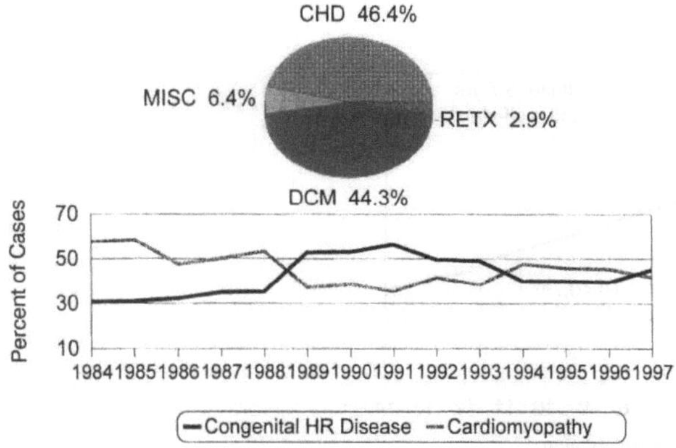

Figure 5. *Pediatric heart transplantation indications and indications by year.*
CHD = *Congenital heart disease*; **RETX** = *retransplantation*; **DCM** = *dilated cardiomyopathy*

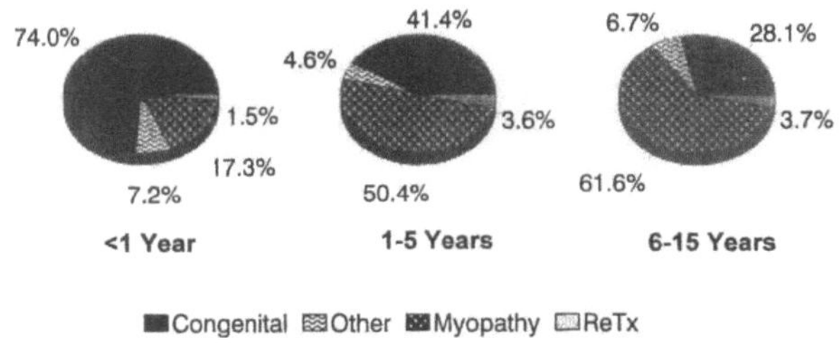

Figure 6. *Pediatric heart transplantation indications by age.* **Retx** = *Retransplantation.*

cardiomyopathy and patients with coronary artery disease. Figures 5 and 6 present the indications for pediatric heart transplantation (age < 16 years), first as overall indications, indications by year for the two major indications, and finally indications by age of the recipient. Congenital heart disease is the most common indication for transplantation in the pediatric population and has been since 1989. As anticipated, congenital heart disease makes up close to 75% of the transplan-tations in the less than 1 year age group, yet less than 30% in the older aged children.

Figure 7 presents the actuarial survival rate after heart transplantation over a 13-year period. The overall 1-year survival rate for heart transplantation is 79%. The patient ½ life (time to 50% survival) is 8.7 years and in those surviving the first year, the patient ½ life is 11.4 years. The falloff in survival is almost a straight line from year 1 through 14, with a constant mortality rate of 4% per year.

The next series of figures represent actuarial survival rates for year of transplantation, recipient age, and retransplantation. Figure 8 demonstrates 5-year actuarial survival rates over the past 17 years broken down in 3-year time blocks. There was a substantial increase in more recent patients, compared with those who underwent transplantation from 1980 to 1985. There is a marginal but statistically significant further increase in survival rates comparing the last 5 years of the 1980s with patients who underwent transplantation from

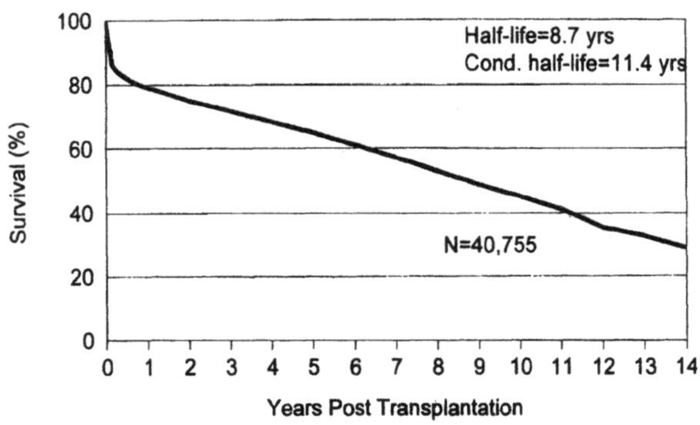

Figure 7. *Total heart transplantation actuarial survival.*

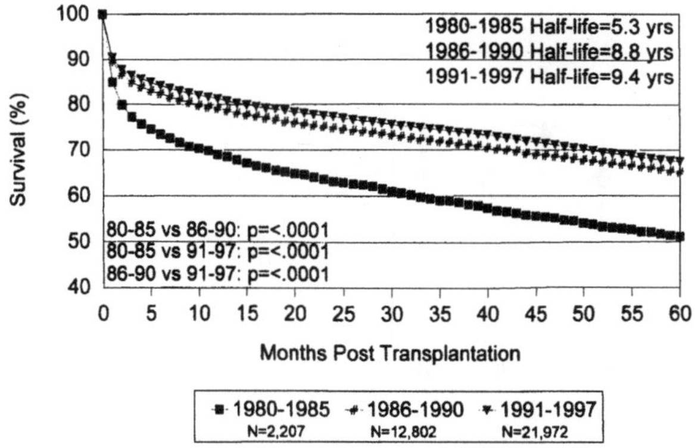

Figure 8. *Adult heart transplantation actuarial survival by era..*

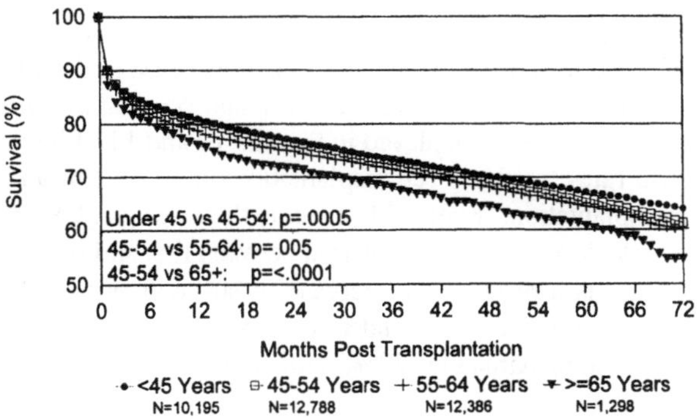

Figure 9. *Adult heart transplantation actuarial survival by age.*

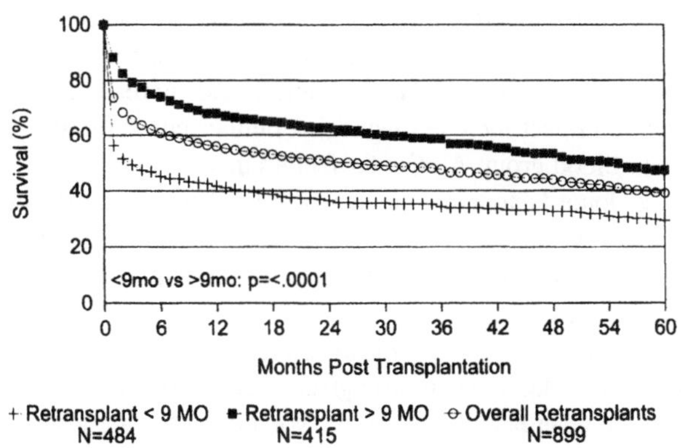

Figure 10. *Adult heart retransplantation actuarial survival.*

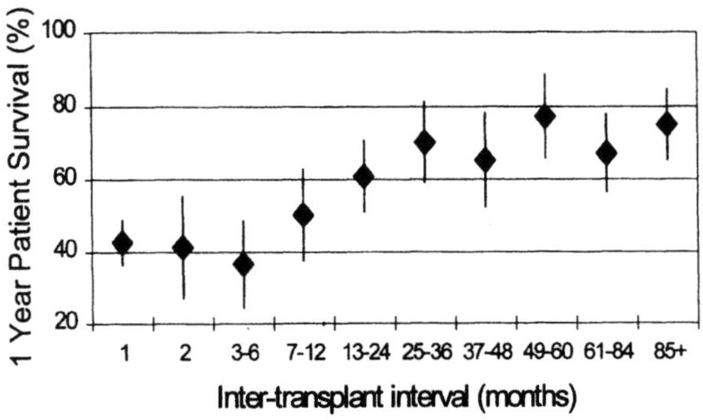

Figure 11. *Adult heart retransplantation 1-year survival by interval from first transplantation.*

1991 onward. Figure 9 demonstrates actuarial survival rates broken down by recipient age group. There is a statistically significant decrease in survival for each increase in decade of life, with a clinically significant decrease in those patients over age 65 years. The actuarial survival rate for adult retransplantation is displayed in Figures 10 and 11. Figure 10 presents 5-year actuarial survival rates for those retransplantations done within and beyond 9 months after the initial transplantation. Figure 11 presents the average (± 95% confidence intervals) 1-year survival rate depending on the interval between first and second transplantation. As can be seen, there is a progressive increase in survival rates with increased time between operations. Those patients who underwent transplantation after 2 years have 1-year survival rates of approximately 70%, still lower than primary transplantation.

Tables I and II show multivariate logistic regression analyses for adult cardiac allograft recipients performed on all patients in the Registry having complete data. In this analysis, the end points are 1- and 5-years survival rates. As has been previously shown in prior Registry reports, the vast majority of risk factors known to affect 1-year mortality persist at the 5-year time point as a result of their profound effects early on. Recipient factors that have a statistically significant negative impact include prior transplantation, requiring a ventricular assist device or ventilator support before transplantation, and increasing age. Recipient factors that have a positive impact include diagnosis of either coronary artery disease or cardiomyopathy and ABO blood group A. Center factors that are negative include low volume, and donor factors include increasing ischemic time, donor sex, and age. In this report (as with last year's report) donor and recipient age, as well as ischemic time, were analyzed as continuous variables and demonstrate a highly statistically significant increasing risk with increasing values.

Figure 12 demonstrates survival rates after pediatric heart transplantation overall and is broken down by age groups. The older age pediatric group has survival rates nearly identical to the adult population, whereas those with the worst outcome are less than 1 year of age. Patients 1 to 5 years of age have intermediate survival rates.

Table 1. Risk factors for 1-year mortality after adult heart transplantation.

Variable	*Odds ratio*	*95% Confidence interval*	*p Value*
Negative recipient factors			
Ventilator	2.66	2.20-3.21	<0.0001
Repeat Tx	2.33	1.80-3.01	<0.0001
VAD	1.49	1.23-1.80	<0.0001
Ctr vol <9 TX/YR	1.3	1.15-1.47	<0.0001
Female donor	1.22	1.11-1.33	<0.0001
Positive recipient factors			
ABO type A	0.9	0.83-0.98	0.01
CAD	0.79	0.68-0.93	0.005
CM	0.71	0.60-0.83	<0.0001
Ischemic time linear			<0.0001
Ischemic time (0)	0.75	0.67-0.83	
Ischemic time (2)	0.93	0.90-0.95	
Ischemic time (4)	1.15	1.09-1.22	
Ischemic time (6)	1.43	1.25-1.64	
Ischemic time (8)	1.78	1.43-2.22	
Recip age (linear)			<0.0001
Recip age 20	0.85	0.69-1.06	
Recip age 30	0.85	0.76-0.94	
Recip age 40	0.89	0.85-0.93	
Recip age 50	1	1.00-1.00	
Recip age 60	1.19	1.11-1.27	
Recip age 70	1.5	1.26-1.79	
Donor age (linear)			<0.0001
Donor age 20	0.89	0.84-0.95	
Donor age 30	0.99	0.99-1.00	
Donor age 40	1.18	1.14-1.22	
Donor age 50	1.48	1.34-1.64	
Donor age 60	1.99	1.59-2.48	

Tx, *Transplantation*; **VAD**, *Vascular assist device;* **Ctr vol**, *center volume*; **CAD**, *coronary artery disease*; **CM**, *cardiomyopathy*; **Recip**, *recipient.* **n** = 17,685

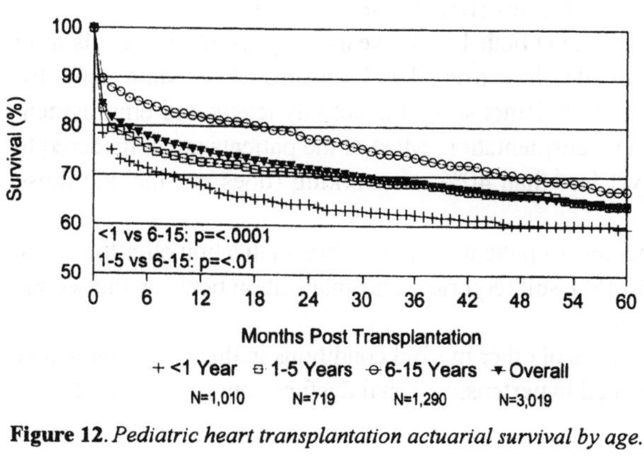

Figure 12. *Pediatric heart transplantation actuarial survival by age.*

Table 2. Risk factors for 5 year mortality after adult heart transplantation

Variable	*Odds ratio*	*95% Confidence interval*	*p Value*
Repeat Tx	3.08	2.34-4.05	<0.0001
Ventilator	1.78	1.40-2.27	<0.0001
Ctr vol <9 Tx/yr	1.29	1.14-1.47	<0.0001
Female donor	1.15	1.04-1.28	0.006
Ischemic time (linear)			<0.0001
Ischemic time (0)	0.77	0.68-0.88	
Ischemic time (2)	0.94	0.91-0.97	
Ischemic time (4)	1.13	1.06-1.21	
Ischemic time (6)	1.37	1.17-1.60	
Ischemic time (8)	1.66	1.29-2.13	
Recip age (linear)			<0.0001
Recip age 20	1.21	0.97-1.51	
Recip age 30	0.99	0.89-1.10	
Recip age 40	0.93	0.89-0.97	
Recip age 50	1	1.00-1.00	
Recip age 60	1.22	1.10-1.31	
Recip age 70	1.71	1.40-2.09	
Donor age (linear)			<0.0001
Donor age 20	0.89	0.83-0.94	
Donor age 30	0.99	0.99-1.00	
Donor age 40	1.19	1.14-1.25	
Donor age 50	1.53	1.34-1.76	
Donor age 60	2.21	1.57-2.82	
Donor age 60	2.21	1.78-2.75	

Tx, *Transplantation*; **Ctr vol**, *center volume*; **Recip**, *recipient*. n = 9,536

Tables III and IV demonstrate the multivariate logistic regression analysis of risk at 1 and 5 years for pediatric heart transplantation. Similar to the adult population, repeat transplantation, ventricular assist device, and ventilator mechanical support carry the greatest risks. Other risk factors include very young age, congenital heart disease, low center volume, and donor age. Interestingly, recipient age risk in the pediatric population is also linear, but in this case, the risk is inversely correlated to age. At 5 years, recipient age is no longer a risk factor, but recipient sex (female) becomes one.

In this year's report, morbidity data at both 1 and 3 years are presented. The data set for these analyses include worldwide data from 1994 onward (U.S. data only for employment status). Figures 13 and 14 demonstrate the activity levels and employment status of patients 1 and 3 years after transplantation. Most of the patients are considered to have no limitations in function, yet less than 40% are working (does not include those retired).

Figure 15 demonstrates the percent of patients requiring hospitalization after the initial transplantation, with approximately 18% still requiring a hospitalization between the second and third years after transplantation.

Figures 16 to 18 outline incidences of other morbid conditions in the first 3 years after transplantation, including drug-treated hypertension, renal dysfunction, drug-treated

Table 3. Risk factors for 1 year mortality in pediatric heart transplantation

Variable	*Odds ratio*	*95% Confidence interval*	*p Value*
Retransplant	2.55	1.44-4.51	<0.0001
IABP/VAD	2.54	1.17-5.51	0.02
Ventilator	1.5	1.24-2.06	0.0003
Congenital	1.41	1.10-2.80	0.006
Ctr vol <9 Tx/yr	1.36	1.08-1.71	0.009
Recip age (linear)			<0.0001
Recip age 0	1.39	1.21-1.61	
Recip age 3	1.2	1.11-1.29	
Recip age 6	1.03	1.01-1.04	
Recip age 12	0.75	0.67-0.85	
Recip age 17	0.58	0.46-0.73	
Donor age (quadratic)			0.003
Donor age 0	1.08	1.03-1.13	
Donor age 10	1	1.00-1.00	
Donor age 20	1.07	1.02-1.12	
Donor age 30	1.33	1.10-1.60	
Donor age 40	1.89	1.24-2.87	
Donor age 50	3.11	0.87-7.86	

IABP, *Intraaortic balloon pump*; **VAD**, *vascular assist device*; **Ctr vol**, *center volume*; **Tx**, *transplantation*; **Recip**, *recipient*
n = 2083.

Table 4. Risk factors for 5 year mortality after pediatric heart transplantation.

Variable	*Odds ratio*	*95% Confidence interval*	*p Value*
Retransplant	3.21	1.40-7.35	0.006
Ventilator	1.47	1.08-2.01	0.02
Diagnosis-cong	1.36	1.03-1.79	0.03
Female recipient	1.31	1.00-1.71	0.05
Donor age (quadratic)			0.03
Donor age 0	1.08	1.01-1.15	
Donor age 10	1	1.00-1.00	
Donor age 20	1.08	1.01-1.15	
Donor age 30	1.34	1.04-1.73	
Donor age 40	1.95	1.10-3.45	
Donor age 50	3.28	1.19-9.08	

Cong, *congenital*; **n** = 1063.

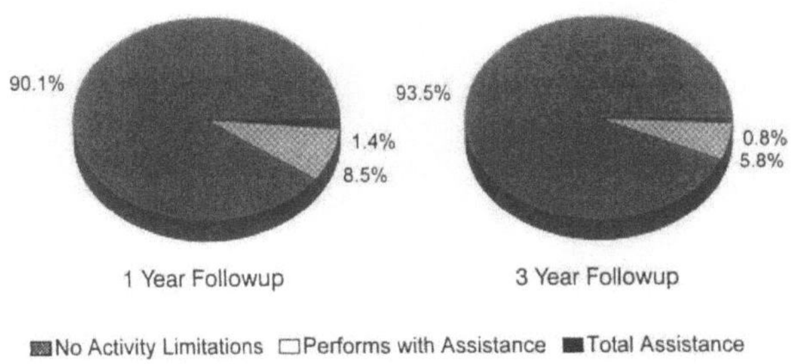

Figure 13. *Heart transplant recipient functional status.*

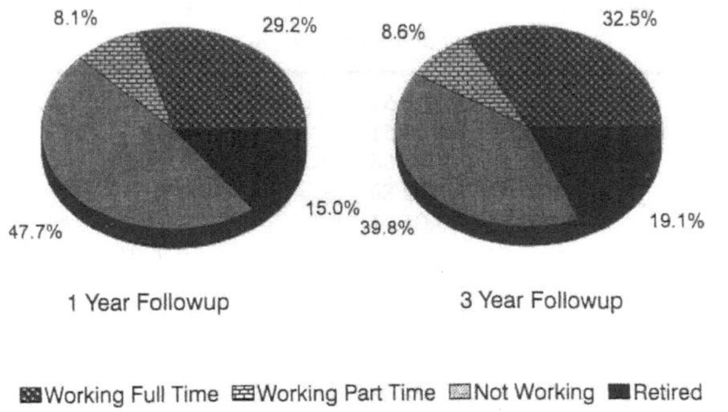

Figure 14. *Heart transplant recipient work status.*

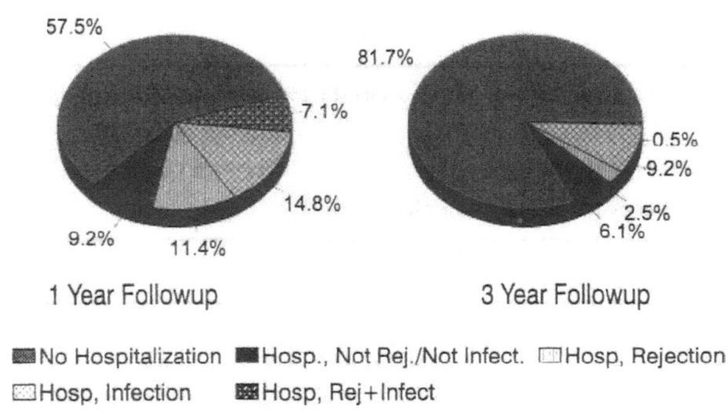

Figure 15. *Rehospitalization after heart transplantation.*

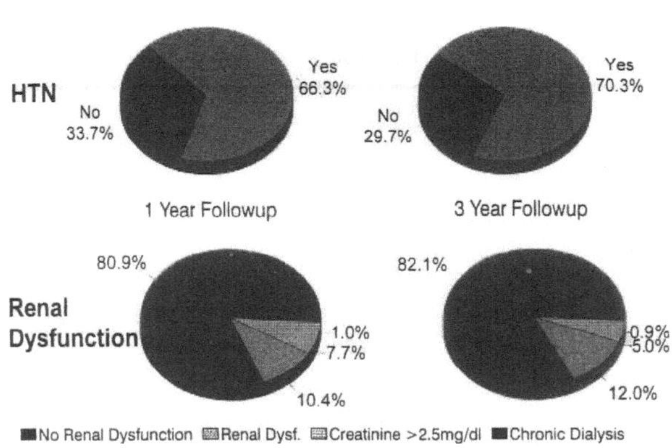

Figure 16. *Hypertension and renal dysfunction after heart transplantation.* **HTN**, *hypertension*

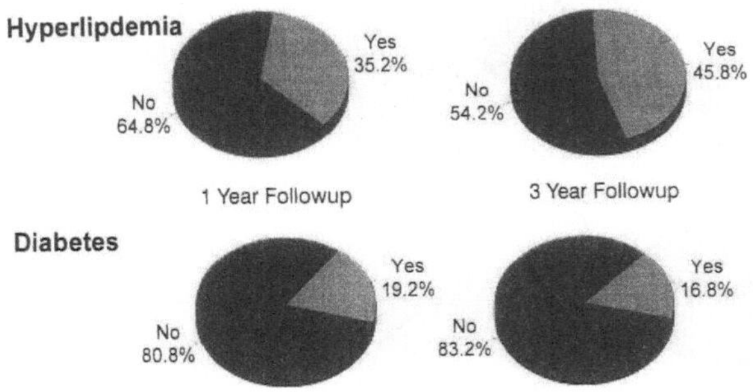

Figure 17. *Hyperlipidemia and diabetes after heart transplantation.*

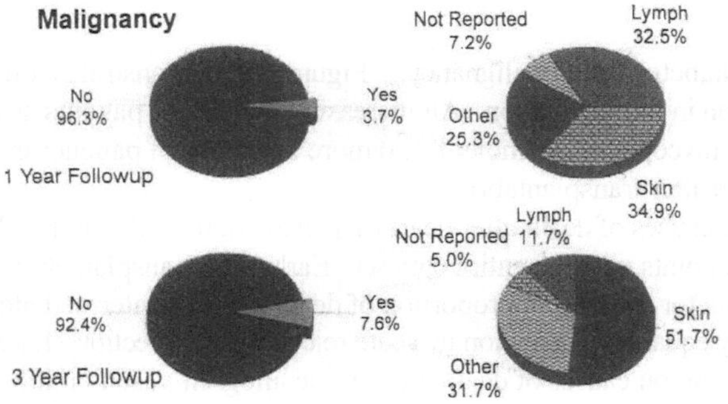

Figure 18. *Malignancy after heart transplantation.*

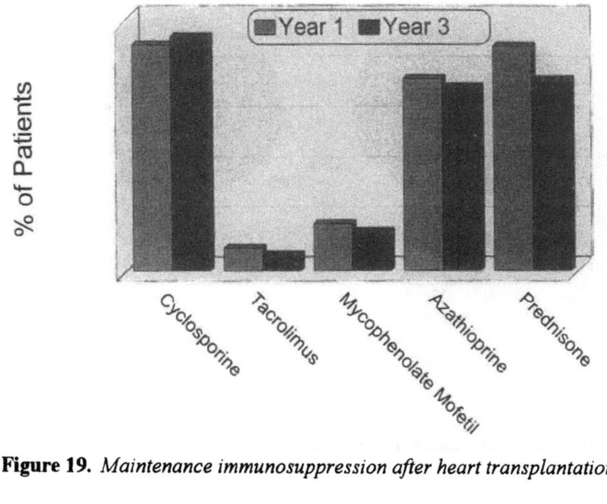

Figure 19. *Maintenance immunosuppression after heart transplantation.*

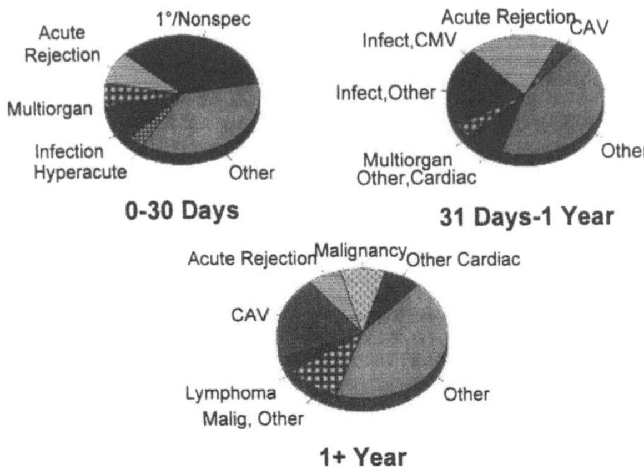

Figure 20. *Heart transplantation cause of death by time after transplantation.* **CMV**, *Cytomegalovirus*, **CAV**, *cardiac allograft myopathy.*

hyperlipidemia, drug-treated diabetes, and malignancy. Figure 19 demonstrates the maintenance immunosuppression in the population. An increasing number of patients are being treated with tacrolimus or mycophenolate mofetil, and more than 75% of patients are still on corticosteroids at 3 years after transplantation.

Figure 20 demonstrates the causes of death after heart transplantation (both adult and pediatric) at three different time points with the entire data set. Early after transplantation, nonspecific graft failure accounts for the largest proportion of deaths. In the intermediate period, there is an approximately equal representation by acute rejection and infection. Late after transplantation the most common causes of death are cardiac allograft vasculopathy, malignancy, and, interestingly, acute rejection. The other category is made up of listed diagnoses not fitting into the more common categories.

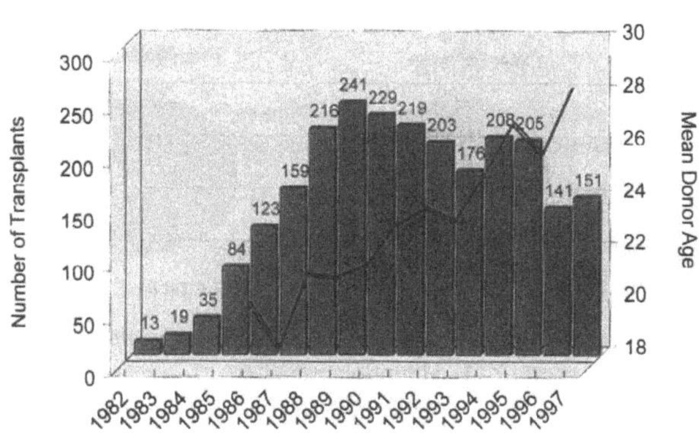

Figure 21. *Heart-lung transplantation volumes and donor age by year.*

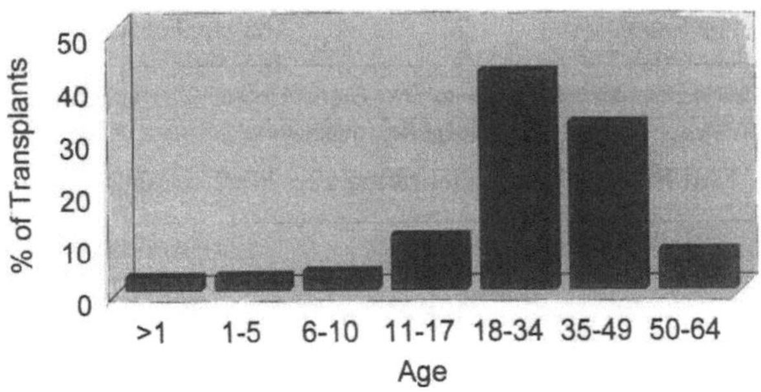

Figure 22. *Age distribution of heart-lung transplant recipients.*

Heart-Lung Tranplantation

Figure 21 shows the number of heart-lung trasnplantations reported to the registry from 1982 to 1997 and the average donor age over this period. The number of heart-lung transplantations peaked in 1989 and has declined thereafter. Similar to heart transplantation, donor age has continued to rise. Figure 22 demonstrates the age distribution for heart-lung transplantation, with clustering between 18 and 49 years.

Figure 23 demonstrates the indications for heart-lung transplantation in the adult population. The three most common indications are pulmonary hypertension, congenital heart disease, and cystic fibrosis.

The 11-year actuarial survival rate for heart-lung transplantation is demonstrated in Figure 24. The 1-year survival rate is approximately 60%, whereas the 11-year survival rate is 21%. The survival ½ life for the entire curve is 2.6 years because of the high first-year mortality rate. The conditional ½ life for those surviving the first year is more than 8.4 years. Tables V and VI demonstrate the multivariate logistic regression analysis of

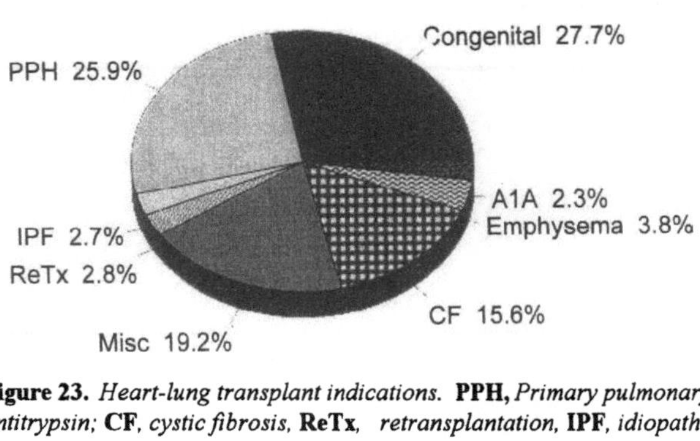

Figure 23. *Heart-lung transplant indications.* **PPH,** *Primary pulmonary hypertension;* **AIA,** *alpha$_1$–antitrypsin;* **CF**, *cystic fibrosis,* **ReTx**, *retransplantation,* **IPF**, *idiopathic pulmonary fibrosis.*

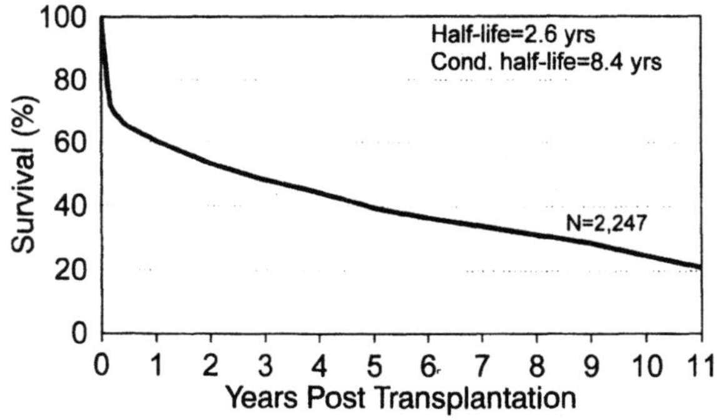

Figure 24. *Heart-lung transplantation actuarial survival.*

Table 5. Risk factors for 1 year mortality after adult heart-lung transplantation

Variable	*Odds ratio*	*95% Confidence interval*	*p Value*
Repeat Tx	5.07	1.25-20.60	0.02
Ctr vol < 5 Tx/yr	1.9	1.27-2.85	0.002
Donor age (linear)			0.004
Donor age 20	0.85	0.76-0.95	
Donor age 30	1.09	1.03-1.15	
Donor age 40	1.39	1.11-1.74	
Donor age 50	1.79	1.20-2.65	
Donor age 60	2.29	1.30-4.02	

Tx, *transplantation;* **Ctr vol**, *center volume.*
n = 527.

Table 6. Risk factors for 3 year mortality in adult heart-lung transplantation

Variable	*Odds ratio*	*95% Confidence interval*	*p Value*
Ventilator	9	1.25-20.60	0.01
Ctr vol <5 Tx/yr	1.7	1.27-2.85	0.02
Donor age (linear)			0.03
Donor age 20	0.87	0.77-0.99	
Donor age 30	1.07	1.00-1.14	
Donor age 40	1.31	1.02-1.69	
Donor age 50	1.61	1.03-2.51	
Donor age 60	1.98	1.05-3.73	

Ctr vol, *center volume*; **Tx**, *transplantation.*
n = 432

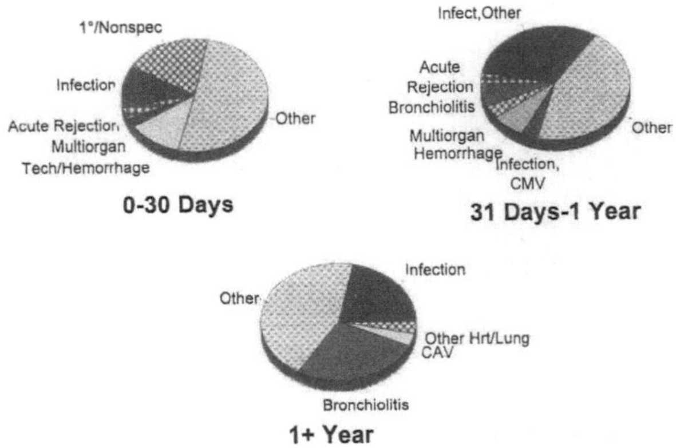

Figure 25. *Heart-lung transplantation cause of death by time after transplantation.* **CMV,** *Cytomagalovirus;* **Hrt,** *heart;* **CAV**, *cardiac allograft vasculaopathy*

risk factors for 1- and 3-year mortality after adult heart-lung transplantation. As shown in previous Registry reports, being on a ventilator before transplantation and low center volume continue to be statistically significant risk factors for death after heart-lung transplantation. As was shown for heart transplantation, the risk according to donor age increases as a continuous variable at both 1 and 3 years (Tables V and VI). Figure 25 demonstrates the most common causes of death after heart-lung transplantation at three different postoperative intervals. Early after transplantation, nonspecific graft failure, infection and technical/hemorrhage factors account for a substantial majority of the deaths. In the intermediate time period, infection is the primary cause, and late after transplantation, infection and bronchiolitis obliterans are the principal causes of death. CAV does account for a small minority of deaths (3%) late after heart-lung transplantation.

Lung Transplantation

Although lung transplantation has enjoyed continued growth through 1993, on the basis of the past 3 years' data, this growth has clearly ceased, again in spite of the use of increasingly older donors (Figure 26). The age distribution for lung transplantation is younger than for heart or heart-lung transplant recipients, primarily because of its use in the cystic fibrosis population (Figure 27). Figure 28 demonstrates the pediatric lung and heart-lung transplantation volumes over the past 14 years. Heart-lung transplantation seems to have been largely abandoned in this patient population, whereas pediatric lung transplantation continues to occur at low but steady rates.

The indications for adult single lung transplantation continue to be dominated principally by chronic obstructive pulmonary disease, whereas cystic fibrosis is the most common indication for double/bilateral lung transplantation, as shown in Figure 29. Idiopathic pulmonary fibrosis and primary pulmonary hypertension are also important

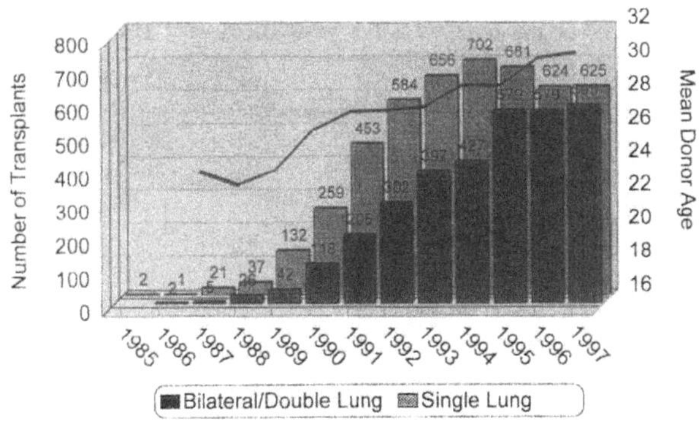

Figure 26. *Lung transplantation volumes and donor age by year.*

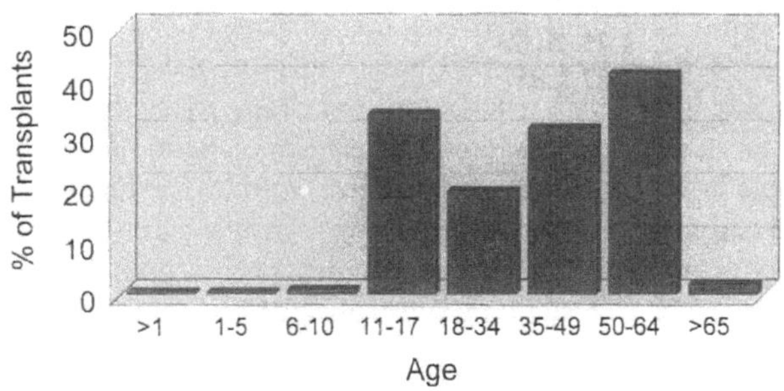

Figure 27. *Age distribution of lung recipients.*

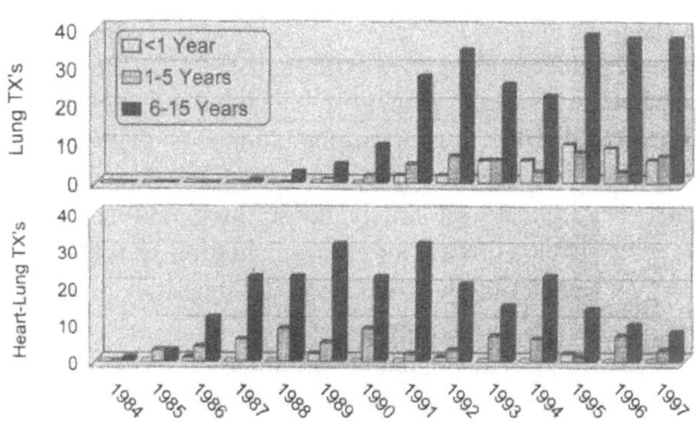

Figure 28. *Pediatric heart-lung/lung transplantation numbers by age and year.*

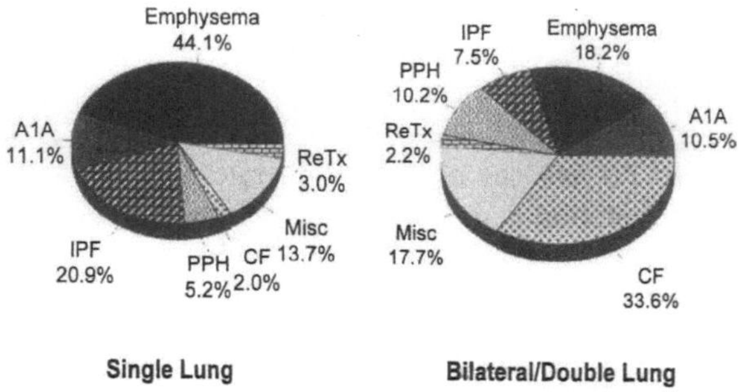

Figure 29. *Adult lung transplantation indications.* **AIA** *alpha$_1$ -antitrypsin*; **Retx**, *retransplantation*; **CF**, *cystic fibrosis*; **PPH**, *Primary pulmonary hypertension*; **IPF**, *idiopathic pulmonary fibrosis.*

indications for these procedures. The indications for pediatric lung and heart-lung transplantation are shown overall and over time in Figure 30 and by the two primary age groups in Figure 31. Congenital heart disease, cystic fibrosis, and primary pulmonary hypertension are the principal indications. Interestingly, retransplantation is used much more frequently in this age group than in adults.

The 7-year actuarial survival rate for all lung transplantations (adult and pediatric) is shown in Figure 32. There is no significant difference in actuarial survival comparing single lung to bilateral/double lung transplantation, with patient half times of 3.6 years and 4.5 years for single and double lung, respectively. For adult transplantation, there is a significant difference comparing lung transplantation performed from 1988 through 1990 compared with later years, but no further improvement after 1991 (Figure 33). Figure 34 demonstrates the effect of recipient age on survival. Patients aged 55 and older had a significantly lower survival than younger recipients.

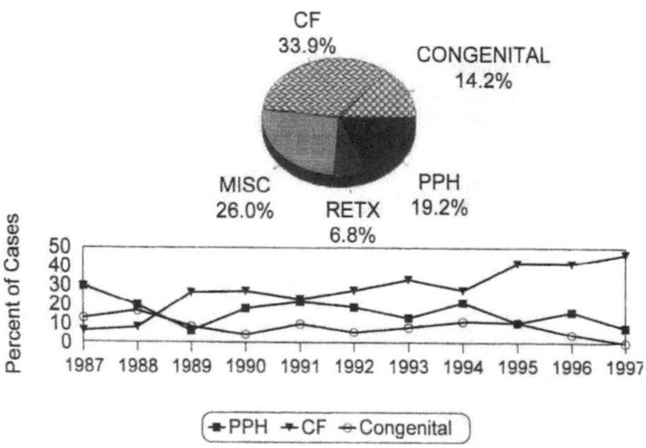

Figure 30. *Pediatric heart-lung/lung transplantation indications and indications by year.* **CF**; *Cystic fibrosis*; **PPH**; *primary pulmonary hypertension*; **ReTx**, *retransplantation.*

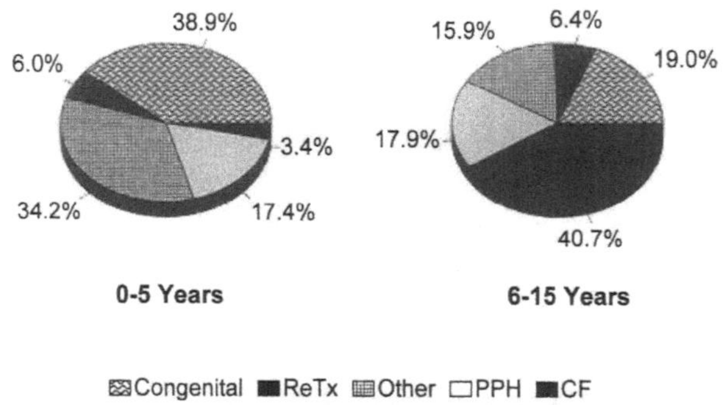

Figure 31. *Pediatric heart-lung/lung transplantation indications by age.* **ReTx,** *retransplantation*; **PPH;** *primary pulmonary hypertension*; **CF;** *Cystic fibrosis.*

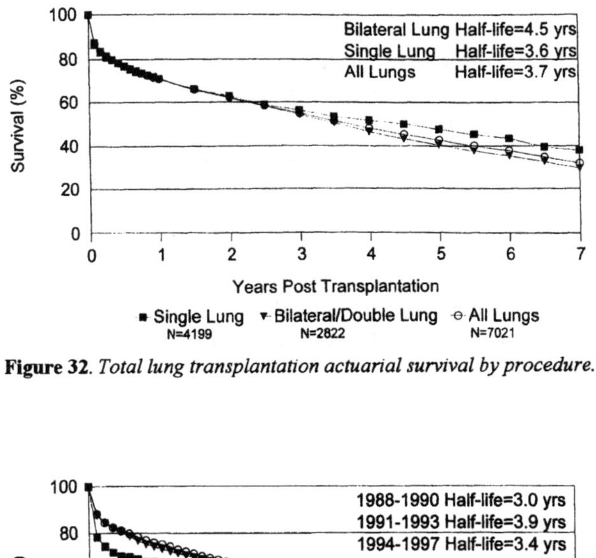

Figure 32. *Total lung transplantation actuarial survival by procedure.*

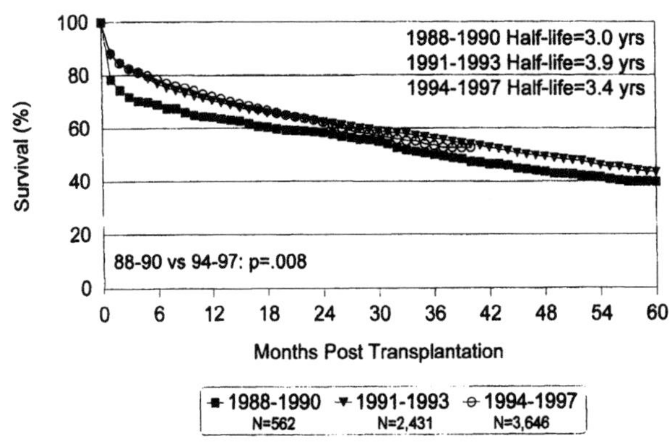

Figure 33. *Total lung transplantation actuarial survival by era.*

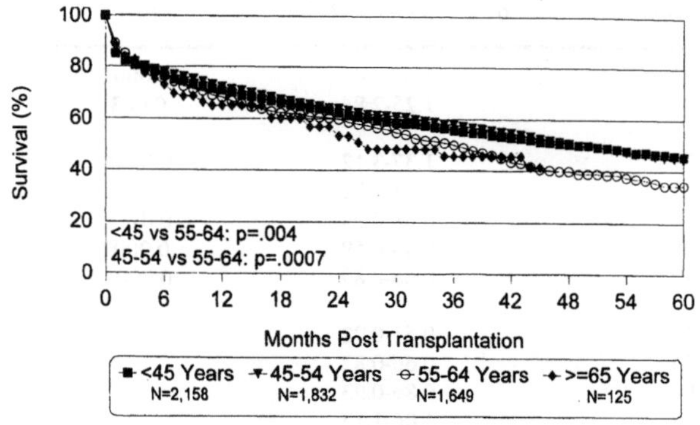

Figure 34. *Adult lung transplantation actuarial survival by age.*

Adult lung and heart-lung transplantation survival rates are presented in Figure 35. The 1-, 2-, and 3-years actuarial survival rates for lung transplantation are 45%, 37%,and 31%, respectively. For heart-lung retransplantation the outcomes are even worse, with survival rates of 33% and 30% at 1 and 2 years, respectively.

Tables VII and VIII present the results of the multivariate logistic regression analyses for risk factors for 1- and 5-year mortality after lung transplantation. Independent predictors of adverse outcome at 1 year include ventilator support, retransplantation, diagnosis other than emphysema, and recipient age. With an increased number of patients in the Registry, donor age is now identified as a significant risk factor in lung transplantation, similar to that seen in heart and heart-lung transplantation. At 5 years outcomes are predicted by retransplantation, underlying diagnoses, and recipient age.

Actuarial survival for pediatric lung and heart-lung transplantation is shown in Figure 36. There are no significant differences in outcomes between these three procedures; however, numbers in all groups are small. Table IX displays the multivariate analysis for 1-year mortality after pediatric lung and heart-lung transplantation.

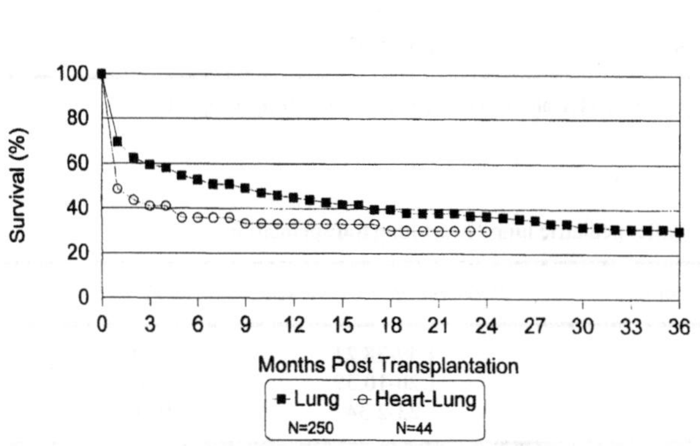

Figure 35. *Adult heart-lung/lung transplantation actuarial survival.*

Table 7. Risk factors for 1-year mortality after adult lung transplantation.

Variable	*Odds ratio*	*95% Confidence interval*	*p Value*
Ventilator	2.39	1.65-3.47	<0.0001
Retransplant	1.88	1.25-2.84	0.003
Diagnoses			
Congenital heart	2.07	1.37-3.12	0.0005
PPH	1.31	1.01-1.71	0.04
A1A	0.74	0.58-0.94	0.01
Emphysema	0.48	0.40-0.59	<0.0001
Female recip	0.77	0.66-0.89	0.0005
Recip age (linear)			<0.0001
Recip age 20	0.6	0.51-0.72	
Recip age 30	0.74	0.66-0.82	
Recip age 40	0.9	0.86-0.93	
Recip age 50	1.09	1.06-1.13	
Recip age 60	1.33	1.21-1.47	
Recip age 70	1.62	1.37-1.92	
Donor age (quadratic)			0.002
Donor age 20	1.07	1.02-1.11	
Donor age 30	1	1.00-1.00	
Donor age 40	1.08	1.03-1.12	
Donor age 50	1.33	1.11-1.58	
Donor age 60	1.87	1.27-2.76	

PPH, Primary pulmonary hypertension; **A1A**, alpha$_1$-antitrypsin deficiency; **Recip**, recipient.
n = 4237

Table 8. Risk factors for 5-year mortality after adult lung transplantation.

Variable	*Odds ratio*	*95% Confidence interval*	*p Value*
Repeat Tx	2.12	1.11-4.06	0.007
IPF	1.68	1.16-2.43	0.01
A1A	0.67	0.48-0.92	0.002
Recip age (linear)			
Recip age 20	1.07	0.68-1.68	
Recip age 30	0.91	0.76-1.10	
Recip age 40	0.92	0.87-0.98	
Recip age 50	1.11	1.04-1.19	
Recip age 60	1.6	1.17-2.18	
Recip age 70	2.74	1.35-5.57	

Tx, Transplantation; **IPF**, idiopathic pulmonary fibrosis; **A1A**, alpha$_1$-antitrypsin deficiency; **Recip**, recipient.
n = 1411.

Table 9. Risk factors for 1-year mortality after pediatric lung / heart-lung transplantation.

Variable	*Odds ratio*	*95% Confidence interval*	*p Value*
Ventilator	13.1	4.49-38.21	<0.0001
Non-white recipient	3.57	1.20-10.59	0.02
Cold ischemic time	1.7	1.23-2.34	0.001

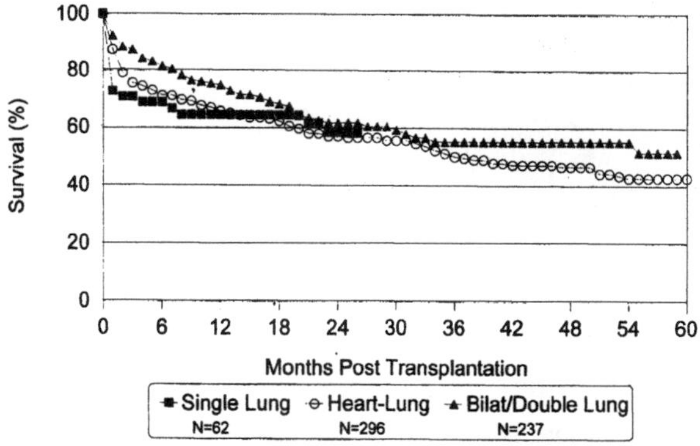

Figure 36. *Pediatric heart/heart-lung transplantation actuarial survival by procedure.*

Independent risk factors include the requirement for mechanical ventilation before transplantation (a 5.56-fold risk), and ABO blood groups of both donor and recipeint. Given the very small numbers, the confidence is wide in these latter two factors, and the predictive ability of these factors needs confirmation.

Figures 37 and 38 demonstrate the activity levels and employment status of patients 1 and 3 years after transplantation. A slightly greater percentage of patients have some limitations compared with those after heart transplantation, although similar percentages

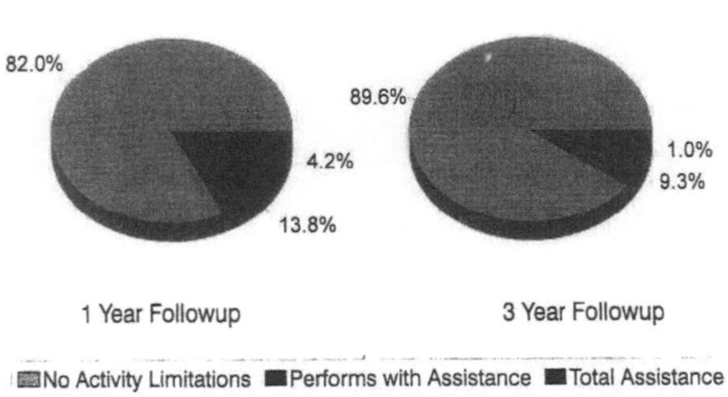

Figure 37. *Lung transplant recipient functional ststus.*

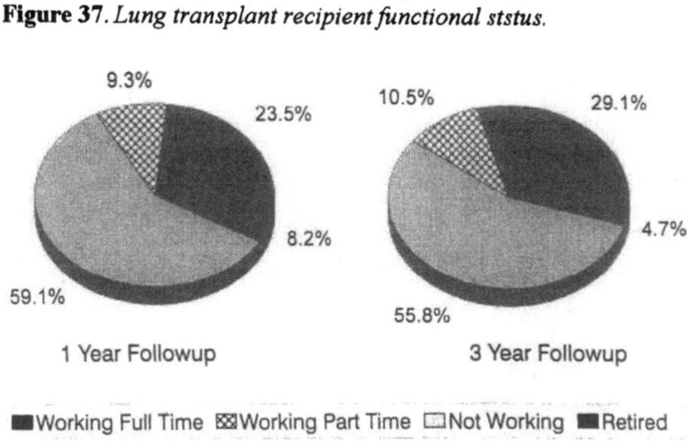

Figure 38. *Lung transplant recipient work status.*

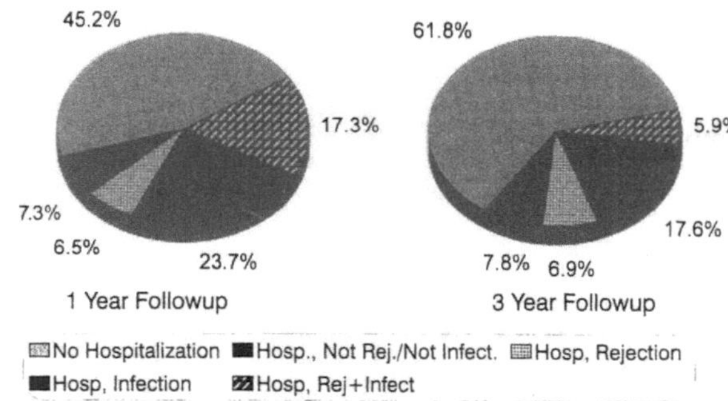

Figure 39. *Rehospitalization after lung transplantation.*

of patients are employed. Figure 39 shows that a significant percentage of patients continue to require repeat hospitalization after lung transplantation, even in the third year after transplantation. Figures 40 to 42 show the prevalence of comorbid conditions in the first 3 years after transplantation, again including drug-treated hypertension, renal dysfunction, drug-treated hyperlipidemia, drug-treated diabetes, and malignancy. Figure 43 demonstrates the maintenance immunosuppression in the population. There is a large proportion of patients receiving tacrolimus after lung transplantation compared with heart transplantation.

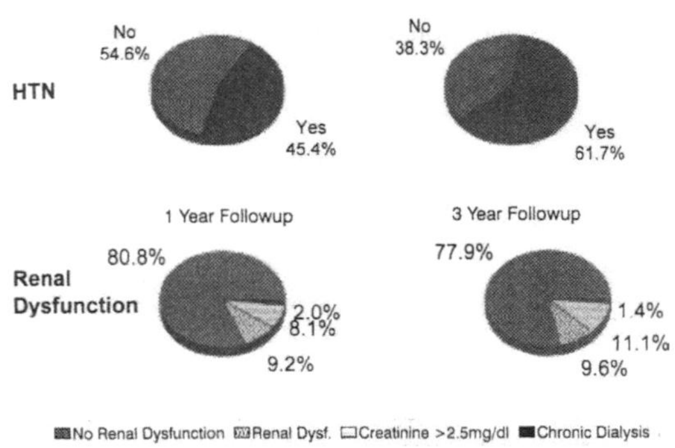

Figure 40. *Hypertension and renal dysfunction after lung transplantation.* **HTN**, *Hypertension.*

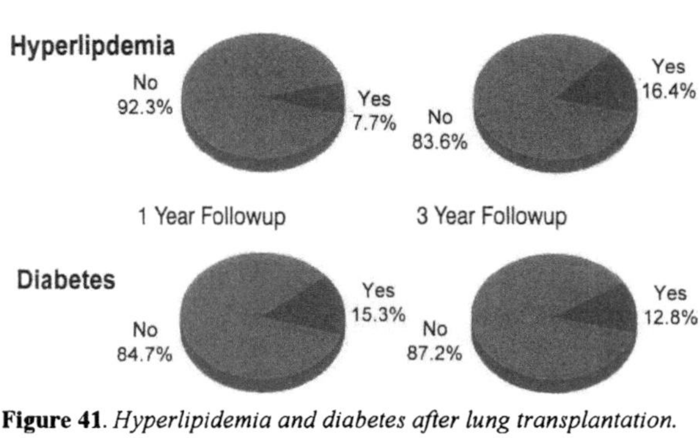

Figure 41. *Hyperlipidemia and diabetes after lung transplantation.*

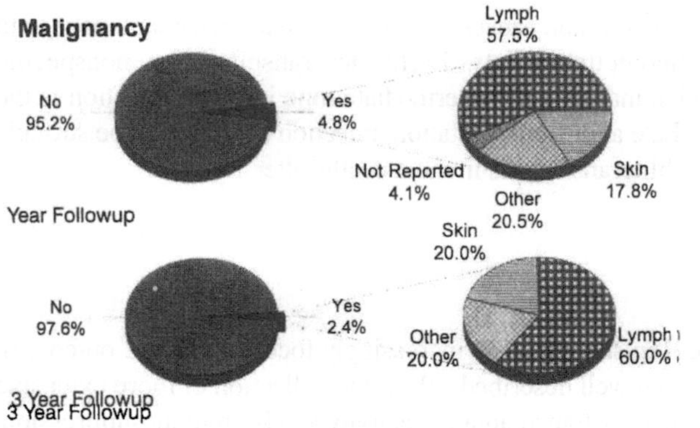

Figure 42. *Malignancy after lung transplantation.*

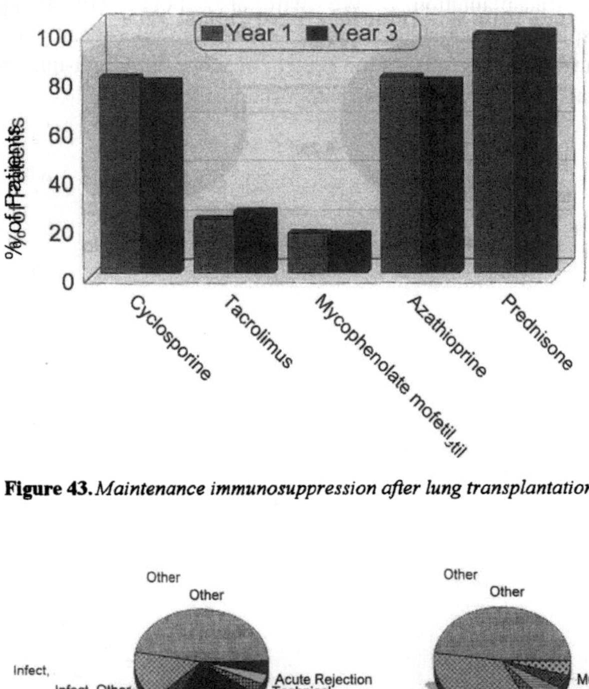

Figure 43. *Maintenance immunosuppression after lung transplantation.*

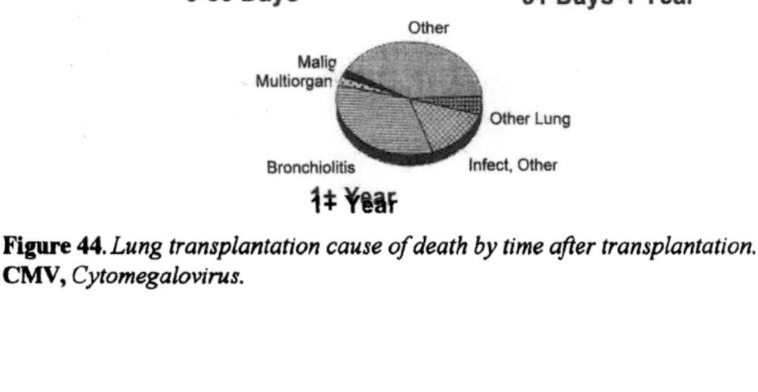

Figure 44. *Lung transplantation cause of death by time after transplantation.*
CMV, *Cytomegalovirus.*

Figure 44 demonstrates the most common causes of death after lung transplantation (both adult and pediatric) at three different time points. Early after transplantation, nonspecific graft failure and infection predominate. In the intermediate time interval, infection is the most common cause of death. Late after transplantation, infection continues to be strongly represented, but bronchiolitis obliterans results in most deaths after 1 years.

Conclusions

As with the previous year the Registry report is increasingly focusing on late outcomes, because early outcomes have been well described. With the collection of more extensive follow-up information, including post-transplantation activity levels, immunosuppression, graft function, and interim hospitalizations, the registry has begun and will continue to focus on morbidity after thoracic transplantation. We will also begin correlating pretransplantation and posttransplantation variables to morbid events, as well as death. We recognize the efforts of the contributing transplantation centers in submitting high-quality data and thank these transplantation programs for their support and cooperation.

7. MECHANICAL CIRCULATORY SUPPORT

Joe Helou and Robert L. Kormos

Introduction

Mechanical cardiac assistance had its origins as an offshoot from the development of cardiopulmonary bypass. Early efforts in the design and development of devices were focused on providing support for the body and the heart during periods of recovery from impaired cardiac function following unsuccessful cardiac surgery and / or acute myocardial infarction. With the recognition that cardiac replacement was needed for end-stage congestive heart failure, research developed along parallel lines with both natural (heart transplantation) and mechanical (total artificial heart) solutions. Therefore, today mechanical circulatory support is used primarily in these two settings: a) for acute onset of myocardial failure that is potentially recoverable (post-cardiotomy or acute myocardial infarction support) and b) for chronic end-stage congestive heart failure which is refractory to traditional medical therapy. The latter setting has the largest potential population of patients that require assistance and help.

Congestive heart failure refers to a clinical syndrome of depressed cardiac output that is unable to meet the metabolic needs of the body. This results in neuro-hormonal compensatory mechanisms (Renin-Angiotensin, Adrenergic and Vasopressin systems) that initially help to restore normal organ perfusion but in the long run are deleterious to both cardiac and end-organ function.

Despite advances in medical and surgical therapies for congestive heart failure, mortality and morbidity remain high.[1] The cost of caring for congestive heart failure patients and their repeated readmissions to hospital places a heavy burden on already scarce health care budgets. When aggressive medical and conventional surgical therapies for severe congestive heart failure no longer provide adequate systemic organ perfusion, several mechanical devices are available to support the failing circulation, in the short or long-term. This support will be provided until sufficient heart function recovers (bridge to recovery) or until a donor heart is available for transplantation (bridge to transplantation).

This chapter will examine the indications and patient selection for mechanical cardiac assist and review the currently available mechanical assist devices in terms of techniques of insertion, peri-operative management, complications and outcomes.

Roy Masters (editor), Surgical Options for the Treatment of Heart Failure, 117-135.

Indications for Mechanical Assist and Patient Selection

The general goals of mechanical cardiac assist are to correct underperfusion of vital organs and to decrease cardiac load. In general patients must be in imminent danger of death or irreversible end-organ damage to be considered for circulatory support. Patients thus are eligible for device insertion if their acute cardiogenic shock persists despite maximal pharmacologic inotropic therapy and support with the intraaortic balloon pump or if their chronic congestive failure is refractory to medical therapy and is not amenable to conventional surgical therapy. The indications for mechanical cardiac assist can thus be generally sub-divided into two categories namely acute and chronic cardiogenic shock and are based on well-defined criteria (Table 1).[2] The acute indications for device insertion include post-cardiotomy cardiogenic shock, acute massive myocardial infarction, acute myocarditis, and severe allograft rejection; whereas the chronic indications include progressive ischemic, dilated idiopathic or valvular cardiomyopathy not amenable to conventional but high-risk surgery.

Table 1: General Criteria for VAD insertion

Hemodynamics	
Cardiac Indexeee	<2L/min/m^2
PCWP and CVP	>18-20 mmHg
SVR	> 2100 dynes-sec/cm^2
MAP	<60 mmHg
Signs of hypoperfusion	
MVO2	<60%
Renal dysfunction	Oliguria (<0.5 ml/kg/hr) and increased creatinine
Metabolic acidosis	
Respiratory failure	Pulmonary edema
Hepatic dysfunction	Elevated liver function tests
Altered mental status	Delirium, agitation or confusion
Maximal medical therapy	

It is very useful and practical to divide potential device candidates into two categories: those in whom the device is used until sufficient cardiac function recovers (bridge to recovery), and those in whom cardiac function is not expected to recover and the device is used to provide circulatory support until a donor heart is available for transplantation (bridge to transplantation).

Several issues have to be considered for post-cardiotomy patients in whom the device is used as a bridge to recovery. Cardiac dysfunction in this setting must be felt to be reversible (e.g. cardiogenic shock secondary to myocardial stunning). A technically unsuccessful operation and a massive peri-operative myocardial infarction make myocardial recovery unlikely, therefore mechanical circulatory support should proceed in these patients only if they are eligible for cardiac transplantation.[3] Similarly, the requirement of biventricular support post-cardiotomy is an indicator of the severity of myocardial dysfunction and peri-operative injury and the success at weaning as well as the survival have been inferior compared to those patients requiring only univentricular support.[4] These patients must therefore meet criteria for cardiac transplantation. Similiarly, because of the high incidence of multi-organ failure and the poor overall survival in patients older than 70 years of age who fail to wean from cardiopulmonary bypass (CPB), device insertion in these patients is relatively contra-indicated.[5] Other exclusionary criteria include severe peripheral vascular disease, uncontrollable septicemia, significant blood dyscrasias and evidence of irreversible end-organ damage.

For post-cardiotomy support weanability rates as high as 40-50 % and hospital discharge rates of 25-35% have been reported. These early results reflect the learning curve with the use of these devices so that current results have improved. The weanability and discharge rates appear to be related to a) the promptness of implantation of the device, b) the age of the patient, c) any delay in implementing biventricular support when univentricular support is inadequate, d) the degree of completed myocardial infarction, and e) preoperative left ventricular function.

Patients receiving mechanical circulatory assist as a bridge to transplantation for chronic heart failure are generally less critically ill than patients selected for support in the setting of acute heart failure. Patients in chronic severe congestive heart failure however have some degree of end-organ dysfunction resulting from chronic tissue underperfusion. They are usually chronically debilitated and suffer from cardiac cachexia as well. In addition these patients are expected to withstand the stress of reoperative surgery (the transplantation) and transplant related complications (infection and rejection). Delaying implantation of the device until irreversible end-organ damage occurs is associated with increased mortality and morbidity. Therefore in these patients, it is imperative that device insertion proceeds early, prior to the development of significant and often irreversible end-organ dysfunction. Timing of device insertion in these patients is often very difficult. Criteria and scoring systems have been developed to stratify these patients and are generally similar to injury severity scores. [6-8]

The timing of implantation of mechanical circulatory support as a bridge to cardiac transplantation depends on a multitude of factors that combine signs of hemodynamic deterioration, threatened end organ dysfunction, and low probability of receiving a transplant before death, as well as the issues of cost effectiveness of long-term hospitalization with medical therapy. Most patients who require mechanical circulatory support demonstrate the persistent need for intravenous inotropic maintenance to assure adequate end-organ perfusion. The need for an intra-aortic balloon pump (IABP) is often an ominous sign and in most transplant centers is not used as ultimate medical therapy as much as a way of stabilizing the patient prior to implant surgery. Subtle signs of low perfusion indicating the need for mechanical support include weight loss, cachexia, decreased level of consciousness, lack of appetite, abdominal bloating or discomfort, constipation or diarrhea, atrial arrhythmias or fever without discernable infection. All of these findings indicate an inflammatory state that co-exists with severe end-stage heart failure and imminent decompensation.

With respect to logistical issues, patients with large body surface areas, those who are blood type "O" and patients who may have been previously sensitized, with the presence of antibodies, will have long waiting times. In these patients, signs of deterioration dictate immediate device implantation.

Device Selection

Once a patient is deemed candidate for mechanical circulatory support, the selection of the device should be individualized and it depends on a number of factors. It is useful to divide the patients into two groups: those receiving mechanical support for acute cardiogenic shock and those receiving support for chronic cardiac dysfunction.

In patients who fail to wean from CPB, every attempt should be made initially to exclude a surgically correctable technical problem. Transesophageal echocardiography in these settings is extremely valuable. The patients rate, rhythm, preload, contractility and afterload all have to be optimized. Should failure to wean from CPB occur despite these measures and despite the establishment of pharmacologic inotropic support, the next step is insertion of an intra-aortic balloon pump. When these procedures are insufficient to separate the patient from the bypass circuit, a number of short and intermediate term mechanical assist devices are available. These include centrifugal pumps, the Abiomed BVS 5000, the Thoratec ventricular assist device (VAD) and the Medtronic Hemopump.

Currently Available Devices

A variety of devices are available for supporting the failing circulation and can be classified into those used for short-term support (hours to days) and those used for longer term support (days to months). Table 2 gives a breakdown of the currently available devices by category.

Table 2. Currently Available Devices

Devices for Short Term Support	*Devices for Longer Term Support*
IABP	Para-corporeal Pneumatic: Thoratec-Implantable
Centrifugal pumps	Pneumatic: IP-HeartMate LVAD
Abiomed BVS 5000	Electric: Novacor LVAS & EV-HeartMate LVAD
Hemopump	Orthotopic: CardioWest TAH

Short-term Support

Intra-Aortic Balloon Pump

The IABP is the most widely used short term circulatory support device. It consists of a balloon catheter positioned in the descending thoracic aorta either via a percutaneous or open femoral artery insertion technique. The proximal tip of the catheter should be positioned 1cm distal to the origin of the left subclavian artery. More distal positioning interferes with renal and mesenteric blood flow. Alternative cannulation sites (ascending aorta and axillary arteries) are available should femoral insertion be impossible due to severe aorto-iliac disease. However, these alternative sites require operative removal of the IABP.

The IABP provides counterpulsation (cyclical inflation of the balloon in ventricular diastole and deflation in systole) i.e. diastolic augmentation and systolic unloading. This improves coronary blood flow and provides afterload reduction without an increase in myocardial oxygen consumption.

The effectiveness of the IABP has been previously demonstrated.[9] It relies however on the presence of native cardiac function and cannot maintain adequate circulation in its absence. In addition, IABP effectiveness is diminished with heart rates more than 120 bpm or in the presence of dysrythmias (e.g. atrial fibrillation).

Complication rates vary from 5 – 35%.[10] Vascular complications predominate and result in ischemia of the extremity distal to the femoral insertion site. This usually resolves upon withdrawal of the IABP but surgical correction is needed in approximately 15% of cases. Risk factors for vascular complications with the IABP include gender, diabetes and hypertension. Other reported complications include infection (1- 20%), iatrogenic aortic dissection, thrombocytopenia, and distal embolization. Although primarily used as post-cardiotomy bridge to recovery, the IABP has been used as bridge to transplantation as well.[11]

Hemopump

The Hemopump is a catheter-mounted axial flow pump that is inserted via the femoral artery or via the thoracic aorta. Two insertions techniques are available; percutaneously (for support needed for < 6 hrs) or via a graft sutured to the femoral artery or the ascending aorta (for support needed for days). The catheter is then advanced through the aortic valve into the left ventricle with the inflow port located in the ventricle and the outflow port in the descending aorta. The catheter tip contains a miniature axial flow pump driven by a small electromagnetic motor. The pump rotates at 17000 – 25000 rpm's and is capable of generating non-pulsatile flows of up to 6 Lpm.

The Hemopump is best suited for short-term support and is thus mainly indicated for supporting patients with acute reversible myocardial dysfunction. It has been successfully used for acute cardiac failure as a bridge to recovery, as well as in chronic cardiac failure as a short-term bridge to cardiac transplantation.[12] In addition this device is being promoted as a substitute for conventional CPB in minimally invasive cardiac surgery as well as to provide support during high-risk PTCA procedures.[13,14] Due to its intra-ventricular position, the Hemopump decompresses the left ventricle, reducing its workload and myocardial oxygen consumption.[15] Unlike the IABP, it provides circulatory support in the absence of native cardiac function, operates independently of cardiac cycle and is therefore unaffected by dysrhythmias. The rates of hemolysis and other blood component damage have not been clinically significant when the device is used for a short period of time. However, hemolysis increases with time and may become clinically significant after extended use. The patients on Hemopump support are systemically heparinized. The potential effects on end-organ function after extended non-pulsatile flow is a limitation. In addition the immobilization of the supported patients hinders their rehabilitation. Therefore this device is solely suitable for support for less than one week.

Contraindications to Hemopump insertion are similar to those of the IABP and include severe aorto-iliac disease, prosthetic aortic valves, aortic stenosis and regurgitation, aortic dissection and aneurysms. In addition, patients with blood dyscrasias and LV thrombi should not be supported with the Hemopump. As well right to left shunting causing severe refractory hypoxemia and mechanical pump failure from entrapment of necrotic myocardial debris in the inlet port have been reported when the Hemopump was used in the setting of post-infarction ventricular septal defect (VSD).

Potential complications include; failure of insertion, mechanical device failure (fracture of the drive cable, peripheral emboli, major vascular injury including iatrogenic aortic dissection, insertion site vascular complications (limb ischemia and pseudoaneurysm formation), ventricular dysrhythmias, myocardial and aortic valve injury.

The Linkoping Heart Center group have used the Hemopump in 24 patients with severe left ventricular dysfunction after coronary artery bypass grafting, achieving a weaning rate of 58%.[16]

Earlier published results revealed a survival to 30 days of 32% in 41 patients supported with the Hemopump.[15] Hemodynamic improvements were noted in all patients and only minimal hemolysis was seen. There were no instances of leg ischemia. However significant inability to insert the pump and mechanical failure rates were noted prompting design modifications.

It is to be noted that the Hemopump device is no longer available for clinical use as of April 1998 (personal communication, Medtronic-DLP). The axial flow pump technology is however being further developed for new and forthcoming cardiac assist devices.

Centrifugal pumps

Centrifugal pumps were first used as alternatives to roller pumps for CPB but because of their simplicity, widespread availability, versatility and low cost, their use has been extended to short-term cardiac assist and extra-corporeal membrane oxygenation (ECMO). However, the limited duration of support, the need for systemic anticoagulation and the associated thromboembolic and bleeding complications as well as the requirement for supervision by specially trained personnel are their main disadvantages. In addition, support by centrifugal pumps have been plagued by the development of severe capillary leak syndrome, especially when the device is used for extended periods of time.

Two centrifugal pumps are currently used for short-term cardiac assist, the Biomedicus Biopump and the 3M Sarns pump. The Biomedicus pump consists of an acrylic pump head with inlet and outlet ports located at 90 degrees to each other. The impeller, consisting of a stack of parallel cones, is driven through magnetic coupling by an external motor. Blood flow is generated by rotation of the impeller and is proportional to the speed of the impeller rotation, generating non-pulsatile flow.

Centrifugal pumps have been mainly used in post-cardiotomy cardiogenic shock either as a bridge to recovery or a bridge to transplantation. Data from the National Registry reveals a rate of weaning or transplantation of 45.7 % with a hospital discharge rate of 25.3%.[17] For those implanted as a bridge to transplantation 68.5% were actually transplanted and 46.9% were discharged. Of those with acute myocardial infarction 26% were either weaned or transplanted and for acute MI. 25.3% of the postcardiotomy patients

were ultimately discharged from the hospital. [17]
Similarly, Noon et al reported their experience with the Biomedicus pump in 172 patients.[18] Of their patients 75% were supported for post-cardiotomy cardiogenic shock and 10% for cardiac allograft failure. Of these, 84 patients (49%) were weaned and 24 patients (20%) were discharged form hospital. Reported complications included bleeding in 60%, renal failure in 44%, respiratory failure in 35% and neurological complications in 33% of patients. The Bad Oeynhausen heart surgery center also reported their seven year experience with the centrifugal pump in 61 patients for both post-cardiotomy and post-infarction cardiogenic shock.[19] Overall 41% were weaned, 16% were transplanted and 36% discharged. Complications included bleeding, multi-organ failure and neurologic events, especially common when support was prolonged, and the most frequent cause of death was multi-organ failure. Use of the Biomedicus pump as a short-term bridge to cardiac transplantation in patients with chronic and deteriorating cardiac failure reveals a successful transplantation rate of 78%.[20]

Abiomed BVS 5000
The Abiomed BVS 5000 system consists of an extra-corporeal, pneumatic, pulsatile cardiac assist device. The pump consists of two polyurethane chambers; a gravity filled "atrial" chamber and a pneumatically driven "ventricular" chamber. It is vertically oriented. Unidirectional flow is maintained by two three-leaflet polyurethane valves, making systemic heparinization mandatory. The device operates in several modes. In the Auto mode, the venous return to the VAD determines the ventricular output. The venous return is in turn augmented by lowering the pump to the floor. Experience with the BVS 5000 in 500 patients from a worldwide voluntary registry was reported in 1996 by Jett.[21] Of these patients 53% were supported for postcardiotomy heart failure and 47% for a variety of other reasons including cardiomyopathy, acute infarction and allograft failure. Most (65%) required biventricular assist devices, with 30% requiring only left and 5% only right ventricular support. Sixty percent (60%) of patients were either weaned from the device or received a transplant. Postcardiotomy patients had a 27% discharge rate, compared with cardiomyopathy patients who had a 40% discharge rate. In addition, complication rates were higher in postcardiotomy patients due to prolonged CPB times and delays prior to device insertion. This highlights the improved survival with early intervention seen in the premarket approval study. The most frequent complication was bleeding (40%) with an overall re-exploration rate of 20%.

Long-Term Support

Thoratec Ventricular Assist Device (VAD)
The Thoratec VAD (Figure 1) is a modified and enhanced version of the Pierce-Donarchy VAD. It is an extra-corporeal, pulsatile, pneumatic VAD. The blood pump is a prosthetic ventricle consisting of a smooth, polyurethane seamless pumping chamber enclosed in a rigid polycarbonate case. Blood flows to the VAD through an atrial or ventricular cannula and from the VAD to the ascending aorta or main pulmonary artery through an arterial

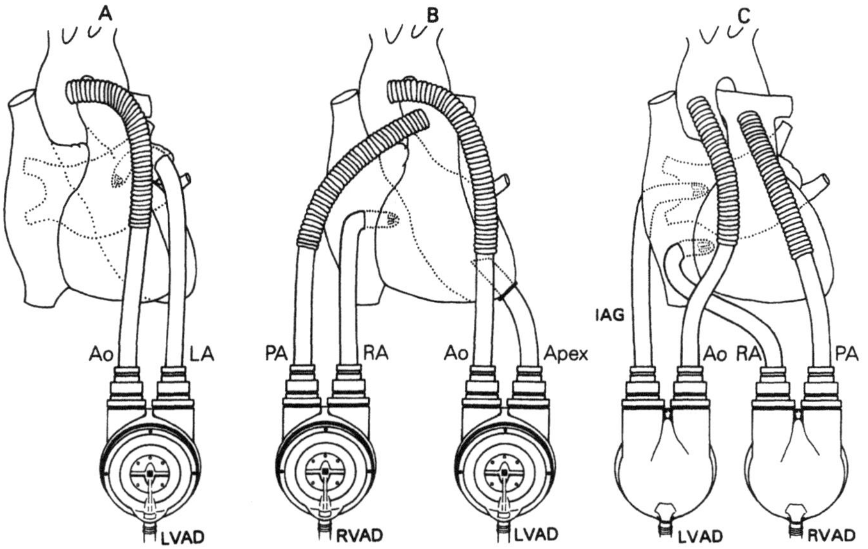

Figure 1: *Thoratec Ventricular Assist System*
Photograph courtesy of Thoratec Laboratories Inc.

graft. Apical ventricular inflow cannulation for LV assist is preferred to left atrial cannulation, as apical cannulation provides higher cardiac output and hence a lower risk of thrombosis in the native heart. In addition the inflow cannula is anchored to thicker and less friable ventricular muscle. Cannulae are passed below the costal margins and connected to the VAD placed para-corporeally on the anterior abdominal wall, thus permitting sternal closure (an advantage over centrifugal pumps). Two mechanical valves maintain unidirectional flow.

The Thoratec VAD is capable of generating 65 ml of stroke volume and flow outputs of up to 7 Lpm. It does so by generating negative and positive pressures to fill and empty the VAD. It operates in one of three modes. In the asynchronous mode, the VAD rate and ejection time are set by the operator. In this mode the VAD operates independently of the supported native heart. In the volume mode, ejection begins as soon as complete VAD filling occurs (fill to empty mode). This is the most commonly used mode of operation because of the automatic pump response to changes in physiological conditions. Finally the synchronous mode is similar in principle to counterpulsation.

The Thoratec VAD is a versatile system capable of providing left (LVAD), right (RVAD) and bi-ventricular (BiVAD) support. Patients supported with systems designed solely for left ventricular support may develop right heart failure and require RVAD support with another system (ie. Hybrid VAD support), adding to the complexity of the setup and patient care. The limitation of the Thoratec device is its extra-corporeal positioning limiting patient's mobility. However, a new portable drive console (the TLC-II) is currently being evaluated in North America. Initial experience in Europe was favorable, allowing greater patient mobility and providing more independence for Thoratec VAD patients.

To date 536 patients worldwide have been supported with the Thoratec VAD as a bridge to transplantation.[22] The age ranged from 8 to 68 yrs and 62% received BiVAD and 38% received either LVAD or RVAD support. Of those supported, 61% underwent cardiac transplantation, with 87% of these being disharged from the hospital. The Thoratec VAD has been used in 151 patients for failure to wean from CPB with 38% being subsequently weaned from VAD support and 58% being discharged from hospital. Duration of support ranged from 1 to 80 days (mean 7 days). Additionally 34 post-cardiotomy patients were considered for transplantation after they failed to wean from VAD support with 70% being transplanted and 75% being discharged.

Novacor LVAS

The Novacor LVAS (Figure 2) is one of two available long-term implantable pulsatile cardiac assist devices. It consists of an implanted pump, a para-corporeal portable control unit and an electromagnetic energy converter. The blood pump is implanted in the anterior abdominal wall and connected to the left ventricle and ascending aorta respectively through inflow and outflow conduits, with custom-designed stented porcine valved conduits maintaining unidirectional flow. Insertion of the Novacor LVAS is performed through a median sternotomy extending to just beyond the umbilicus. Prior to the establishment of

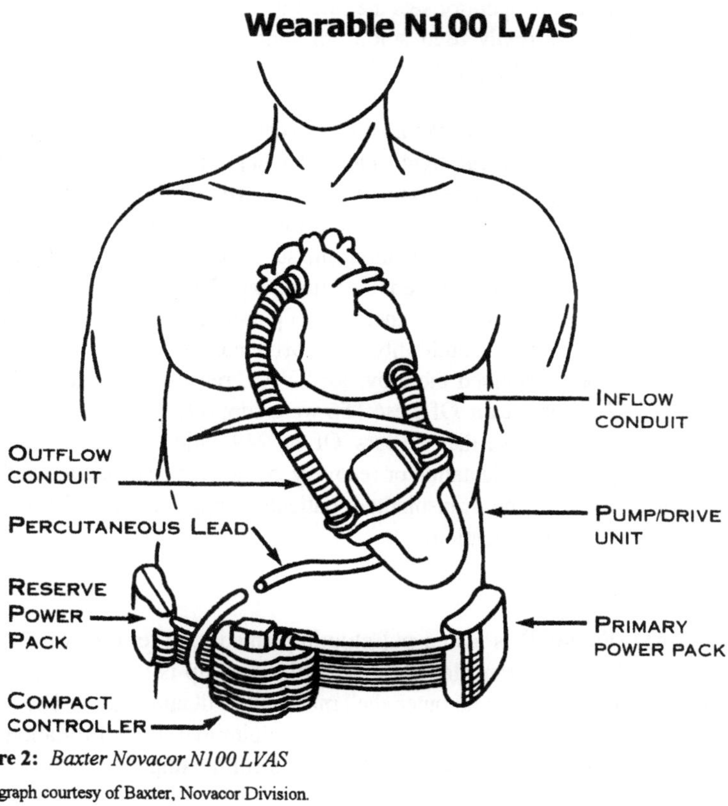

Figure 2: *Baxter Novacor N100 LVAS*

Photograph courtesy of Baxter, Novacor Division.

CPB, a preperitoneal pocket is created posterior to the left rectus abdominis muscle where the pump is positioned. The outflow graft is then brought along the diaphragm and is anastomosed end to side to the ascending aorta using a partial clamp. Upon establishment of CPB, the apex of the left ventricle is exposed and a series of circumferential pledgeted sutures are sewn around the apex and through an apical sewing ring. The sutures are then tied and a stab incision is made at the center of the sewing ring. A core of apical myocardium is then cut using a circumferential blade and removed. The apical cannula is then introduced and the purse-string suture of the apical sewing ring is tied. The skirt of the apical cannula is then circumferentially sewn to the apical sewing ring. The pump is activated and de-aired through the outflow graft.

The Novacor LVAS pump is comprised of a dual pusher-plate sac-type blood pump encapsulated in a fiberglass reinforced polyester shell. The pump has a maximum stroke volume of 70 cc's and can generate flows exceeding 10-12 L / min. The wearable controller provides power and automatic control through a percutaneous lead and air vent. This untethered configuration provides the patient with substantial mobility and autonomy.

The Novacor LVAS may be operated in one of three modes. In the synchronized mode, the pump diastole coincides with the cardiac systole, thus providing effective counterpulsation and maximal unloading of the left ventricle. In the fill to empty mode, the pumping rate depends on the filling rate of the device. This maximizes cardiac output. Finally in the fixed rate mode, the operator sets the rate and volumes.

The Novacor LVAS is currently used solely for long-term mechanical bridge to transplantation. Anticoagulation with heparin and aspirin ultimately converted to warfarin and aspirin is required.

Similar to the HeartMate LVAD, the Novacor LVAS can only provide mechanical left ventricular support; should mechanical right ventricular support be required, another ventricular assist device system has to be used. While right ventricular failure has been reported in up to 20% of LVAD recipients, most of these patients can be managed with hemodynamic optimization and pharmacologic inotropic support. Less than 5% of patients supported with the Novacor LVAS have required mechanical right ventricular assist (personal communication). Patient selection is therefore of paramount importance. Another disadvantage of the Novacor lies in the audibility of the drive mechanism.

To date 970 patients have received the Novacor LVAS, representing a cumulative clinical experience of 267 patient years. Of these 156 were supported for > 6 months, 40 for more than one year and 8 for more than 2 years. Of the 949 patients who received the Novacor LVAS as a bridge to transplantation or recovery, 57% were transplanted and 3% were weaned, respectively. Of the transplanted patients, approximately 90% were discharged home (personal communication).

HeartMate LVAD

The HeartMate LVAD (Figure 3) is also a pulsatile implanted long-term cardiac assist device used solely as a bridge to transplantation. The blood pump is made of a flexible polyurethane diaphragm housed in a rigid outer shell made out of titanium alloy. The blood contacting surfaces are uniquely designed to promote pseudointimal lining formation and to reduce the risk of thromboembolism and hemolysis, thus eliminating the

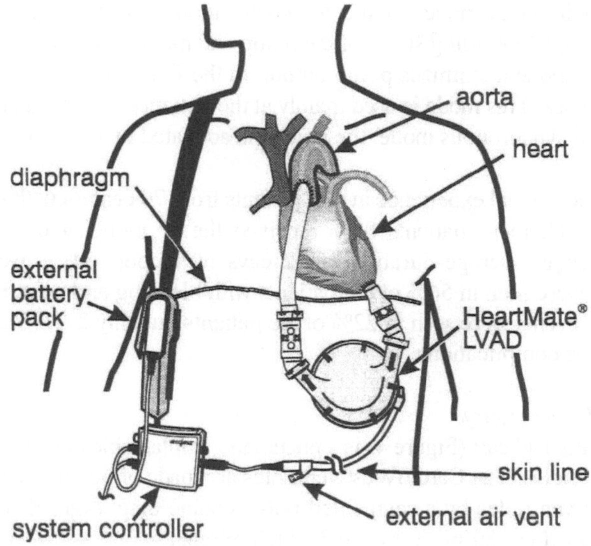

Figure 3: *TCI HeartMate LVAS*

Photograph courtesy of Thermo CardioSystems Inc.

need for anticoagulation. Unidirectional flow is maintained with porcine valves housed in the inlet and outlet Dacron graft conduits.There exist two HeartMate models, an implantable pneumatic (IP) and a vented electric (VE) model. Both models consist of the same pusher plate blood pump and are implanted in the same abdominal location. They differ mainly in their method of pump actuation. The VE-HeartMate LVAS is electrically powered by a wearable rechargeable battery pack, whereas the IP-HeartMate LVAS receives its pneumatic power from an external drive console. The VE model therefore allows for greater patient mobility. A new portable console for the IP-HeartMate that can be pulled on wheels or worn with a shoulder strap has recently been introduced and tested. Portable batteries allow for up to 8 hrs of uninterrupted operation. This new driver substantially increases the mobility of patients supported with the pneumatic HeartMate LVAD.

Implantation of the HeartMate LVAD is done on CPB through a median sternotomy that is extended to the umbilicus. Following the removal of a core of apical left ventricular myocardium with a circular knife, the inlet cannulae is inserted and sewn to the LV apex with interrupted pledgeted sutures. It is then passed through the diaphragm. The outlet graft is brought over the diaphragm and is anastomosed end to side to the ascending aorta. The inlet and outflow grafts are then attached to the device that is positioned intra-abdominally or in a preperitoneal pocket in the left upper quadrant. The drive line (IP and VE HeartMate) and air vents line (VE HeartMate) are then tunneled subcutaneously to the left lower quadrant and exit at that site to be connected to the drive console or the external battery pack.

Both the VE and IP HeartMate models have a maximal stroke volume of 85cc's and are thus capable of generating flows of up to 12 and 10 Lpm respectively. They can both be operated in the automatic and fixed-rate modes. In addition, the IP-HeartMate can be operated in the external synchronous mode. In the automatic mode, the flow rate is continuously adjusted according to the filling status of the pump and maintains an average stroke volume of 75cc's. This mode maximizes pump output. In the fixed rate mode, the operator sets the rate and volumes. This mode is used mainly at the initiation of mechanical support. Finally in the external synchronous mode, the system is activated by the patient's R wave.

Poirier reported worldwide clinical experience in 482 patients from 70 centers with the HeartMate LVAD in 1997.[23] Of these patients 89% received the IP model and 11% received the VE model. After an average duration of 72 days of support 64 % were transplanted. Adverse events were seen in 56% of the patients with bleeding and infection predominating. Neurological events were seen in 22% of the patients but only 2-3% were device-related thromboembolic complications.

CardioWest Total Artificial Heart (TAH)

The CardioWest C-70 total artificial heart (Figure 4) is a pneumatic, implantable device that totally replaces the failing ventricles. The CardioWest ventricles are made of polyurethane. Blood is propelled out of the ventricles by a segmented polyurethane diaphragm that is displaced forward by compressed air during systole and which retracts

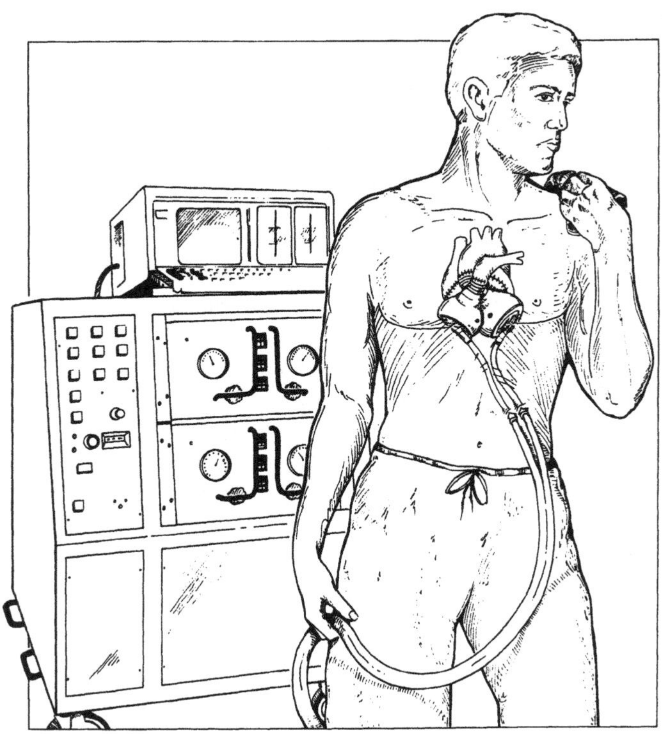

Figure 4: *Cardiowest TAH*
Photograph courtesy of CardioWest

during diastole allowing prosthetic ventricular filling. The TAH is capable of providing flows up to 10 Lpm.

Implantation of the TAH should be considered for patients in severe biventricular failure with rupture of the interventricular septum as a bridge to transplantation. Enthusiasm for the TAH has diminished due to higher incidence of complications with the TAH, the obligatory cardiac transplant associated with its use and the advent of more versatile VAD's.

Between 1993 and 1996, 79 patients underwent placement of the CardioWest TAH worldwide.[24]. The most common indications for orthotopic TAH insertion were cardiomyopathy and ischemic heart disease. A total of 55 patients (70%) were transplanted of which 50 survived (91% of patients transplanted) and were discharged home. There were 255 adverse events representing a mean complication rate of three events per patient. Most frequent complications were renal failure, infection, bleeding, hepatic and respiratory failure. Neurologic events occurred in 13% of patients and 26.5% of patients died during mechanical support. The most common cause of death was multiple organ failure. The mean duration of implant was 34 days (range 0-186 days) and the mean age of the group was 45 years (range 16-62 years).

In a 1996 review, Arabia et al compared the outcomes of patients supported with the four most commonly used long-term VAD's including the Novacor LVAS, the TCI HeartMate LVAD, the Thoratec VAD and the CardioWest TAH.[25] A total of 1,286 devices (28% Novacor LVAS, 39% TCI Heartmate, 29% Thoratec VAD and 4% CardioWest TAH) were implanted worldwide for circulatory support since 1984. A total of 776 (60%) patients were transplanted and 88.5% of those transplanted were eventually discharged home. The individual success rate for bridge to transplant and subsequent discharge home for each device was as follows: Novacor LVAS 91%; TCI Heartmate LVAD 89%; Thoratec LVAD 93%, Thoratec BiVAD 81% and CardioWest TAH, 92%.

Post-operative Care and Complications

The post-operative care for patients on ventricular assist devices falls under two broad categories: a) Routine post-operative cardiac surgical care and b) care specific to the ventricular assist device used. Post-operatively the patient is weaned from the ventilator if hemodynamically stable, if there is no active bleeding and if ventilatory weaning parameters are met. This is usually done within 24-48 hours. Withdrawal of inotropic support is dictated by requirements for right ventricular. In general inotropic support for the right ventricle can be discontinued within 5-7 days but, occasionally with marginal right ventricular function, up to two weeks of inotropic support has been required. The type of device used dictates anticoagulation requirements. For those that require anticoagulation some form of intravenous Dextran is usually started within 2 to 4 hours of surgery when bleeding subsides. After chest tube losses have decreased, intravenous heparin and enteric-coated aspirin are often then started and then the Dextran is discontinued, Coumadin and low dose aspirin ultimately replace intravenous heparin. Patients supported with the HeartMate LVAS usually require no anticoagulation but practices vary. Should anticoagulation be used, it is usually in the form of low dose ASA and dipyridamole.

Patients receive 3-5 days of intravenous antibiotics following device implantation for infection prophylaxis. Subsequently antibiotics are administered selectively and only with evidence of infection.

There is special emphasis on nutritional support and physical rehabilitation. These patients often are are chronically debilitated and cachectic. Nutritional support is of great importance in the rehabilitation of these patients and plays an important role in their preparation for the cardiac transplant and the attendant risks of immunosupression. The patients are also started on an active physical exercise regimen, initially in the form of short walks and ultimately in the form of treadmill exercises.

As these patients recover their need for close medical care decreases and some patients can be discharged home with close follow-up while awaiting transplantation.

Bleeding and Blood Product Administration

Bleeding remains the most common initial complication in mechanically supported patients.[26] Risk factors include pre-operative liver congestion and failure, prolonged CPB times and its attendant hemostatic defects and previous surgery. Up to 25% of recipient of devices require re-operation for bleeding. Use of serine protease inhibitors has reduced the bleeding complications and the need for re-exploration and its administration is recommended. [27] Use of leukocyte-poor blood components and HLA-matched platelet donor helps to prevent HLA alloimmunization.

RV Failure

The effect of left ventricular assistance on right ventricular function is controversial and has both beneficial and detrimental effects.[28] A reduction in right ventricular afterload due to relief of passive pulmonary hypertension during LVAD support has a positive effect on right ventricular function. This effect usually overwhelms the loss of contractility produced in the right ventricle secondary to the septal shift caused by decompression of the left ventricle. In cases where blood flow through the pulmonary circulation is compromised, this effect will be lost and right ventricular dysfunction predominates. This occurs in situations that increase pulmonary vascular resistance including pneumothorax, hemothorax, adult respiratory distress syndrome, sepsis, severe preoperative inflammatory state and when massive blood transfusion are required. In general, the more severe the shock and multi-organ dysfunction before implantation, the more likely right ventricular dysfunction will be seen after LVAD implantation. In general right ventricular failure occurs in up to 20% of LVAD recipients and is usually manifested by decreased VAD output associated with increased central venous pressure (CVP). The differential diagnosis includes tamponade. Right ventricular failure can be managed with optimization of right side filling pressures, inotropic support and pulmonary vasodilators, including inhaled nitric oxide. Should these treatment modalities fail, mechanical support is indicated. This can be achieved with the use of short or intermediate term VAD's such as centrifugal pumps, the Abiomed BVS 5000 or the Thoratec VAD. While the need for right ventricular support after LVAD insertion cannot be completely predicted prior to the LVAD implantation predictors of the need for RVAD support include a) evidence of depressed right ventricular function b) the patient's clinical status c) elevated and fixed pulmonary vascular resistance and d) low pulmonary arterial pressures in the presence of overt right ventrrricular failure. [29 - 32] The importance of early recognition of right ventricular failure or its potential after LVAD insertion is to be stressed. RVAD insertion at the time of LVAD implantation is associated with fewer complications as compared to its insertion a few days later. If RVAD support is judged to be probable based on the above predictors, then choosing a versatile system capable of biventricular assist (such as the Thoratec VAD or the Abiomed BVS 5000) is recommended.

Infection Complication

Infectious complications remain a significant cause of morbidity and mortality in mechanically supported patients.[33,34] The predisposing factors include previously established infection, chronic cardiac cachexia and malnutrition, immobilization, presence of prosthetic material, transcutaneous drive lines, colonization from indwelling urinary catheters, endotracheal tubes, central venous catheters and re-exploration for bleeding. Pre-operative antibiotic prophylaxis, meticulous sterile technique, aggressive treatment of documented infections and the minimization of invasive procedures are in order to decrease the rate of infectious complications.[35-37]

Post implant infections are also related to the length of stay in the intensive care unit on inotropic support before device implantation and to the acuteness of patient presentation. The relative incidence of mediastinitis and pump pocket infection has been remarkably low in the current era reaching levels of 3-5%. However, the incidence of blood borne infection varies greatly from center to center and has ranged from 15% to 55%, with the most serious of these being fungal endocarditis. The incidence of driveline infection is approximately 25% in most series, and accounts for 35% of readmissions in patients who are ultimately discharged with implantable VADs. Although the mortality from driveline infection in and to itself is not excessive, the morbidity and effects on quality of life are noticeable. Finally, there is an undetermined incidence of blood stream infection from chronic driveline infection. The mortality of bloodstream infection is close to 50% and is a known aggravating factor for thromboembolic events. However with the exception of device endocarditis, infectious complications are generally not associated with a poorer outcome.[34,35] Patients who remained infection-free during VAD support had outcomes similar to those that had documented, and adequately treated, infections during mechanical support. The overall survival, success of transplantation and post-transplant infection rates were similar in the two groups.

Thromboembolic Complications

Mechanical cardiac assist devices, similarly to any other mechanical device in contact with blood, activate the coagulation cascade and result in thrombus formation and thromboembolism, often with devastating results. Despite rigorous anticoagulation regimens, thromboembolic complications are reported in up to 30 % of mechanically supported patients. This is compounded by the associated anticoagulation related hemorrhage. The TCI-HeartMate with its pseudointimal formation eliminates the blood-prosthetic material interface and has had lower incidence of thromboembolic complications.

Cardiac Dysrhythmias

Cardiac dysrhythmias are common in patients with advanced cardiac dysfunction and remain so after VAD implantation. The etiology of myocardial irritability is related to increased arrhythmogenecity associated with ventricular dilatation and scarring, ongoing ischemia, high dose inotropic support and sympathetic system overdrive. Malignant ventricular arrhythmias in patients with BiVAD is usually of no consequence.[38] In LAVD patients, the ventricular tachyarrhythmias are usually hemodynamically tolerated early on after device implantation, but chronically in euvolemic patients or in patients who are somewhat dehydrated, noticeable drops in cardiac output and exercise tolerance will be noticed. Ventricular fibrillation on the other hand contributes to significant decreases in LVAD output and need to be aggressively treated with cardioversion /defibrillation and anti-arrhythmic agents.[39] As a general rule, patients who present with ischemic cardiomyopathy who pre-implantation have an automatic implantable cardiac defibrillator (AICD) should have that defibrillator reactivated after implant surgery.

Patent Foramen Ovale and Other Indracardiac Shunts

A patent foramen ovale is present in up to 25% of the population and should be closed at the time if VAD implantation to eliminate the risk of severe intracardiac shunting. This complication should be kept in mind and ruled out should severe refractory hypoxemia develop post LVAD insertion.

Multi-Organ Failure

Multi-organ failure remains the most common cause of death in patients with mechanical circulatory support. It is the result of pre-insertion factors including the severity of pre-operative cardiac dysfunction and secondary end-organ damage, the presence of pre-insertion cardio-respiratory arrest and the persistence of post-insertion low output states. Earlier institution of circulatory support before the development of irreversible end-organ damage results in lower morbidity and mortality from multi-organ failure.

The recovery of end organ function following device implantation in those patients that showed demonstrable impairment of pre-operative renal or hepatic function is dependent upon expeditious biventricular support. Studies with the Thoratec Biventricular Assist System show that indeed patients with biventricular support recover renal and hepatic function more quickly when the right-sided filling pressures have been decreased and the requirement for inotropic support is withdrawn.

Ventricular Recovery and Device Weaning

Long term ventricular unloading may improve cardiac function sufficiently enough to allow for device removal. It has been shown that LVAD supported hearts have normalization of myocardial fiber orientation, regression of ventricular hypertrophy and reversal of dilatation.[40, 41] The potential for myocardial recovery is dependant on a number of factors including age, the etiology of the cardiac dysfunction and its natural history, pre-existing ventricular function, and associated co-morbid illnesses. Studies have suggested that recoverability of myocardium on a ventricular assist device in the long term will most likely depend upon the degree of fibrotic change present in the myocardium. In addition, it is felt that patients with ischemic cardiomyopathy are less likely to show recoverability as compared to those with either inflammatory or idiopathic changes. Currently, most reports of recoverability in the chronic phases of ventricular assist device support are still anecdotal and remain to be evaluated. Evaluation of myocardial recovery still remains under development, however some combination of evaluation by cardiac catheterization, echocardiography and exercise testing may be the best combination. During cardiac catheterization with device support reduced to minimally tolerable levels, one should see preservation of mixed venous oxygen saturation and cardiac index with low filling pressures. Under those same conditions echocardiography should demonstrate a slight increase in ejection fraction as the heart is filled with evidence of maintenance of blood pressure, with improved left and right ejection fractions. Finally, with reduced ventricular support a patient should be able to demonstrate a peak $V0_2$ of 15 or greater during a sub-maximal exercise study. Although these criteria hold for the withdrawal of support in chronic patients, post cardiotomy support withdrawal is usually dictated by preservation of cardiac index, blood pressure and hemodynamics with improved echocardiographic findings on transesophageal echocardiography

Summary and Future Outlook

Significant advances have been made in the treatment of end-staged heart failure with mechanical support of the failing circulation becoming a mainstay of therapy for acute and chronic cardiogenic shock. Totally implantable pulsatile assist devices will certainly be a reality in the not-so distant future. Transcutaneous power (TET) and remote device control will allow for untethered and out of hospital patient rehabilitation. As such the quality of life of such supported patient will be improved and costs for caring for these patients will be reduced. Indeed as a treatment for end-satge heart failure long-term permanent assist devices may supplant cardiac transplantation, with its limitations in terms of organ availability and complications.

References

1. Massie BM et al. Survival of patients with congestive heart failure: past, present and future prospects. Circulation 1987; 75: (suppl) IV 11-9.
2. Norman JC et al. Prognostic indices for survival during post-cardiotomy intra-aortic balloon pumping. J Thorac Cardiovasc Surg 1977; 74 : 709-14.
3. Jett GK. Postcardiotomy support with ventricular assist devices: selection of recipients. Sem Thorac Cardiovasc Surg 1994; 6:136-9.
4. Castells E et al. Ventricular circulatory assistance with the Abiomed system as a bridge to heart transplantation. Transplant Proc 1995; 27: 2343-5.
5. Wareing TH et al. Postcardiotomy mechanical circulatory support in the elderly. Ann Thorac Surg 1991; 51: 443-7.
6. Farrar DJ et al. Preoperative predictors of survival in patients with Thoratec ventricular assist devices as a bridge to heart transplantation. J Heart Lung Transplant 1994; 13: 93-101.
7. Swartz MT et al. Risk stratification in patients bridged to cardiac transplantation. Ann Thorac Surg 1994; 58:1142-5.
8. Oz MC et al. Screening scale predicts patients successfully receiving long-term implantable left ventricular assist devices. Circulation 1995; 92 (Suppl): II-1169.
9. O'Connell JB et al. Effect of peri-operative hemodynamic support on survival after cardiac transplantation. Circulation 1988; (Suppl II):III-78.
10. Alcan KE et al. Current status of intra-aortic balloon counterpulsation in critical care cardiology. Crit Care Med 1984; 12: 489-95.
11. Birovljev S et al. Heart transplantation after mechanical circulatory support: four years experience. J Heart Lung Transplant 1992; 11: 240-6.
12. Lonn U et al. Hemopump treatment in patients with post cardiotomy heart failure.Ann Thorac Surg 1995; 60: 1067-71.
13. Mack MJ et al. Video-assisted coronary bypass grafting on the beating heart. Ann Thorac Surg. 1997; 63 (6 Suppl): S100-3.
14. Ferrari M et al. PTCA with the use of cardiac assist devices: Risk stratification, short- & long- term results. Cath & Cardiovasc Diagnosis 1996; 38:242-8.
15. Wampler RK et al. Treatment of cardiogenic shock with the Hemopump left ventricular assist device. Ann Thorac Surg 1991; 52: 506-13.
16. Peterzen B et al. Postoperative management of patients with Hemopump support after coronary artery bypass grafting. Ann Thorac Surg 1996; 62(2): 495-500..
17. Joyce LD et al. Experience with generally accepted centrifugal pumps: Personal and collective experience. Ann Thorac Surg 1996; 61(1): 287-90.
18. Noon GP et al. Clinical experience with the Biomedicus centrifugal ventricular support in 172 patients. Artif Organs 19 (7): 756-60.
19. El-Banayosy A et al. Seven years of experience with the centrifugal pump in patients in cardiogenic shock. Thorac Cardiovasc Surgeon 1995; 43: 347-51.
20. Bolman III RM et al. Circulatory support with a centrifugal pump as a bridge to cardiac transplantation. Ann Thorac Surg 1989; 47:108-12.
21. Jett GK. ABIOMED BVS 5000: experience and potential advantages. Ann Thorac Surg 1996; 61(1): 301-4
22. Thoratec VAD system. Monograph of clinical results. Thoratec Laboratories. December 1998
23. Poirier VL. The HeartMate left ventricular assist system: Worldwide clinical experience. Eur J Cardiothor Surg 1997; 11: S39-S44.
24. Arabia FA et al. International experience with the CardioWest total artificial heart as a bridge to heart transplantation. Eur J Cardiothor Surg 1997; 11: S5-S10.
25. Arabia FA et al. Success rates of long-term circulatory assist devices used currently for bridge to heart transplantation. ASAIO Journal 1996; 42: M542-M546.
26. Goldstein DJ et al. Use of Aprotinin in LVAD recipients reduces blood loss, blood use and perioperative mortality. Ann Thorac Surg 1995; 23:1063-68.
27. Copeland JG III. Thromboembolism and bleeding: clinical strategies. Ann Thorac Surgery 1996; 61(1): 376-7.
28. Farrar DJ. Ventricular interactions during mechanical circulatory support. Sem Thorac & Cardiovasc Surg 1994; 6(3):163-8.
29. Kormos RL et al. Evaluation of right ventricular function during clinical left ventricular assistance.

Trans Am Soc Artif Intern Organs 1989; 35: 547-550.
30. Pennington DG et al. The importance of biventricular failure in patients with post-operative cardiogenic shock. Ann Thorac Surg 1985; 39:16-26.
31. Kormos RL et al. Transplant candidate's clinical status rather than right ventricular function defines need for univentricular versus biventricular support. J Thorac & Cardiovasc Surg 1996; 111(4): 773-82.
32. Pavie A et al. Physiology of univentricular versus biventricular support. Ann Thorac Surg 1996; 61:347-9.
33. Myers TJ et al. Frequency and significance of infections in patients receiving prolonged LVAD support. ASAIO Transactions 1991; 37(3): M283-5.
34. Argenziano M. et al. The influence of infection on survival and successful transplantation in patients with left ventricular assist devices. Journal of Heart & Lung Transplantation 1997; 16(8): 822-31.
35. Fischer SA et al. Infectious complications in left ventricular assist device recipients. Clinical Infectious Diseases 1997; 24(1): 18-23.
36. McCarthy PM et al. Implantable LVAD infections: Implications for permanent use of the Device. Ann Thorac Surg 1996; 61:359-65.
37. Holman WL et al. Infections during extended circulatory support: University of Alabama at Birmingham experience 1989-1994. Ann Thorac Surg 1995; 61: 366-71.
38. Farrar D et al. Successful biventricular circulatory support as a bridge to cardiac transplantation during prolonged ventricular fibrillation and asystole. Circulation 1989; 80 (Suppl):III 147-151.
39. Oz MC et al. Malignant ventricular arrhythmias are not well tolerated in patients receiving long-term left ventricular assist devices. J Am Coll Cardiol 1994; 24:1688-91.
40. Scheinin S et al. The effect of prolonged left ventricular support on myocardial histopathology in patients with end-stage cardiomyopathy. ASAIO Journal 1992; 31: M271-4.
41. Jacquet L et al. Evolution of human cardiac myocyte dimension during prolonged mechanical support. J Thorac Cardiovasc Surg 1991; 101: 256-9.

8. DYNAMIC CARDIOMYOPLASTY

Vinay Badhwar, David Francischelli, and Ray C-J. Chiu

Introduction

Dynamic cardiomyoplasty (DCMP) is in the final stages of a clinical trial to evaluate it as a surgical alternative for the management of end-stage heart failure. This procedure is conceptually based upon imparting the contractile force of the patient's own skeletal muscle to perform cardiac assistance. It is accomplished by wrapping the latissimus dorsi muscle (LDM) around the failing heart and, by means of an implantable cardiomyostimulator, stimulating the muscle to contract in synchrony with cardiac systole. DCMP has been proposed as an alternative and bridge to transplantation in selected patients. Compared with other surgical options in heart failure this approach has a number of advantages. Cardiomyoplasty obviates the donor organ dependency and immunosuppression of transplantation. This totally implantable form of biomechanical assist, also avoids the power constraints and thromboembolic risks experienced with mechanical assist devices. The LDM can be utilized with little or no loss of shoulder function, and the DCMP procedure itself costs significantly less than other surgical options for the treatment of heart failure.

This chapter will outline the historical progress and biologic basis for skeletal muscle powered assist, delve into the physiologic mechanisms of DCMP, and summarize the techniques and current clinical experience with DCMP. Future perspectives on DCMP and other forms of biomechanical cardiac assist will also be discussed.

Historical Development

The idea of using skeletal muscle to augment cardiac function was introduced in the 1930s, when a muscle graft was used to repair traumatic ventricle defects.[1,2] Some early clinicians attempted to use the vascularity of a muscle graft as a source of exogenous myocardial blood supply.[3-5] It was not until 1959, that the notion of utilizing stimulated skeletal muscle as a means of cardiac assistance was introduced by Kantrowitz and McKinnon.[6] They wrapped a pedicled portion of diaphragm around the distal aorta and stimulated it in diastole to achieve hemodynamic assist by means of counterpulsation.

In the 1960's, as investigators began applying muscle to treat myocardial pathology such as aneurysms, the use of stimulated skeletal muscle to perform biomechanical cardiac

Roy Masters (editor), Surgical Options for the Treatment of Heart Failure, 137-156.

assistance became plausible.[7] During this era, important obstacles such as sub-optimal muscle stimulation and rapid fatiguability hindered its clinical development. It was not until the late 1970s and early 1980s that these limitations were overcome with the discovery of burst stimulation for optimal muscle contraction, and the concept of myo-transformation to impart fatigue resistance.[8 - 10] These steps paved the path for progressive experimental work on DCMP which culminated in 1985 with the first successful clinical cases performed by Carpentier and Chachques in Paris, followed closely by others.[11 - 14] Since then, nearly 1,000 cases of DCMP have been performed worldwide, and a Phase III multi-center randomized controlled trial is in progress in North America.

Biological Principles Governing Skeletal Muscle Assist

During early investigations with stimulated muscle to perform the functions of cardiac assist or repair, it became clear that certain biological obstacles had to be overcome. First, it was noted that skeletal muscle fatigued rapidly when it was unceasingly stimulated. Second, concerns were raised as to how changes in the geometric shape and stretch of a muscle would effect is contractile performance. Finally, it was observed that when single electrical impulses were delivered to the muscle, as from the early pacemakers, the force of contraction was insufficient to provide any meaningful hemodynamic benefit. With ongoing study into the plausibility of muscle as a form of biomechanical assistance, three key concepts emerged: the principles of transformation, conformation, and burst stimulation.

Transformation

Skeletal muscle is comprised of variable amounts of oxidative slow twitch (Type I) and glycolytic fast twitch (Type II) fibers. Early work with cross-innervation studies of muscle preparations, noted that certain fiber types could be altered through changes in neural signals.[7] In 1976, this essential concept was elaborated on by Salmons and Sreter who demonstrated that mixed Type I and II fatigue-prone skeletal muscle fibers could be morphologically altered into a totally Type I fatigue resistant muscle by repeated low frequency electrical stimulation.[15] This ability to phenotypically alter fiber composition and confer fatigue resistance to skeletal muscle is known as transformation.

Histochemical analysis of this reproducible phenomenon revealed that after chronic electrical stimulation, the fast skeletal myosin isoforms found in the non-transformed muscle were replaced by slow skeletal myosin, similar to that found in cardiac muscle.[16] Furthermore, stains for myofibrillar ATPase also demonstrated a complete phenotypic alteration from light stained mixed fibers, to all slow-twitch dark-stained fibers (Figure 1). The mechanisms behind this process seems to involve a switch to aerobic metabolic processes and genetic alterations in expressing the type of myosin protein found. Along with corroborating experimental evidence, these studies confirmed that with directed electrical stimulation, a biochemical and physiological transformation of skeletal muscle into a fatigue-resistant power source, was indeed possible.[17 - 19]

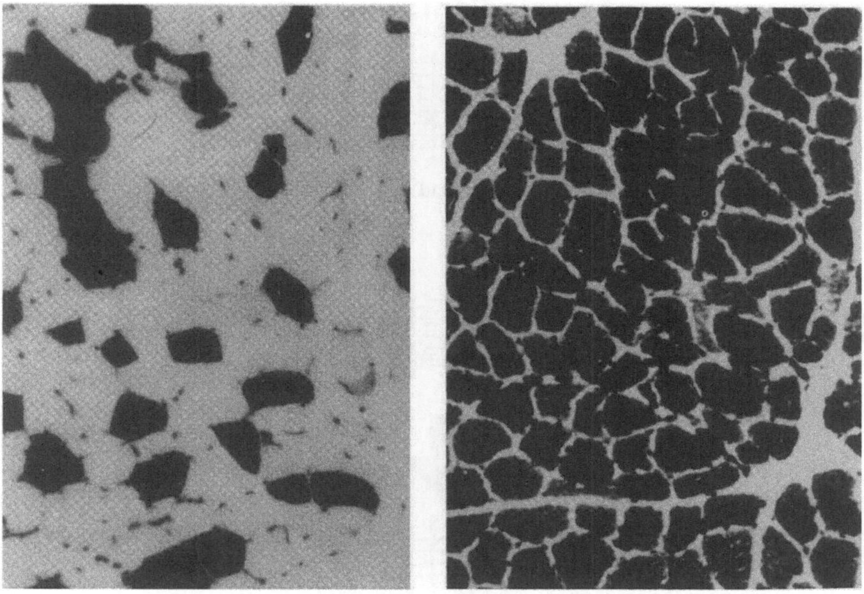

Figure 1. *Photomicrographs documenting histochemical changes of LDM during electrical transformation. Myofibrillar ATPase stains at pH of 4.6: NT, nontransformed; T, transformed after 4 weeks of low frequency electrical stimulation. Light fibers are Type II, glycolytic, fast-twitch, and fatigue prone. Dark fibers are Type I, oxidative, slow-twitch, and fatigue resistant.*

From Ianuzzo CD, et al,[16] with the permission of the publisher

Conformation

Early in the development of cardiomyoplasty and muscle assist, it was noted that skeletal muscle performance followed the principles of a Frank-Starling functional curve similar to those that govern myocardial function.[20] This posed the question as to the ideal stretch or orientation of the muscle wrap in order to optimize performance. It was observed that in cardiomyoplasty, within weeks after the latissimus dorsi was wrapped around the heart, the muscle adapted to the change in orientation by altering its geometric shape to conform to that of the epicardial surface; a phenomenon that persisted even after the native heart was removed. This ability of 'conformational change' was found to be associated also with the deletion or addition of sarcomeres in an attempt to restore optimal resting tension.[21-23] This permits the skeletal muscle fibers to alter their length in order to restore resting tension, thus preserving the molecular interaction of the actin and myosin chains within the sarcomere itself (Figure 2). By studying the effect of preload on muscle wrap function, Gealow et al found that through this process of conformation, muscle could adapt over time to generate an optimum pressure at a fixed preload.[24] This illustrated that muscle has the unique ability to conform functionally as well as morphologically.

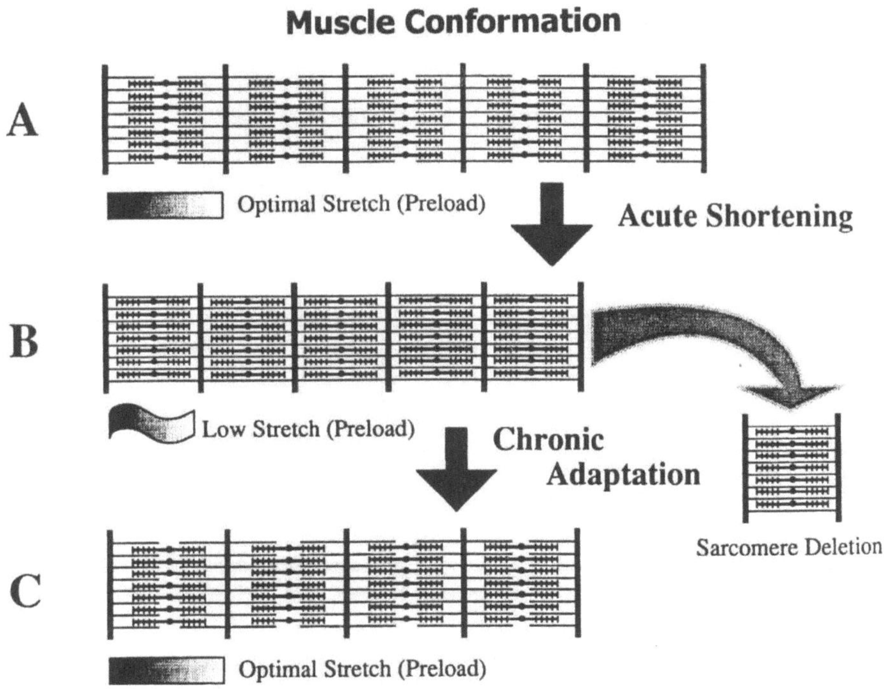

Figure 2. *Muscle conformation. Schematic representing ability of muscle to conform by altered sarcomere expression. When muscle is brought from its optimal stretch (A), to a state of altered preload (B), deletion of sarcomere units occur in order to restore the optimal resting tension (C).*

From Li CM, et al,[55] with permission of the publisher.

Burst Stimulation

Skeletal muscle and cardiac muscle differ in their response to electrical stimuli. In response to a single electrical impulse, the myocardium functions as a unique all-or-none contractile syncytium due to its specialized conduction system and the presence of intercalated disks. In comparison, the contractile response of skeletal muscle is a reflection of individual motor units. Therefore, a single electrical impulse stimulates only a few motor units at a time and results merely in a muscle twitch.[25] In 1980, it was shown that by adding a burst of stimuli in the form of a pulse train, it became possible to markedly increase the recruitment of motor units and induce a summation of twitches into a graded full contractile response.[9] Based on these experimental studies, a burst frequency of 30 Hz appeared to achieve the maximum recruitment of skeletal muscle units.[26, 27] This resulted in the construction of the first burst or pulse train myostim-ulator synchronizable to the cardiac cycle, which was the precursor to the cardiomyostimulators currently used in DCMP.

Choice of Latissimus Dorsi

Other muscles have been used for circulatory support in experimental animals, including the pectoralis major, rectus abdominus, psoas, and serratus anterior.[28 - 30] Though the principles of transformation, conformation, and burst stimulation can be universally applied to any skeletal muscle system, the latissimus dorsi has emerged as the muscle of choice over others due to some important advantages.[31, 32] Its large surface area originates from the thoracolumbar fascia and inserts by means of a tendinous extension onto the proximal humerus. It is supplied primarily by a single thoracodorsal neurovascular pedicle which makes manipulation of the muscle relatively forgiving in terms of viability and functionality. Furthermore, being in close proximity to the heart, the LDM is indulgent to transthoracic mobilization without compromising arm or shoulder function.

Mechanisms of Cardiomyoplasty

The initial vision for the mechanism of DCMP was simply that of direct cardiac massage. Conceptually, the bimanual open compression of the heart would be replaced with a synchronized skeletal muscle to perform this direct systolic squeeze to eject blood out of the ventricles. If this was the only mechanism behind the functional benefit of DCMP, then hemodynamic parameters such as ejection fraction (EF) and cardiac output (CO) would correlate directly with outcome. However, based on clinical and experimental evidence, this has not been the case. Though some investigators have shown a beat to beat improvement in hemodynamic assistance upwards of 20 to 40%, clinical experience with DCMP has found that measurable quantitative hemodynamic improvements have been inconsistent or modest at best.[33, 34] In spite of this, it is reported with virtual unanimity that patients experience significant improvements in their functional status and symptoms of heart failure.[35 - 37] In an attempt to explain this paradox, investigators have evaluated different fiber orientations of the muscle wrap and examined different measurable parameters such as aortic flow velocity, dP/dt, and segmental wall motion, in order to show a hemodynamic benefit of LDM contraction during systole.[38, 39] After cardiomyoplasty, though many report significant systolic augmentation over pre-operative baseline, stimulator on/off studies have failed to reveal a consistent hemodynamic difference. This disparity between the irrefutable body of clinical evidence supporting a quality of life benefit, and observations of only marginal improvements in hemodynamic parameters with stimulation of the cardiomyoplasty wrap, has led to the exploration of other mechanisms to explain the effects of cardiomyoplasty in heart failure.

Using a pressure-volume loop to study the effects of DCMP, it was revealed that in addition to a systolic benefit, cardiomyoplasty actually decreased myocardial wall stress during systole.[40] This myocardial sparing effect was confirmed when direct measurements of transmural pressure gradients were performed in DCMP.[41] During compression by the muscle wrap, a significant decrease in the mean ventricular wall stress was detected. It was observed that this effect could allow for augmentation of ventricular function without compromising myocardial oxygen consumption or coronary blood flow.[42] Since we know that in response to injury, the myocardium undergoes progressive dilatation as an adaptive response to altered wall stresses, the effect of a muscle wrap could conceptually protect myocytes from overt functional stress and thereby prevent the myocardial dilatation.[43] This so called 'girdling' effect of cardiomyoplasty to provide a passive constraint to progressive ventricular dilatation, has been recently observed experimentally as well as clinically.[44 - 46] Furthermore, studies comparing adynamic and dynamic muscle wraps to controls, reveal a significant benefit even when the wrap is left unstimulated.[47, 48]

The important role of ventricular remodeling in heart failure is increasingly being recognized. This has led to new treatment options attempting to reverse this histopathologic process.[49 - 52] Medically, one approach has been to attack the renin-angiotensin system to induce afterload reduction. As described in his book, newer surgical options also enjoy experimental and clinical success by addressing the remodeling process. This is accomplished either by unloading the ventricle to permit histologic myocardial recovery as with mechanical assist devices, or by directly changing ventricular architecture as with aneurysm repair, valve surgery, and partial ventriculectomy.[53, 54] Recently, through emerging evidence on passive ventricular constraint in cardiomyoplasty, and with a better understanding of the pathophysiology of heart failure, the concepts of the 'girdling' and 'myocardial sparing' have provided a potential explanation on how the reversal of the remodeling process is accomplished in DCMP (Figure 3).[46]

Surgical Technique

Preoperative Evaluation

Once the patient has been medically evaluated for DCMP, proper physical and mental preparation of the patient is essential. After a thorough medical discussion with the patient and his family, a complete preoperative assessment may require evaluation by an anesthesiologist, physiotherapist, social worker, or psychologist as indicated. The patient should also be properly examined to ensure that the latissimus dorsi is intact and is of appropriate size. The patient's preoperative nutritional state should be optimized where possible since operating on deconditioned patients with severe cardiac cachexia not only may affect operative morbidity, but may result in a gross mismatch of LDM to the failing

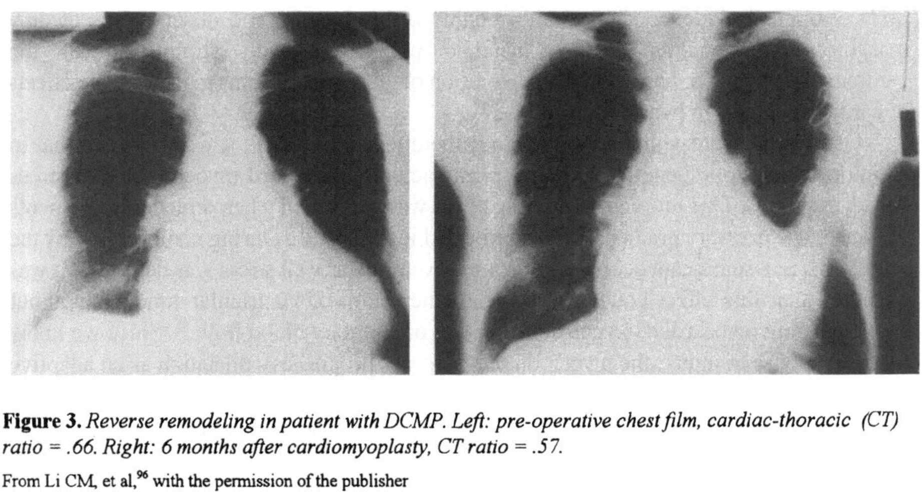

Figure 3. *Reverse remodeling in patient with DCMP. Left: pre-operative chest film, cardiac-thoracic (CT) ratio = .66. Right: 6 months after cardiomyoplasty, CT ratio = .57.*

From Li CM, et al,[96] with the permission of the publisher

heart.[56] For these patients, use of exercise programs and anabolic steroids to strengthen the LDM has been proposed.[57]

For optimal results with DCMP, current investigational indications include patients with New York Heart Association (NYHA) class III symptoms, left ventricular ejection fraction (LVEF) of >20%, and maximal oxygen consumption (VO2) of >15ml/kg/min.[58] Caution should be exercised when considering patients with previous cardiac or thoracic procedures as extensive adhesions may increase the technical difficulty and risk to these fragile patients. Although absolute contraindications are still being disecussed, patients in terminal NYHA class IV failure have a higher operative mortality and should be avoided. Furthermore, even though some patients with ejection fractions as low as 10% have survived and shown benefit, clinical experience has revealed a higher risk in patients with high pulmonary vascular resistance, VO2<10ml/kg, and low LVEF.[34]

Operative Approach

As with other surgical approaches to heart failure, the safe and effective performance of DCMP requires a dedicated team of medical professionals accustomed to the delicate needs of heart failure patients. This team should include nurses, physiotherapists, cardiologists, anesthesiologists, intensivists, and surgeons. Though DCMP can be performed safety and with minimal morbidity off pump, a primed circuit and perfusionist should also be on stand-by should cardiopulmonary bypass be urgently required. The procedure described below is one which is most commonly employed, a technique originally described by Carpentier, with a few possible modifications.

The key steps to the operation are: LDM mobilization and trans-thoracic delivery, muscular and myocardial lead placement, the peri-ventricular muscle wrap, and cardiomyostimulator insertion (Figure 4).

Anesthesia is administered using a double lumen endotracheal tube, without muscle relaxants so as to allow for LDM testing during the procedure.[59] The patient is first positioned in the right lateral decubitus position, and after identification of the appropriate landmarks, the left LDM is approached through an incision starting superiorly from the posterior axillary line along its antero-lateral anatomic border. The LDM is then atraumatically dissected from the chest wall with preservation of its thoracodorsal neurovascular pedicle. The assistance of a plastic surgeon experienced in latissimus dorsi harvesting could be a useful resource during flap preparation.[60] The LDM is then detached from its ligamentous humeral insertion, two intramuscular leads are weaved across its proximal margin, and optimal contraction thresholds are ascertained. A mini thoracotomy incision is performed in the second interspace and a 6cm portion of the third rib is resected. Through this window, the LDM is then placed into the thoracic cavity while care is taken to preserve the orientation and avoid tension of the intact neurovascular pedicle. The ligamentous insertion of the LDM is then affixed to the periosteum of the second or third rib with a non-absorbable heavy suture. The skin is closed after the placement of subcutaneous drains.

The patient is then repositioned and a median sternotomy is performed. The left pleura is opened and the LDM is retrieved while preserving proper orientation of the neurovascular pedicle. It is recommended that the pericardium be entered just medial to

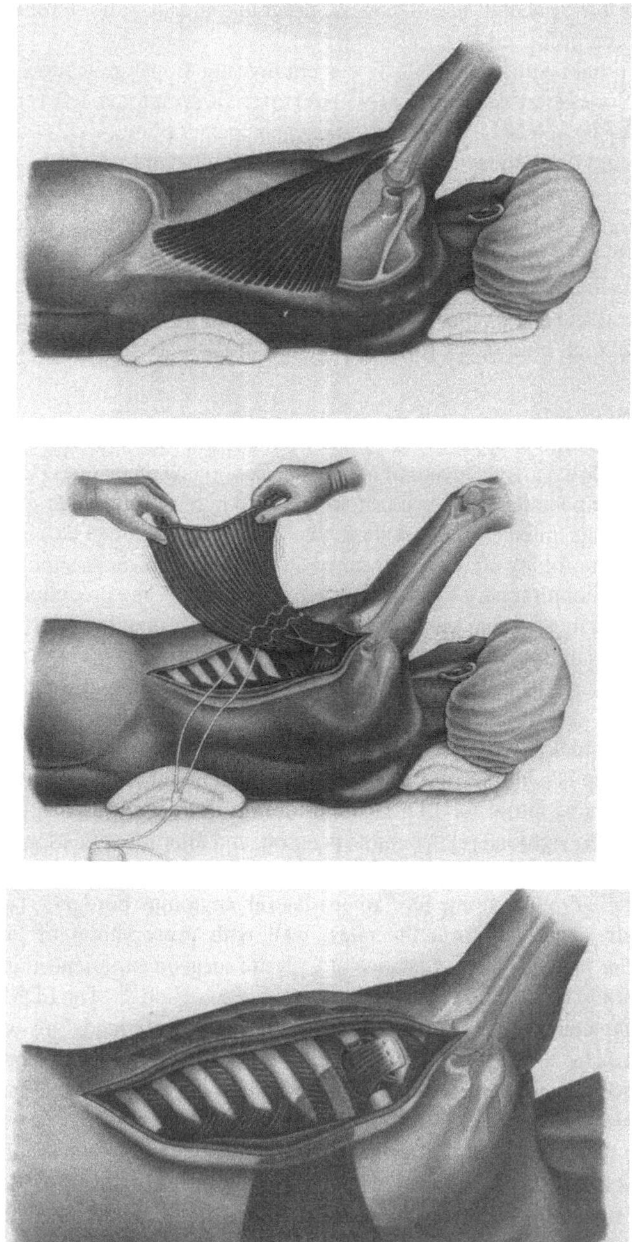

Figure 4. *Surgical techniques for left latissimus DCMP*. **A.** The patient is positioned in the left thoracotomy position, and the LDM is detached while preserving the thoracodorsal neurovascular bundle. **B.** Intramuscular electrodes are placed proximally on the LDM. **C.** The muscle is delivered into the left chest by means of a thoracic window, and the ligamentous insertion is secured to the rib periosteum.

From Chiu RCJ,[97] with the permission of the publisher

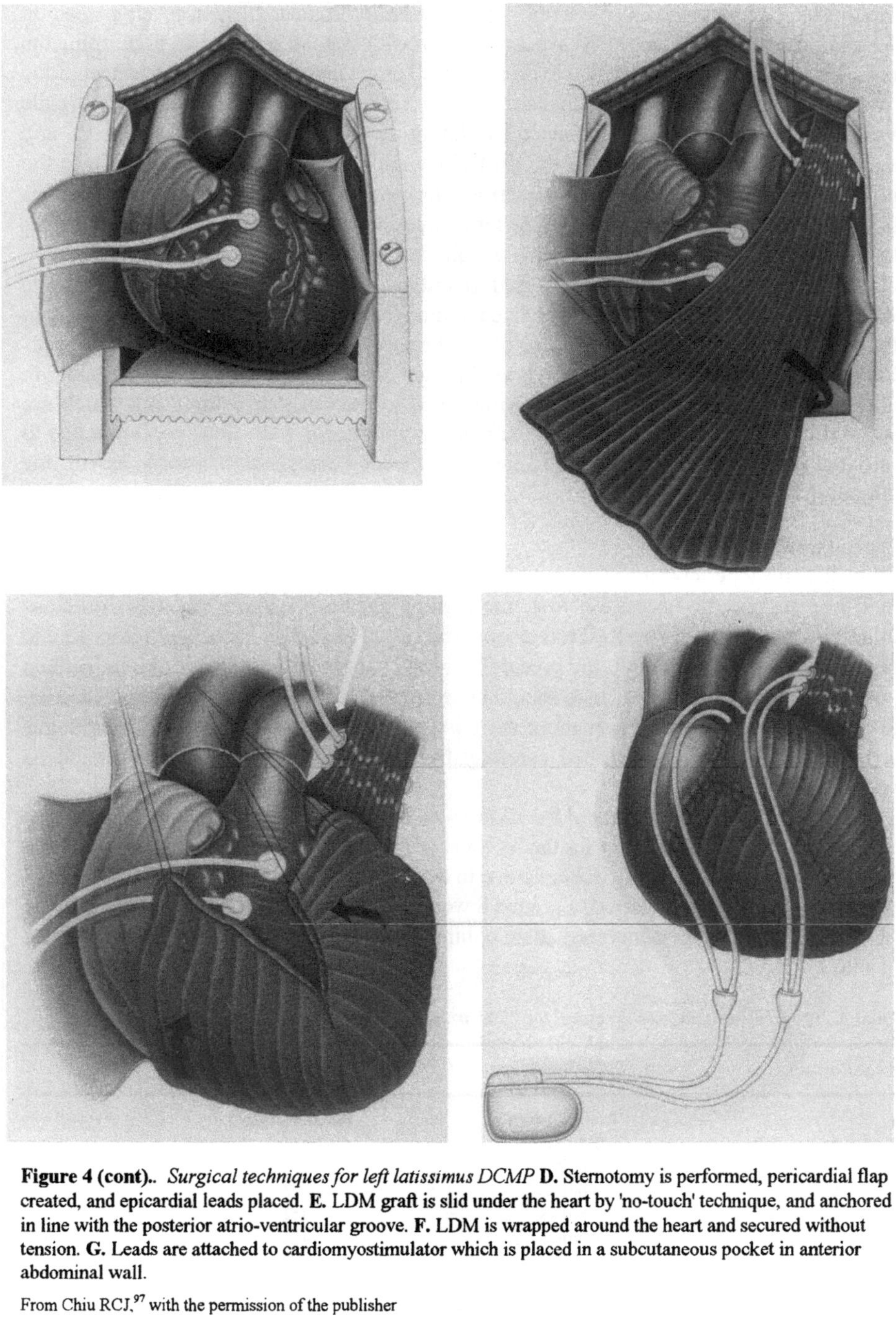

Figure 4 (cont).. *Surgical techniques for left latissimus DCMP* **D.** Sternotomy is performed, pericardial flap created, and epicardial leads placed. **E.** LDM graft is slid under the heart by 'no-touch' technique, and anchored in line with the posterior atrio-ventricular groove. **F.** LDM is wrapped around the heart and secured without tension. **G.** Leads are attached to cardiomyostimulator which is placed in a subcutaneous pocket in anterior abdominal wall.

From Chiu RCJ,[97] with the permission of the publisher

the left phrenic nerve in order to facilitate the harvest of a pericardial flap should one be required to complete the muscle wrap. Two epicardial leads are then securely placed on the right ventricle to ensure LDM synchronization with systolic sensing. In performing the muscle wrap, it is a good practice to do so by utilizing a myocardial 'no-touch' technique in order to minimize arrhythmias that are often associated with manipulation of these fragile ventricles. This can be accomplished by sliding the muscle posterior to the heart, and anchoring it with two sutures to the posterior pericardium; one just to the left of the pulmonic valve, and the other at the inferior vena cava-right atrial junction.[61] The LDM is then folded around the heart from posterior to anterior, and the edges are sutures together to form the completed cardiomyoplasty. As alluded to earlier, should the edges not readily oppose, a pericardial patch could be used to bridge the defect. It should be noted that the wrap does not need to be overly tight since optimal resting tension will be restored within four to six weeks due to the process of conformational change, discussed previously. Finally, the epicardial and muscle leads are brought out below the xiphoid and the sternum is re-approximated. The leads are then attached to the cardiomyostimulator which are secured in a subcutaneous pocket in the anterior abdominal wall. It is good practice to interrogate the cardiomyostimulator to ensure unimpeded transmission, prior to leaving the operating theatre.

Post-Operative Care

Immediate postoperative management is best administered in an intensive care unit. Should inotropic support be necessary, first line therapy should consist of phosphodiesterase inhibitors and forms of afterload reduction. The use of high dose vasoconstrictors should be avoided if possible, due to the precarious blood supply of the LDM in the immediate postoperative period.[60] Vigilance should be exercised during intravenous administration to avoid fluid overload. Throughout the postoperative recovery, atrial and ventricular arrhythmias should be controlled carefully by medical or electrical cardioversion as necessary.

The LDM is left unstimulated for 10 to 14 days while the patient recuperates from the operation.[62-64] This is to allow for the recovery of the distal portion of the muscle graft that has been rendered transiently ischemic due to division of collaterals during the dissection. After this vascular delay period, a graded 8 week protocol of stimulation is applied to the LDM to induce transformation and attain optimal burst capacity for maximal cardiac assist (Table 1).

Table 1. *Progressive stimulation protocol for LDM transformation after cardiomyoplasty*

Week Post-op	*Pulse Number*	*Stimulation Ratio*
1 + 2	No stimulation	No Stimulation
3 + 4	1 pulse	1:2
5 + 6	2 pulses	1:2
7 + 8	3 pulses	1:2
9	4 pulses	1:2
10	5 pulses	1:2
11	6 pulses	1:2
12 +	Pulse Train	1:2

Cardiomyostimulator Programming

Cardiomyostimulators function by sensing the electrocardiographic R wave, and after a programmed delay, a burst or pulse train is delivered to the skeletal muscle. A guideline for optimal stimulation parameters may include a pulse train amplitude of 3-6 V, frequency of 30Hz, and duration of 125ms. In current cardiomyostimulators, both burst parameters and synchronization delay can be programmed as a percentage of the RR interval in order to allow the stimulator to automatically adapt to changing heart rates. Stimulation voltage requirements can be estimated by axillary palpation of the extrathoracic portion of the muscle graft, or by visualization using ultrasonography or.fluoroscopy. As there are subtle variations in the hemodynamic needs between patients, the synchronization delay is best optimized using echocardiography.[65] This permits the timing of contraction and relaxation so as not to interfere with diastolic filling. A muscle wrap that contracts prematurely may inadvertently augment a previously asymptomatic element of mitral regurgitation common to patients with dilated cardiomyopathy. Therefore, echocardiography is used to fine-tune the synchronization delay so that the LDM contraction is timed with mitral valve closure. Doppler measurements of aortic root velocity may be used to further optimize hemodynamic performance by adjusting the delay period to maximize aortic flow.

Although a muscle stimulation to heart rate ratio of 1:1 was formerly used, current recommendations are to set the assist ratio at 1:2.[58] This has come about for a few main reasons. If the muscle does not have sufficient time to relax, such as with increasing heart rates at a 1:1 setting, a degree of diastolic impairment may result. Chronic stimulation studies have revealed that the LDM can be damaged as a result of overstimulation which can result in decreased efficiency to perform cardiac assist.[66-68] At higher contraction rates there is decreased time for muscle perfusion which may contribute to progressive muscle fatigue and ischemia. Chronic studies have revealed that overstimulation of LDM grafts can lead to ischemia, fatty degeneration, fibrosis, and eventually atrophy.[69-71] By optimizing stimulation to a 1:2 ratio, LDM function can be preserved without significant change in hemodynamic assist. Recent investigation is taking this a step further, indicating that perhaps we do not even have to continuously stimulate the muscle 24 hours a day.[72] It has been suggested that intermittent stimulation limited to waking hours could provide the systolic assist when most needed, while preserving the function of the graft when it is not. Further investigation is required to determine if the application of intermittent stimulation would provide superior cardiac assistance due to the overall health of the muscle graft.

Lessons Learned from Cardiomyoplasty Clinical Trials

For over a decade, Medtronic Inc. has coordinated a multi-center trial approved by the U.S. Food and Drug Administration (FDA) to evaluate the cardiomyostimulators and leads used in DCMP. It is interesting to note that due to the FDA's rigorous process of device evaluation, cardiomyoplasty has become, by serendipity, one of the few innovative surgical procedures to actually undergo the scrutiny of a randomized controlled trial.[73] Stemming from an experimental entity to the encouraging success of index cases, most new surgical procedures are catapulted into clinical practice after only a brief process which usually amounts to trial and error. Cardiomyoplasty, however, has reaped the rewards of completing a Phase I and II clinical trial through a maturation of technique and a renewed understanding into its physiological mechanisms. It is currently amid the final randomized multi-center Phase III component of the FDA trial.

Phase I of the cardiomyoplasty trial was carried out to explore procedure feasibility, case selection criteria, patient outcome, and safety of the cardiomyostimulator. In an attempt to address these questions, 118 patients from 14 centers, with varying degrees of heart failure severity, were assessed from July 1985 to April 1991. Over 80% of patients surviving past 3 months attested to a symptomatic and quality of life benefit after DCMP, as manifested by a mean improvement of 1.6 NYHA functional classes.[74] Improvement in hemodynamic parameters were not as evident, however. Major lessons learned from this trial were that moribund patients and those with NYHA functional class IV status had a poorer outcome and higher mortality as compared to NYHA class III patients. Similar findings were seen in patients with LVEF values of <20% and VO2 <10ml/kg/min.[75] Operative mortality was 38% for class IV and 12% for class III patients. Twelve month survival was 12% for class IV and 78% for class III. The information gained from this trial guided future patient selection and prompted further study into the mechanisms and optimization of stimulation protocols for DCMP.

The Phase II trial was set out to determine the efficacy and safety of the procedure and included 68 patients from May 1991 to September 1993, who had DCMP performed in 8 centers; 5 in the United States, 2 in Canada, and 1 in Brazil. Data from the Phase I trial guided patient selection to NYHA class III patients refractory to medical management. This non-randomized cohort were compared to medically treated case matched controls, and was comprised of 31% ischemic and 69% idiopathic dilated cardiomyopathy patients. The perioperative mortality in this trial was reduced to 12%, with an average LVEF increase of 15%. Over 85% of surviving patients had an improvement in their quality of life and functional status (Figure 5). When compared to controls, the overall ICU stay in the treatment group was also found to be significantly less. The notable findings of functional improvement and decreased ICU stay implied an overall cost savings to society. This prompted a Phase III randomized controlled trial, approved by the FDA, to further evaluate this inference.

The Cardiomyoplasty-Skeletal Muscle Assist Randomized Trial (C-SMART) is a multi-center Phase III study that was established to ascertain if DCMP has a benefit over conventional medical therapy for heart failure. As of this writing, 101 patients have been randomized; 54 in the cardiomyoplasty arm, and 47 in the medical treatment arm. To date there has been only 1 operative mortality (<2.5%), which incidentally occurred in a patient that crossed over from the medical arm one year after randomization, as permitted by the FDA trial guidelines. In previous years, explanations for the operative mortality included the technical learning curve of performing DCMP. However, it should be noted that 3/4 of the procedures done as part of the C-SMART trial have been in centers that have had no prior clinical experience with DCMP. This improvement in operative mortality is thought to be due to refined patient selection, avoidance of associated cardiac procedures during DCMP, and standardized follow up (Figure 6). Current results reveal an improvement in functional status and symptoms after DCMP that parallel the results

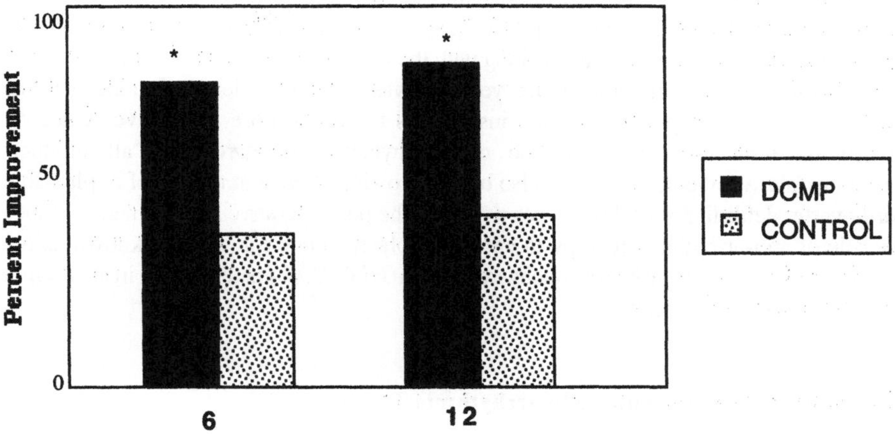

Figure 5. *Improved NYHA functional class from cardiomyoplasty. Data from Phase II FDA study revealing symptomatic improvement in NYHA class in DCMP vs. controls at 6 and 12 months (6 months: 79% vs. 49%; 12 months: 84% vs. 52% for DCMP vs. medically treated controls respectively, p<0.01)*

From Furnary AP et al,[58] with the permission of the publisher

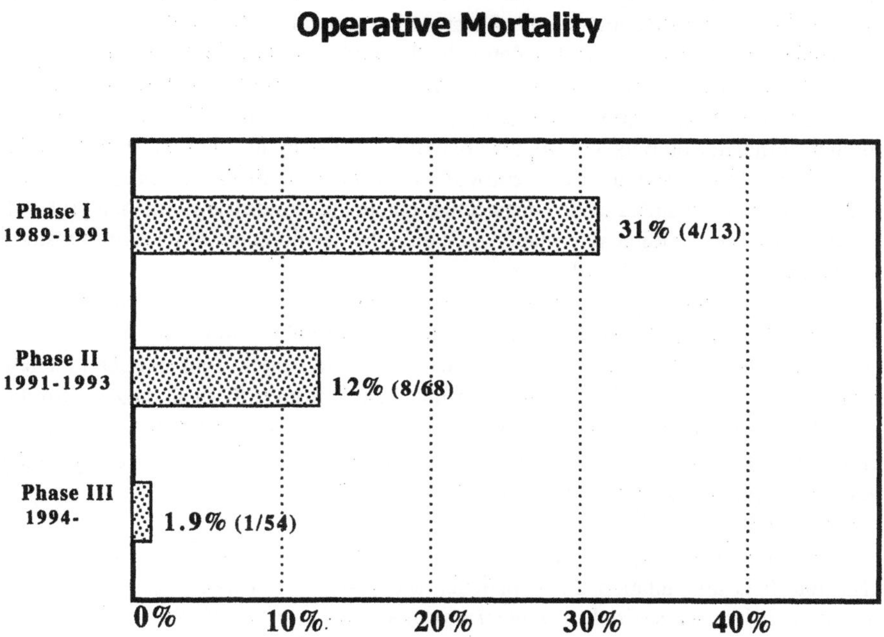

Figure 6. *Reduced operative mortality in cardiomyoplasty. Compiled data from FDA clinical trials revealing reduction of 30 day operative mortality.*

Courtesy of Medtronic, Inc.

seen in the earlier trials.[76] To date, after an average follow up of 12 to 14 months, the total deaths in the medical treatment group is 26% as compared to 17% in the cardiomyoplasty group. When these were scrutinized along with the total deaths since 1985, only a minority were found to occur from pump failure, yet there was a high prevalence of sudden cardiac death.[75, 76] This has prompted some institutions to take a more aggressive stance on arrhythmia prevention with the use of prophylactic amiodarone in all of their cardiomyoplasty patients. There has also been a growing interest in the use of implantable cardioverter defibrillator (ICD) devices as part of the post-operative management.[77] Since the role of anti-arrhythmic therapy in cardiomyoplasty is unclear, a study known as the Combined Cardiomyoplasty-Anti-tachyarrhythmia Trial (CAT) is underway in an attempt to better address this question.

Cardiomyoplasty and Anti-tachyarrhythmia Therapy

The relationship between heart failure and arrhythmias has been widely described, although not fully understood.[78 - 80] Indeed in most heart failure studies, 40 to 50% of total mortality is contributed to sudden cardiac death.[81, 82] The use of ICD in patients with heart failure has been advocated as a method of mitigating this problem.[83] Although most cardiomyoplasty patients experience functional improvements, there remains a notable arrhythmic mortality.[84, 85] By implanting an ICD into DCMP patients, it was hypothesized that both the mechanical and electrical components of heart failure could be addressed.[86]

Initial concerns that muscle stimulation by the cardiomyostimulator would be sensed by the ICD resulting in faulty arrhythmia detection, were addressed by animal studies.[87] It was found that under normal conditions, not only does the ICD not sense the cardiomyostimulator outputs, but the cardiomyoplasty system does not interfere with the ability of the ICD to detect and treat ventricular aberrance. Defibrillation thresholds were found to be acceptable and remained distinct throughout the muscle transformation protocol. This paved the way for clinical implants, including the development of a feasibility study currently underway in the United States.[77]

Patients who are eligible for this combined therapy are admitted from one of 3 categories: a) an ICD patient who developed heart failure and would benefit from DCMP; b) a DCMP patient who developed arrhythmias and would benefit from an ICD; c) a new patient who has received neither therapy but would benefit from both. In all patients, careful testing at implant and during follow up visits are performed to ensure that each device operates without interfering with the other. This testing follows guidelines set for implanting dual chamber pacemakers in conjunction with an ICD or a cardiomyostimulator.[88 - 90]

As of this writing, approximately 30 patients worldwide have received a combined DCMP and ICD implantation. In all patients, acceptable defibrillation thresholds were obtained, most by means of only a single transvenous lead inserted into the right ventricle. To date, no patients have had a postoperative complication due to device interaction. Approximately one third of these patients received at least one anti-tachyarrhythmia treatment by the ICD that terminated a potentially fatal arrhythmia.[91]

Though its efficacy in heart failure has yet to be determined, it has been suggested that an ICD has a survival benefit over antiarrhythmic drugs in patients who have had a prior episode of ventricular fibrillation or sustained ventricular tachycardia.[92] Preliminary results from combined cardiomyoplasty / ICD patients have revealed that this combination is technically feasible, the addition of an ICD can prevent potentially fatal arrhythmias, and that perhaps the population that may benefit from DCMP could be expanded to include NYHA class III patients with an indication for ICD insertion.

Future Perspective

Throughout the historical development of DCMP, critical information was gained on the plasticity of skeletal muscle to effectively perform the work of circulatory assist. Through growing understanding of governing biological principles, we now realize that if efficiently harnessed, skeletal muscle has the potential to serve as a significant biomechanical power source. This power source could theoretically be utilized for a variety of mechanical human applications.

Mechanical ventricular assist device development is entering a new era of miniaturization and efficiency in order to cope with the growing needs of the population. A major technological obstacle to a mandate of total implantability, is finding an appropriate long-term internal power source. Recently, skeletal muscle has been proposed as such a power source.[93] Investigators are evaluating the biomechanical characteristics of muscle in order to integrate this implantable energy source with the present technology of mechanical ventricular support systems.[94] Preliminary data on the power output of different configurations, reveals that if harnessed efficiently, skeletal muscle may actually be able to power some of the electrical ventricular assist systems used today.[95] Perhaps in the future, the hybridization of muscle and machine will lead to a totally implantable ventricular assist system for prolonged use.

As for cardiomyoplasty, it appears that its maturation as a clinical entity has been an education in the clinical trial process itself. The valuable information gained from its critical appraisal has refined patient selection, surgical technique and indications, and has created an evidence based niche for its application to the management of heart failure. However, unlike most new surgical procedures, since cardiomyoplasty has been subjected to the rigorous environment of the randomized controlled trial, its widespread clinical application has become dictated by the stringent procedures that govern the distribution of the cardiomyostimulator device. There is no doubt that an evidence based critical evaluation of any new treatment will result in patient benefit. However, unlike a randomized control trial for a new medication, there is no ethically sound "placebo" operation when this process is applied to the evaluation of a surgical procedure. This illustrates the unique adversity that C-SMART is facing. Recruitment appears to be impeded by slow physician referral who sport the "too well", "too sick" phenomenon.[73] Another problem faced is one of patient crossover and the refusal of randomization. After all, once the patient has been mentally prepared for the procedure and then is randomized to medical treatment, it becomes quite distressing; especially if their symptoms deteriorate as the evidence suggests. Though there may not be any deficiency in the procedure itself, these points bring up the unique difficulties that need to be addressed in studies, such as C-SMART, that contrast medical to surgical treatments.

Information from the Phase I and II trials and preliminary data from C-SMART, has revealed that DCMP has proven to be of significant benefit to NYHA III patients refractory to medical therapy. If the current randomized study can be completed in spite of the recruitment difficulties, cardiomyoplasty could be poised to take its place with other innovative procedures in the armamentarium of the heart failure surgeon.

Acknowledgements

This work was supported by an operating grant from the Medical Research Council of Canada.

References

1. DeJesus FR. Breves consideraciones sobre un caso do herida penetrante del coranda. Bol Assoc Med PR 1931;23:380
2. .Leriche R, Fontaine R. Essai experimental de traitement de certains infarctus de myocarde et de l'aneurisme de coeur par un graffe de muscle strie. Bull Soc Natl Chir 1933;59:229.
3. Beck CS. The development of a new blood supply to the myocardium by operation. Ann Surg 1935;102:801.
4. Griffith GC, Bates W. A ventricular perforation in transplanting a new blood supply. New Int Clin 1938;2:17.
5. Weinstein M, Shafiroff BG. Grafts of free muscle transplants upon the myocardium. Science 1946;104:410.
6. Kantrowitz A, McKinnon WMP. The experimental use of the diaphragm as an auxiliary myocardium. Surg Forum 1959;9:266.
7. Buller AJ, Eccles JC, Eccles RM. Interactions between motoneurons and muscles in respect of the characteristic speeds of their responses. J Physiol 1960;150:417.
8. Von Recum A, Stule JP, Hamada O, et al. Long-term stimulation of a diaphragm muscle pouch. J Surg Res 1977;23:422.
9. Drinkwater DC, Chiu RCJ, Modry D, et al. Cardiac assist and myocardial repair with synchronously stimulated skeletal muscle. Surg Forum 1980;31:271.
10. Macoviak JA, Stephenson LW, Armenti F, et al. Electrical conditioning of in situ skeletal muscle for replacement of myocardium. J Surg Res 1982;32:429.
11. Chachques JC, Carpentier A, Chauvaud S. Development of a non-tiring stimulation of the latissimus dorsi flap to replace myocardium. Artif Organs 1984;8:379.
12. Chachques JC, Mitz V, Hero M. Experimental cardioplasty using the latissimus dorsi muscle flap. J Cardiovasc Surg 1985;26:457.
13. Carpentier A, Chachques JC. Myocardial substitution with a stimulated skeletal muscle: first successful clinical case. Lancet 1985;8440:1267.
14. Magovern GJ, Park SB, Magovern GJ Jr, et al. Latissimus dorsi as a functioning synchronously paced muscle component in the repair of a left ventricular aneurysm. Ann Thorac Surg 1986;41:116.
15. Salmons S, Sreter FA. Significance of impulse activity in the transformation of skeletal muscle type. Nature 1976;263:30.
16. Ianuzzo CD, Hamilton N, O'Brien PJ, et al. Biochemical transformation of canine skeletal muscle for use in cardiac-assist devices. J Appl Physiol 1990;68:1481.
17. Armenti F, Bitto T, Macoviak JA, et al. Transformation of canine diaphragm to fatigue-resistant muscle by phrenic nerve stimulation. Surg Forum 1984;35:259.
18. Frey M, Thom H, Gruber H, et al. The chronically stimulated psoas muscle as an energy source for artificial organs. Eur J Surg Res 1984;16:232.
19. Koller R, Girsch W, Huber L, et al. Experimental in situ conditioning of the atissimus dorsi muscle for circulatory assist by multichannel stimulation. Artif Organs 1994;18:523.
20. Kochamba G, Chiu RCJ. The physiologic characteristics of transformed skeletal muscle for cardiac assist. Trans Am Soc Artif Organs 1987;33:404.
21. Hill AB, Li C, Tchervenkov C, et al. Dynamic cardiomyoplasty for hemodynamic support during acute pulmonary hypertension. J Thorac Cardiovasc Surg 1992;103:1200.
22. Tardieu C, Tabary JC, Tardieu G, et al. Adaptation of sarcomere numbers to the length imposed on the muscle. Adv Physiol Sci 1981;24:99.
23. Herring SW, Grimm AF, Grimm BR,. Regulation of sarcomere number in skeletal muscle: a comparison of hypothesis. Muscle and Nerve 1984;7:161.
24. Gealow KK, Solien EE, Bianco RW, et al. Conformational adaptation of muscle: implications in cardiomyoplasty and skeletal muscle ventricles. Ann Thorac Surg 1993;56:520-6.
25. Carlson FD, Wilkie DR. Mechanical Aspects of Muscular Contraction. Muscle Physiology. Englewood Cliffs, NJ: Prentice-Hall Inc, 1974:25-51.
26. Chiu RCJ, Walsh GL, Dewar ML, et al. Implantable extra-aortic balloon assist powered by transformed fatigue-resistant skeletal muscle. J Thorac Cardiovasc Surg 1987;94:694.
27. Li C, Hill AB, Desrosiers C, et al. A new implantable pulse burst generator for skeletal muscle powered aortic counterpulsation. Trans Am Soc Artif Intern Organs 1989;35:620-5.
28. Frey M, Thom H, Gruber H, et al. The chronically stimulated psoas muscle as an energy source for artificial organs: an experimental study in sheep. In: Chiu RCJ, ed. Biomechanical Cardiac Assist: Cardiomyoplasty and Muscle-Powered Devices. Mount Kisco, NY: Futura Publishing Co. Inc., 1986.

29. Arnold PG, Piaroloero RC, Waldorf JC. The serratus anterior muscle: intrathoracic and extrathoracic utilization. Plastic Reconstr Surg 1983;73:240.
30. Wijnberg DS, Hensen ABG, Grandjean PA, et al. The rectus abdominis cardiomyoplastic procedure: preliminary results. Artif Organs 1994;18:529.
31. Perier P, Acar C, Chachques JC. Anatomy of the Latissimus Dorsi Muscle: I. Description. In: Carpentier A, Chachques JC, Grandjean PA, eds. Cardiomyoplasty. Mount Kisco, NY: Futura Publishing Co. Inc., 1991:63-8.
32. Radermecker MA, Triffaux M, Fourny J, et al. Anatomical rationale for use of atissimus dorsi flap during the cardiomyoplasty operation. Surg Radiol Anat 1992;14:5.
33. Hagege A, Desnos M, Fernandez F, et al. Clinical study of the effects of latissimus dorsi muscle flap stimulation after cardiomyoplasty. Circulation 1995;92:II210.
34. Carpentier A, Chachques JC, Acar C, et. al. Dynamic cardiomyoplasty at seven years. J Thorac Cardiovasc Surg 1993;106:42.
35. Orghetti-Mario SA, Romano W, Bocchi EA, et al. Quality of life after cardiomyoplasty. J Heart Lung Transplant 1994;13:271.
36. Furnary AP, Swanson JS, Grunkemeier G, et al. Lessons learned before and after cardiomyoplasty: risk sensitive patient selection and post procedure quality of life. J Card Surg 1996;11:200.
37. Tasdemir O, Kucukaksu SD, Vural KM, et al. A comparison of the early and midterm results after dynamic cardiomyoplasty in patients with ischemic or idiopathic cardiomyopathy. J Thorac Cardiovasc Surg 1997;113:73.
38. Kao RL, Christlieb IY, Magovern GJ, et al. The importance of skeletal muscle fiber orientation for dynamic cardiomyoplasty. J Thorac Cardiovasc Surg 1990;99:134.
39. Schreuder J, van der Veen F, van der Velte E, et al. Beat-to-beat analysis of left ventricular pressure-volume relation and strokevolume by conductance cathteter and aortic modelflow in cardiomyoplasty patients. Circulation 1995;91:2010.
40. Lee KF, Dignan RJ, Parmar JM, et al. Effects of dynamic cardiomyoplasty on left ventricular performance and myocardial mechanics in dilated cardiomyopathy.J Thorac Cardiovasc Surg 1991;102:24.
41. Chen F, Aklog L, deGuzman B, et al. New techniques measures decreased transmural myocardial pressure in cardiomyoplasty. Ann Thorac Surg 1995;60:1678.
42. Kawaguchi O, Goto Y, Futaki S, et al. Mechanical enhancement and myocardial oxygen saving by synchronized dynamic left ventricular compression. J Thorac Cardiovasc Surg 1992;103:573.
43. Pfeffer MA, Braunwald E. Ventricular remodeling after myocardial infarction: experimental observations and clinical implications. Circulation 1990;81:1161.
44. Capouya ER, Gerber RS, Drinkwater DC, et al. Girdling effect of nonstimulated cardiomyoplasty on left ventricular function. Ann Thorac Surg 1993;56:867.
45. Kass DA, Baughman K, Pak P, et al. Reverse remodeling from cardiomyoplasty in human heart failure external constraint versus active assist. Circulation 1995;91:2314.
46. Oh JH, Badhwar V, Chiu RCJ. Mechanisms of dynamic cardiomyoplasty: current concepts. J Cardiac Surg 1996;11:194.
47. Mott BD, Oh JH, Misawa Y, et al. Mechanisms of cardiomyoplasty: comparative effects of adynamic versus dynamic cardiomyoplasty. Ann Thorac Surg 1998;65:1039.
48. Oh JH, Badhwar V, Mott BD, et al. The effects of prosthetic cardiac binding and adynamic cardiomyoplasty in a model of dilated cardiomyopathy. J Thorac Cardiovasc Surg 1998;116:48
49. Fazio S, Sabatini D, Capaldo B, et al. A preliminary study of growth hormone in the treatment of dilated cardiomyopathy. N Engl J Med 1996;334:809.
50. McDonald KM, Rector T, Carlyle PF, et al. Angiotensin-converting enzyme inhibition and beta-adrenoreceptor blockade regress established ventricular remodeling in a canine model of discrete myocardial damage. J Am Coll Cardiol 1994;24:1762.
51. Katz AM. Cardiomyopathy overload: a major determinant of prognosis in congestive heart failure. N Engl J Med 1990;322:100.
52. Cohn JN. Structural basis for heart failure; ventricular remodeling and its pharmacological inhibition. Circulation 1995;91:2504.
53. Scheinn SA, Capek P, Radovancevic B, et al. The effects of prolonged left ventricular support on myocardial histopathology in patients with end-stage cardiomyopathy. ASAIO J 1992;38:M271.
54. McCarthy JF, McCarthy PM, Starling RC, et al. Partial left ventriculectomy and mitral valve repair for end-stage congestive heart failure. Eur J Cardiothorac Surg 1998;13:337.
55. Li CM, Chiu RCJ. The mechanisms and optimization of programming. In: Brachman J, Stephenson LW, eds. Current Clinical Practices in Dynamic Cardiomyoplasty. New York: Futura Publishing, 1997:1-55.

56. Mott BD, Misawa Y, Lough JO, et al. Clinico-pathological correlation of dynamic cardiomyoplasty. Can J Cardiol 1996;11:133E.
57. Fritzsche D, Krakor R, Asmussen G, et al. Anabolic steroids (Metenolone) improve muscle performance and hemodynamic characteristics in cardiomyoplasty. Ann Thorac Surg 1995;59:961.
58. Furnary AP, Jessup M, Moreira LFP. Multicenter trial of dynamic cardiomyoplasty for chronic heart failure. J Am Coll Cardiol 1996;28:1175.
59. Robinson RJS, Truong DT, Odim JNK, et al. Dynamic cardiomyoplasty.J Cardiothorac Vasc Anesth 1992;16:476.
60. Chiu RCJ. Cardiomyoplasty. In: Edmunds H Jr., ed. Cardiac Surgery in the Adult. New York: McGraw-Hill, 1997:1491-504.
61. Chiu RCJ, Odim JNK, Blundell PE,. Dynamic Cardiomyoplasty. In: Kapoor AS, Laks H, eds. Atlas on Heart and Lung Transplantation. New York: McGraw Hill, 1994:25-36.
62. Mannion JD, Velchik M, Hammond R, et al. Effects of collateral blood vessel ligation and electrical conditioning on blood flow in dog latissimus dorsi muscle. J Surg Res 1986;47:332.
63. Chachques JC, Carpentier A. Post-op management in cardiomyoplasty. In: Carpentier A, et al, eds. Cardiomyoplasty. Mount Kisco, NY: Futura, 1991:131-8.
64. Carroll SM, Carroll CM, Stremel RW, et al. Vascular delay of the latissimus dorsi muscle: an essential component of cardiomyoplasty. Ann Thorac Surg 1997;63:1034.
65. Helou J, Misawa Y, Stewart J, et al. Optimizing "delay period" for burst stimulation in dynamic cardiomyoplasty. Ann Thorac Surg 1995;59:74.
66. Hudlicka O. Anatomical changes in chronically stimulated skeletal muscles. Semin Thorac Cardiovasc Surg 1991;3:106.
67. El Oakley RM, Jarvis J, Barman D, et al. Factors affecting the integrity of latissimus dorsi muscle grafts: implications for cardiac assistance from skletal muscle. J Heart Lung Transplant 1995;14:359.
68. Ianuzzo CD, Ianuzzo SE, Locke M, et al. Preservation of the latissimus dorsi muscle during cardiomyoplasty. J Card Surg 1996;11:99.
69. Kalil-Filho R, Bocchi E, Weiss RG, et al. Magnetic resonance imaging evaluation of chronic changes in latissimus dorsi cardiomyoplasty. Circulation 1994;90:II102.
70. Ianuzzo CD, Ianuzzo SE, Carson N, et al. Cardiomyoplasty: degeneration of the assisting skeletal muscle. J Appl Physiol 1996;80:1205.
71. Davidse JH, van der Veen F, Lucas CM, et al. Structural alterations in the latissimus dorsi muscles in three patients more than 2 years after a cardiomyoplasty procedure. Eur Heart J 1998;19:310.
72. Kashem MA, Chiang BY, Ali A, et al. Preliminary report on continuous stimulation vs. intermittent stimulation of latissimus dorsi muscle in chronic canine model of cardiomyoplasty. Basic Appl Myol 1998;8:231.
73. Li CM, Chiu RCJ. The importance and limitations of prospective randomized studies for new, evolving surgical procedures: lessons from the dynamic cardiomyoplasty trial. Pacing Clin Electrophysiol 1996;19:2035.
74. Mott BD, Austin LL, Chiu RCJ. Dynamic cardiomyoplasty: multicenter clinical trials. In: Cooper DKC, ed. The Transplantation and Replacement of ThoracicOrgans. Boston: Kluwer Academic Publishing, 1996:767-73.
75. Furnary AP, Chachques JC, Moreira LF, et al. Long-term outcome, survival analysis, and risk stratification of dynamic cardiomyoplasty. J Thorac Cardiovasc Surg 1996;112:1640.
76. Magovern GJ, Simpson KA. Clinical cardiomyoplasty: review of the ten-year United States experience. Ann Thorac Surg 1996;61:413.
77. Chekanov VS, Deshpande S, Schmidt DH. Cardiomyoplasty combined with implantation of a cardioverter defibrillator. J Thorac Cardiovasc Surg 1997;114:489.
78. Middlekauff HR, Stevenson WG, Warner-Stevenson L, et al. Syncope in advanced heart failure: high risk of sudden death regardless of origin of syncope. J Am Coll Cardiol 1993;21:110.
79. Larsen L, Markham J, Haffajee CI. Sudden death in idiopathic dilated cardiomyopathy: role of ventricular arrythmias. Pacing Clin Electrophysiol 1993;16:1051.
80. Brachmann J, Hilbel T, Grunig E, et al. Ventricular arrhythmias in dilated cardiomyopathy. Pacing Clin Electrophysiol 1997;20:2714.
81. Packer M. Sudden unexpected death in patients with congestive heart failure: a second frontier. Circulation 1985;72:681.
82. NHLBI. Report of the task force on research in heart failure. Bethesda, MD: US Department of Health and Human Services, publication No. PB95-129045, 1994

83. Borggrefe M, Chen X, Martinez-Rubio A, et al. The role of implantable cardioverter defibrillators in dilated cardiomyopathy. Am Heart J 1994;127:1145.
84. Bocchi EA, Moriera LFP, de Moraes AV, et al. Arrhythmias and sudden death after dynamiccardiomyoplasty. Circulation 1994;90:II-107.
85. Chachques JC, Berrebi A, Hernigou A, et al. Study of muscular and ventricular function in dynamic cardiomyoplasty: a ten-year follow up. J Heart Lung Transplant 1997;16:854.
86. Thakur RK, Chow LH, Guiraudon GM, et al. Latissimus dorsi dynamic cardiomyoplasty: role of combined ICD implantation. J Card Surg 1995;10:295.
87. Francischelli D, Peterson D, Stein P, et al. Cardiomyoplasty and defibrillator: a combined treatment for heart failure. In: Carpentier A, Chachques JC, Grandjean P, eds. Cardiac Bioassist. Armonk, NY: Futura Publishing, 1997:417-28.
88. Spotnitz HM, Ott GY, Bigger JT, et al. Methods of implantable cardioverter-defibrillator-pacemaker insertion to avoid interactions. Ann Thorac Surg 1992;53:253.
89. Calkins H, Brinker J, Veltri EP, et al. Clinical interactions between pacemakers and automatic implantable cardioverter-defibrillators. J Am Coll Cardiol 1990;16:666.
90. Francischelli DE, Gealow KK, Cerkvenik J, et al. Combined cardiomyoplasty/DDD bradycardia therapies. ASAIO J 1994;24:42.
91. Schlepper M, Neuzne J, Pitschner HF. Implantable cardioverter defibrillator: effect on survival. Pacing Clin Electrophysiol 1995;18:569.
92. The Antiarrhythmics versus Implantable Defibrillators (AVID) Investigators. A comparison of antiarrhythmic-drug therapy with implantable defibrillators in patients resuscitated from near-fatal ventricular arrhythmias. N Engl J Med 1997;337:1576.
93. Farrar DJ, Reichenbach SH, Hill JD. In vivo measurements of skeletal muscle in a linear configuration powering a hydraulically actuated VAD. ASAIO J 1994;40:M309.
94. Whalen RL, Bowen MA, Lim GW, et al. A skeletal muscle powered ventricular assist device. ASAIO J 1996;25.
95. Badhwar V, Badhwar RK, Oh JH, et al. Power generation from four skeletal muscle configurations: design implications for a muscle powered cardiac assist device. ASAIO J 1997; 43:M651.
96. Li CM, Chiu RCJ: Surgical ventricular remodelling: Pathophysiological basis for cardioreduction (Batista) operation. Heart Failure Review 1997;2:71.
97. Chiu RCJ: Using skeletal muscle for cardiac assistance. Science and Medicine (Scientific American), 1994; Nov/Dec:68.

9. PARTIAL LEFT VENTRICULECTOMY

Richard J. Kaplon and Patrick M. McCarthy

Introduction

End-stage heart failure currently affects 1% of people under 55 years old, 9% of people over 80 years old, and is expected to continue to increase in prevalence.[1] Despite improvements in pharmacologic management of heart failure with newer agents such as angiotensin-converting enzyme inhibitors or beta-blockers such as carvedilol, approximately 25% of patients die while awaiting heart transplantation.[2-4] Even with attempts at expanding the donor pool through "alternate recipient lists", the limited number of hearts available for transplantation has plateaued.[5, 6] Ventricular-assist devices (VAD) have been effective as bridges to transplantation for those patients refractory to medical therapy, however, present use of VADs as destination therapy remains investigational.[7-9] Clinical attempts at cardio-myoplasty and xenotransplantation have, thus far, been generally disappointing.[10, 11]

Batista's Experience

Based on his observations regarding the inter-relationship of heart mass and radius, Dr. Randas Batista developed the procedure he termed "partial left ventriculectomy" (PLV). In order to maintain a normal relationship, an increase in ventricular cavitary radius must lead to an increase in ventricular wall mass. When radius increases without an appropriate increase in mass, dilatation leads to clinical heart failure. According to the law of Laplace, intraventricular pressure is proportional to mural tension and inversely related to chamber radius. Batista reasoned that reducing the radius by excising part of the ventricular wall would diminish mural tension, improving overall left ventricular (LV) function and decreasing myocardial oxygen consumption.

Batista first presented this work as a case report of a 34 year-old patient with New York Heart Association (NYHA) class IV heart failure who underwent PLV.[12] The patient's ejection fraction (EF) rose from 17% pre-operatively to 44% at 2 months. Batista reported performing 154 similar such procedures during the following year; however, due to the socioeconomic circumstances of his practice, meaningful follow-up of these patients was unavailable. The primary etiologies of the end-stage heart failure for which Batista operated were Chagas', ischemic and dilated cardiomyopathies (CM).

Roy Masters (editor), Surgical Options for the Treatment of Heart Failure, 157-164.

Batista brought his procedure to the United States, collaborating with Dr. Thomas Salerno.[13] At their combined institutions, they performed 120 PLV's. The profiles for those patients being operated on in Brazil were the same as previously described; the primary indication for surgery in Buffalo was dilated (viral or idiopathic) CM, with or without valvular involvement. Patients undergoing surgery in Buffalo included elderly patients or patients otherwise not transplant candidates. In the combined series from Buffalo and Brazil, patients underwent PLV alone (n=40), PLV plus valve replacement (n=51), PLV plus bypass (n=10), PLV plus autotransplantation (to reduce left atrial size to control atrial fibrillation; n=7), PLV plus others (n=12). In Brazil, most patients had an Alfieri mitral valve repair, whereas in Buffalo, most patients underwent mitral valve replacement with a tissue prosthesis.[14] Patients in this group had a mean age of 53 years; 80% were male; all were in NYHA functional class IV; all had EF's < 20%. From this experience, the 30 day mortality was 22% and 2 year mortality was approximately 45%. Ten percent of patients showed no improvement in NYHA functional class; however, 57% of survivors were in class I and 33% were in class II at follow-up. Again, complete follow-up of the Brazilian patients was not available.

The Cleveland Clinic Experience

Recognizing the potential benefit of Batista's procedure, we undertook a prospective study to critically evaluate the clinical benefits of ventricular volume reduction. Initially we chose only transplant candidates in NYHA functional class III or IV despite maximal medical therapy, with an LV end-diastolic diameter (LVEDD) greater than 7 cm on at least one recent echocardiogram. Choosing from primarily transplant candidates accomplished two goals: (a) patients not improved by the PLV could be relisted for transplantation and patients failing post-operatively could be bridged with a VAD; (b) transplant patients not undergoing PLV would serve as an appropriate control population compared to patients undergoing cardioreduction. After the excessive media reports surrounding the "Batista procedure", we received thousands of referrals for PLV; however, during the year that ensued we selected and performed 57 PLV's with mitral valve repair/replacement.[15]

Patients had a mean age of 53 years and 42 were male. Fifty-five patients were diagnosed pre-operatively with idiopathic dilated CM; one patient had valvular CM and one patient had familial CM. We chose to not include patients suffering ischemic CM or those with extensive myocardial scarring or fibrosis, believing that creating a smaller heart that remained scarred would not improve function. We perform a modification of the Dor aneurysmectomy for patients with ischemic cardiomyopathy, placing an endocardial patch to reduce ventricular volume.[16] Fifty-four patients were awaiting transplantation; the remaining three were denied transplantation because of age or co-morbidities. Thirty-five patients were in NYHA class IV failure; the 21 patients in NYHA class III failure had an average of 2 hospital admissions for heart failure prior to surgery, and had previously been class IV. One patient was supported by the Heartmate LVAD (Thermocardiosystems, Inc., Woburn, MA) for 88 days but had developed a device infection requiring explantation. In addition to maximal medical therapy, 23 (40%) patients required inotropic support pre-operatively and 3 required intra-aortic balloon counterpulsation.

Pre-operative echocardiography documented severe ventricular dysfunction (EF 14.4+/-7.7%) and marked ventricular dilatation (LVEDD 8.4+/-1.1 cm; LV end-diastolic volume (LVEDV) 254+/-85ml) in all patients. Mitral regurgitation (MR) was 2.8+ (range 0 to 4+). Even with 40% of patients on inotropic support, pre-PLV hemodynamics showed severe ventricular compromise (cardiac index (CI) 2.2+/-0.7 $l/min/m^2$) with elevated filling pressures (pulmonary artery pressures: 51+/-12 systolic, 36+/-8 mean, 27+/-8 diastolic mmHg; left atrial pressures: 24+/-8 mmHg). Peak oxygen consumption (MVO2) was 10.6+/-3.9 ml/kg/min.

Our technique for PLV gradually evolved from Batista's initial method working with the heart beating and using the Alfieri mitral repair stitch.[17] We performed the operation using cardiopulmonary bypass with antegrade and retrograde cold blood cardioplegia. While we continued to use the Alfieri mitral repair in most cases, we incorporated the use of a posterior annuloplasty ring to support mitral leaflet approximation and reduce annulus size commensurate with ventricular reduction.[18] We now routinely use a No. 26 Cosgrove-Edwards ring (Baxter-Edwards, Irvine, CA) to undersize the dilated mitral annulus.

The ventriculectomy resection comprises the lateral wall of the left ventricle in the circumflex coronary artery distribution (Figure 1). We begin our incision approximately 2 cm lateral to the left anterior descending coronary artery (LAD) and 3 cm proximal to the apex. This is extended along the anterior papillary muscle to a point approximately 2 cm from the mitral annulus. Divided marginal branches of the circumflex coronary artery are oversewn. Returning to the apex of the heart, the incision is extended to 3 cm parallel to the LAD and carried along the posterior papillary muscle to connect to the initial incision, thus creating an excised wedge of ventricle between the papillary muscles.

The goal of the ventricular excision is to restore near-normal LVEDD. This is determined by the relation of the circumference of a circle to its diameter: every 3.14 cm

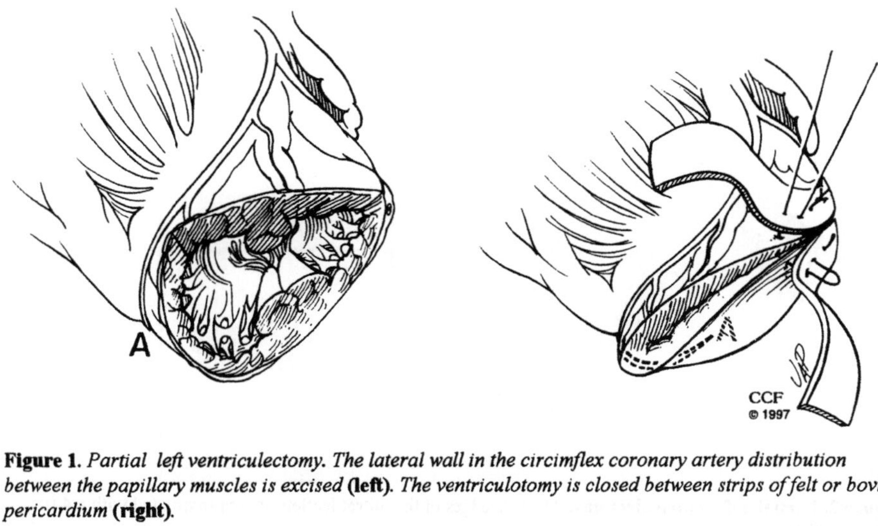

Figure 1. *Partial left ventriculectomy. The lateral wall in the circimflex coronary artery distribution between the papillary muscles is excised* **(left).** *The ventriculotomy is closed between strips of felt or bovine pericardium* **(right).**

Reproduced with permission from McCarthy PM, Starling RC, Wong et al. Early results with partial left ventriculectomy. J Thorac Cardiovasc Surg 1997;114:756

(π cm) of LV wall resected (i.e. circumference) reduces LVEDD by 1 cm. The limitation of the resection, therefore, is the papillary muscles. If intra-papillary LV wall resection was not adequate to reduce LVEDD to near-normal, papillary muscles were resected, more ventricular wall excised, and the papillary heads reimplanted. Since the anterior wall and septum do most of the work post-operatively, we preferentially resect the posterior papillary muscle.

With the ventricle open, the Alfieri mitral valve repair is performed. The anterior and posterior mitral leaflets are approximated at the central portion of their free edges with a single 4.0 Ethibond suture (Figure 2). The ventriculotomy is closed in three layers with strips of soft felt or bovine pericardium to distribute tension evenly along the suture line (Figure 1). After the cross clamp is removed, tricuspid valve repair can be performed as needed.

All patients were evaluated intraoperatively with transesophageal echocardiography. Fifty-five patients underwent concomitant Alfieri mitral valve repair, 51 with ring annuloplasty; two patients required mitral valve replacement for intrinsic mitral leaflet pathology. A De Vega tricuspid annuloplasty was performed in 33 (58%) patients and one patient required a Cosgrove-Edwards ring for 4+ tricuspid regurgitation. Five patients required coronary artery bypass grafting, one required aortic valve repair and one needed aortic valve replacement. Eleven patients required LVAD placement perioperatively for low cardiac output. The technique for LVAD insertion was similar to our previous reports.[19]

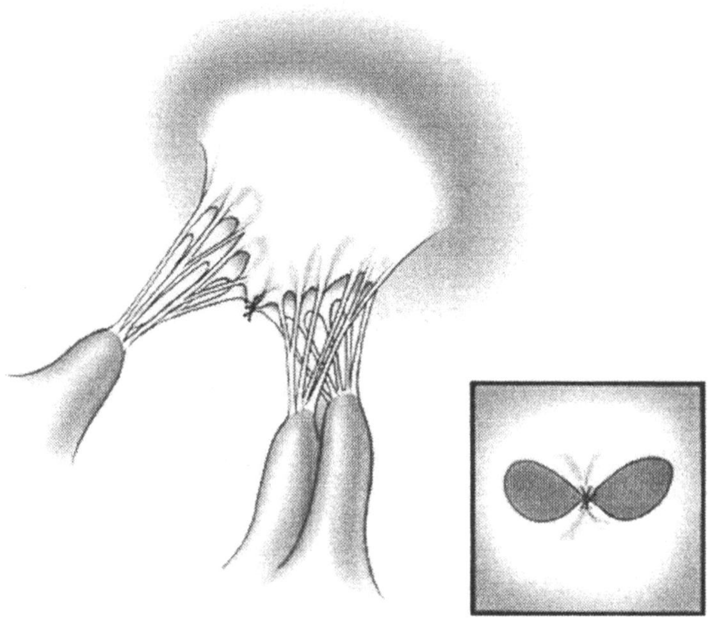

Figure 2. Partial left ventriculectomy. The free edges of the mitral leaflets are approximated with a 4.0 suture (Alfieri repair).

Reproduced with permission from McCarthy PM, Starling RC, Wong et al. Early results with partial left ventriculectomy. J Thorac Cardiovasc Surg 1997;114:756

Because of reports of high risk of sudden death due to arrhythmias, all patients were maintained on amiodarone post-operatively.[13] Further, because we have seen a high incidence of left atrial thrombus, all patients are now placed on warfarin sodium (Coumadin).

Post-operatively, six patients required relisting for transplantation.[15] Five have been transplanted and one is still waiting. Of the eleven patients requiring LVAD placement, two died, six were transplanted and two are still waiting. One patient improved and the LVAD was explanted. There were two early and seven late deaths. Both early deaths occurred in patients supported on LVADs. Three patients died suddenly between three and nine months post-operatively. These were likely due to arrhythmias, despite amiodarone therapy. Three late deaths were due to progression of heart failure and one was due to right ventricular failure after transplantation. Hospital mortality was 3.5% and one year actuarial survival was 82.1+/-5.5%.

At 3 month follow-up, most patients were symptomatically improved (Table 1). The NYHA class, EF, LVEDD, LVEDV, MR and MVO2 were all significantly better, only cardiac index did not change.

In total, 24 patients were considered "failures" of therapy: 11 required LVAD placement, 6 required relisting for transplantation, and seven non-LVAD patients died.[15] The only factor that was associated with failure was age < 40 years, however, more detailed analysis of this subgroup revealed only that this appeared to be a sicker group of patients preoperatively.[15] As compared to patients older than 40, the younger group had more UNOS status 1 patients (81.8% vs. 30.4%), more patients in NYHA class IV failure (90% vs. 56.5%) and had a greater pre-operative inotrope requirement (72.7% vs. 32.6%). Age itself did not appear to be a factor.

Table 1. *Cleveland Clinic Experience. Pre-operative and 3 month results.*

Parameter	*Pre-operative (mean ± SD)*	*Post-operative 3 months (mean ± SD)*	*"p" value*
NYHA Class	3.7	2.2	
EF	14.4±7.7 %	23.2±10.7%	<.001
LVEDV	254±85 ml	179±73 ml	<.001
LVEDD	8.4±1.1 cm	6.3 ±0.9 cm	<.001
MR	2.8 ±1.1	0.65±0.8	<.001
MVO2	10.6±3.9 ml/kg/min	15.3±4.5 ml/kg/min	<.001
CI	2.2 ±0.7 l/min/m^2	2.2 l/min/m^2	

NYHA, New York Heart Association
EF, Ejection Fraction
LVEDV, Left Ventricular End Diastolic Volume;
LVDD, Left Ventricular End Diastolic Dimension
MR, Mitral Regurgitation
MV02, Peak Oxygen Consumption, CI, Cardiac Index

Discussion

These early results from our experience are encouraging. Our one-year actuarial survival of 82% compares favorably with 79% one-year actuarial survival for all heart transplants reported in the International Society of Heart and Lung Transplantation 1997 registry report.[6] Similarly, other centres have begun to report favorable outcomes with PLV.

Angelini, et al., report their experience with 14 patients undergoing PLV.[20] Unlike the patients treated at the Cleveland Clinic, their population was older (mean age 65 years), more heterogeneous in terms of etiology of CM (eight idiopathic, 5 ischemic, one valvular), and 13 were not considered transplant candidates. Nonetheless, they report an in-hospital survival of 78%, and only one late death, likely due to an arrhythmia. Patients in this series experienced a significant increase in CI from 1.9 l/min to 2.7 l/min.

The mechanism by which PLV benefits patients remain controversial. In comparison to Batista's, Salerno's and Angelini's experience, our patients did not demonstrate a major improvement in CI. Nonetheless, in all series, survival was better than the expected one-year survival of similar patients otherwise managed medically.[21] In a multiple compartment elastance model attempting to stimulate PLV, Dickstein, et al., found that diastolic changes offset improvement in systolic function.[22] They believe that, according to the Frank-Starling relationship, overall pump function is, at least short-term, depressed after PLV. Their argument, however, is based on excision of ventricular mass. As Chanda, et al., point out, the goal of the Batista operation is to reduce ventricular *volume*, not mass.[23] Since ventricular mass does not increase proportionally with chamber dilatation, volume reduction surgery should decrease wall stress and improve overall cardiac function.

Another area of controversy regarding the mechanism of improvement seen with PLV is the role of mitral valve reconstruction in these patients. Bolling, et al., demonstrate that mitral repair in patients with severe ventricular function and 4+ MR can be performed with reasonable survival and good ventricular functional improvement.[24] They performed ring-annuloplasty mitral repair in 48 patients, all of whom had pre-operative 4+ MR, were receiving maximal medical therapy and were in either NYHA class III or IV failure. In their study, one and two year actuarial survivals were 82% and 71%, respectively. EF improved from 17+/-3% to 26+/-8%, and NYHA functional class was reduced from 3.9+/-0.3 to 2.0+/-0.6. In comparison to patients undergoing PLV, however, Bolling notes that his patients have more severe MR (4+ vs 2.8+ in our experience), better ventricular function, smaller LV size and less inotropic requirement. While Bolling's work offers one possible mechanism of improvement seen with PLV, further study is required to better understand the effect of volume reduction on the left ventricle.

Conclusion

Even with these early successes with PLV, caution must be exercised with regard to the future of this procedure, as stated in the Society of Thoracic Surgeons position paper.[25] Experience with this operation is limited, with only short-term results published in peer-review journals. Patient selection, a factor that we consider critical to outcome, has varied among institutions. While some groups have chosen to perform PLV on non-transplant patients, we believe that failures of PLV should be transplant or LVAD candidates. Other institutions have elected to include ischemic CM as an indication for PLV; we prefer to perform a modified Dor procedure for this entity. Our early clinical impression is that routine use of Dobutamine echocardiography, PET scans and cardiac MRI will help to determine which patients will most benefit from cardioreduction. We believe that the future of this operation will rest with objective scientific scrutiny, performed by multidisciplinary teams, at centres dedicated to the management and care of heart-failure patients.

References

1. O'Connell JB, Bristow MR. Economic impact of heart failure in the United States: time for a different approach. J Heart Lung Transplant 1994;13:S107-12.
2. Clark AL, Coats AJ. New evidence for improved survival in chronic heart failure. Clin Cardiol 1994;17(2):55-8.
3. Packer M, Bristow MR, Cohn JN, et al. The effect of carvedilol on morbidity and mortality in patients with chronic heart failure. N Engl J Med 1996;334:1349-55.
4. Saxon LA, Stevenson WG, Fonarow G, et al. Predicting death from progressive heart failure secondary to ischemic or idiopathic dilated cardiomyopathy. Am J Cardiol 1993;72(1):62-5.
5. Laks H, Scholl FG, Drinkwater DC, et al. The alternate recipient list for heart transplantation: Does it work? J Heart Lung Transplant 1997;16:735-42.
6. Hosenpud JD, Bennett LE, Berkeley KM, Fiol B, Novick RJ. The registry of the International Society for Heart and Lung Transplantation: Fourteenth official report - 1997. J Heart Lung Transplant 1997;16:691-712.
7. Frazier OH. First use of an untethered, vented electric left ventricular assist device for long-term support. Circulation 1994;2908-14.
8. Portner PM,. Oyer PE, Pennington DG, et al. Implantable left ventricular assist system: bridge to transplantation and the future. Ann Thorac Surg 1989;47:142-50.
9. McCarthy PM, Young JB, Smedira NG, Hobbs RE, Vargo RL, Starling RC. Permanent mechanical circulatory support with an implantable left ventricular assist device. Ann Thorac Surg 1997;63:1458-61.
10. Chiu RC-J. Cardiomyoplasty. In: Edmunds LH, editor. Cardiac surgery in the adult. New York: McGraw-Hill;1997: 1491-504.
11. Lin SS, Platt JL. Immunologic barriers to xenotransplantation. J Heart Lung Transplant 1996;15:547-55.
12. Batista RJV, Santos JLV, Takeshita N, Bocchino L, Lima PN, Cunha MA. Partial left ventriculectomy to improve left ventricular function in end-stage heart disease. J Card Surg 1996;11:96-7.
13. Batista RJV, Verde J, Nery P, et al. Partial left ventriculectomy to treat end-stage heart disease. Ann Thorac Surg 1997;64:634-8.
14. Fucci C, Sandrelli L, Pardini A, Torracca L, Ferrari M, Alfieri O. Improved results with mitral valve repair using new surgical techniques. Eur J Cardiothorac Surg 1995;9:621-7.
15. McCarthy JF, McCarthy PM, Starling RC, et al. Partial left ventriculectomy and mitral valve repair for end-stage congestive heart failure. Eur J Cardiothorac Surg 1998;in press.
16. Dor V. Left ventricular aneurysms: the endoventricular circular patch plasty. Sem Thorac Cardiovasc Surg 1997;9(2):123-30.
17. McCarthy PM, Starling RC, Wong J, et al. Early results with partial left ventriculectomy. J Thorac Cardiovasc Surg 1997;114:755-65.
18. Cosgrove DM, Arcidi J, Rodriguez L, Stewart WJ, Powell K, Thomas JD. Initial experience with the Cosgrove-Edwards annuloplasty system. Ann Thorac Surg 1995;60:449-504.
19. McCarthy PM, Wang N, Vargo RL. Preperitoneal insertion of the Heartmate 1000 IP implantable left ventricular device. Ann Thorac Surg 1994;57:634-8.20.
20. Angelini GD, Pryn S, Mehta D et al. Left ventricular volume reduction for end-stage heart failure. Lancet 1997;350:489.
21. Cowie MR, Mosterd A, Wood DA, et al. The epidemiology of heart failure. Eur Heart J 1997;18:208-25.
22. Dickstein ML, Spotnitz HM, Rose EA, Burkhoff D. Heart reduction surgery: An analysis of the impact on cardiac function. J Thorac Cardiovasc Surg 1997;113:1032-40.
23. Chanda J, Kuribayashi R, Abe T. Batista operation for dilated cardiomyopathy: A physiologic concept. J Thorac Cardiovasc Surg 1998;115:261.
24. Bolling SF, Pagani FD, Deeb GM, Bach DS. Intermediate-term outcome of mitral reconstruction in cardiomyopathy. J Thorac Cardiovasc Surg;115:381-8.
25. Replogle RL, Kaiser GC, Cohn LH, et al. Left ventricular reduction surgery. Ann Thorac Surg 1997;63:909-10.

10. XENOTRANSPLANTATION

Farah N.K. Bhatti and John Wallwork

Introduction

While transplantation is an established form of treatment for many end stage disease processes that lead to heart failure, the number of transplants performed is limited by a relative lack of donor organs. This has led not only to a levelling off in heart transplant activity world-wide, but actually to a decrease in the number of operations performed in 1995 and 1996, despite the use of older organ donors each year. Although waiting lists are kept artificially low by patient selection, the disparity between growing waiting lists and falling transplant numbers continues to widen leading to a proportion of people dying whilst awaiting transplant. In the United Kingdom in 1996, of people waiting for a heart, only 63% were transplanted, and 14% died while waiting.[1] Figures from the United Network for Organ Sharing (UNOS) at the end of 1996 show a similar situation, with 3700 people waiting for a heart transplant in the U.S.A., 2343 transplants being performed, and 744 deaths on the waiting list. The mismatch between the waiting lists and transplants actually performed is depicted, for all organs, in Figure 1.[2]

Potential Solution to Donor Shortage

A number of approaches can be applied to try and resolve this issue. Firstly, optimal utilization must be made of those organs that are available and this includes strategies such as multiorgan donation and coordination of transplant services to minimize organ wastage. Secondly, the development of artificial organs and tissues that could be implanted permanently would alleviate the need for human donor organs. There are a number of left ventricular assist devices available and these have been used as both to allow recovery of the heart as well as a bridge to transplantation (the latter use, of course, delays but does not prevent the need for a donor heart). Total artificial hearts are also a focus of active research; whilst theoretical benefits include helping the organ shortage situation and the avoidance of long term immunosuppressive therapy, problems such as haemolysis, thromboembolism, line infection and developing portable power sources all need addressing. Finally, xenotransplantion, the transplantation of organs between different species, could provide a solution to the problem. The main advantage of xenotransplantation would be the provision of a readily available supply of organs to meet the demand, and perhaps being

Roy Masters (editor), Surgical Options for the Treatment of Heart Failure, 165-173.

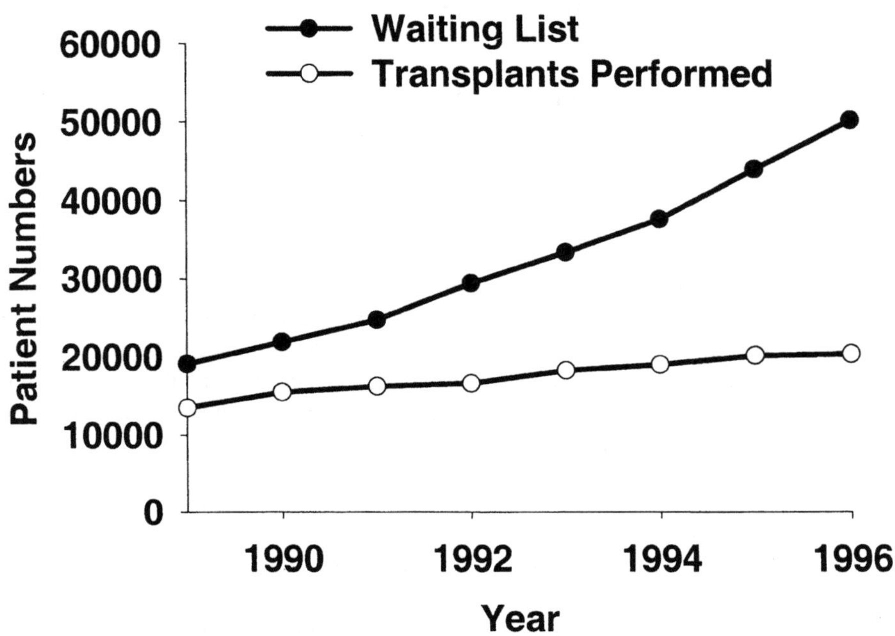

Figure 1 *Numbers of Patients on Waiting Lists for Transplantation & Number of Transplants Performed: USA Data is shown for all organs in the United States. The increasing disparity between the steadily growing waiting list and the relatively static number of transplants performed can be seen.*

able to widen the eligibility criteria to join the transplant waiting list. Additional benefits would include practical considerations such as performing planned procedures with shorter ischaemic times.

Historical Overview of Cardiac Xenotransplantation

There are 8 accounts in the literature of humans receiving xenogeneic hearts.[3] From the first documented attempt at cardiac xenotransplantation by Hardy in 1964 to the last case of Baby Fae performed by Bailey at Loma Linda in 1984, none has been particularly successful. In five of the cases, non-human primate donors were used (chimpanzees and baboons) in either an orthotopic or heterotopic position; all failed either due to an inability to support the circulation or due to vascular rejection, although one patient did survive out to 20 days before death occurred. In three reports, all in 1968, sheep and pig hearts were used; none of these organs survived beyond a few minutes. The world experience is summarised in Table 1.[3]

Table 1. *Clinical Experience in Cardiac Xenotransplantation.* **Summary of the experience of cardiac xenotransplantation in man. Both concordant and discordant species combinations have been attempted, but prolonged life-supporting xenograft survival has not been achieved.**

DATE	SURGEON	DONOR	SURVIVAL OF GRAFT
1964	HARDY	CHIMPANZEE	2 HOURS
1968	COOLEY	SHEEP	STOPPED IMMEDIATELY
1968	ROSS	PIG	4 MINUTES
1968	ROSS	PIG	STOPPED IMMEDIATELY
1969	MARION	CHIMPANZEE	"RAPID FAILURE"
1977	BARNARD	BABOON	5 HOURS
1977	BARNARD	CHIMPANZEE	4 DAYS
1984	BAILEY	BABOON	20 DAYS

Pigs As Donors

Pigs appear to be suitable as donors of organs for human use due to anatomical and physiological similarities.[4] Factors such as the large litter sizes produced and the short gestation period also make breeding in large numbers a viable option. Pigs can also be bred in specified pathogen free (SPF) conditions, thus allowing the health status of the animal to be guaranteed. In ethical terms, pigs are bred in their many millions as a food source so it is difficult to argue against their use to save human life.

Transplantation between widely disparate species such as pig and man, however, results in rapid and violent rejection of the graft in a matter of minutes to hours.[5] It is this phenomenon, known as hyperacute rejection (HAR), that defines pig and man as a discordant species combination and has prevented the successful use of porcine organs for transplantation.

Immunological Barriers

The key components of HAR are the presence of naturally occurring antibodies that recognise antigens on the donor cell surface leading to activation of the complement system and organ destruction. The predominant xenoantigen is the gal (alpha 1,3) gal epitope that is present on the cell surfaces of all mammals except man, old world monkeys and the great apes. The latter group of primates have preformed antibodies against this epitope and therefore hyperacutely reject organs from donor species such as the pig. Histologically HAR is characterised by microvascular thromboses, haemorrhage and oedema; deposition of the terminal components of the complement system can be demonstrated immunohistochemically.

Three approaches have been attempted to overcome HAR of pig organs when transplanted into primates. Firstly, one can attempt to remove the natural antibodies pretransplantation, by immunoadsorption for example.[6] This strategy, however, offers only a temporary reduction in antibody levels. Secondly one can alter the nature of the antigen to try and prevent its recognition. This has been done by removing the galactose terminal of the gal (alpha 1,3) gal epitope or by replacing it with a different sugar residue.[7] Although "gal knockout" mice have been produced, this has not, so far, been a successful strategy in pigs. The third, and potentially most promising, approach is that of circumventing the recipient's complement system.

Complement inhibition

The complement system consists of over thirty proteins that circulate in an inactive form. Activation of the system, either by the classical (antigen-antibody mediated) or the alternative pathway, leads to the generation of C3b by C3 convertase and then membrane attack complex (MAC). There exist, however, a number of molecules that serve to prevent self-damage on activation of the complement system; these molecules are termed regulators of complement activity (RCAs) and are species specific.[8] Three membrane bound RCAs in man are decay accelerating factor (DAF), membrane cofactor protein (MCP) and CD59. It was postulated, and then confirmed in vitro, that incorporation of a human RCA (for example human DAF) into the cell surface of a non-human mammalian species might afford it some protection against damage by human complement.[9] This then led to the production of pigs expressing hDAF on their cell surface at Imutran Ltd in Cambridge.

Generation of Pigs Transgenic for hDAF

The first stage in the generation of hDAF transgenic pigs was the microinjection of an 6.5 kB hDAF minigene construct into the male pronucleus of a fertilised pig ovum harvested from a pregnant sow, and its reimplantation into a sow that was synchronous in oestrus cycle with the ovum donor.[10,11] Using this technology, 49 hDAF transgenic pig were produced that had incorporated between 1 and 30 copies of the construct into their genome. These pigs were then characterised in term of protein expression and it was found that some founder lines expressed higher amounts of hDAF in their organs than was found in human control tissue. Equally importantly, the transgenic manipulation had no adverse effects on the pigs in terms of general well being, growth, sexual maturity and reproduction. A founder line with good expression of hDAF in the heart was used to breed pigs for the cardiac studies described below.

Ex-vivo Perfusion Experiments

A working heart model was used in which hearts from hDAF transgenic pigs, non-transgenic pigs (positive controls) and rhesus monkeys (negative controls) were perfused with human blood. It was demonstrated that the hDAF transgenic pig hearts functioned superiorly to non-transgenic control pig hearts and had a cardiac performance similar to the rhesus hearts.[12] Furthermore, markers of myocardial damage, such as creatine phosphokinase remained low in the hDAF transgenic pig hearts and the rhesus hearts while rising significantly in the control pig hearts. Only the non-transgenic pig hearts showed any evidence of HAR histologically.

In Vivo Cardiac Studies

The next stage was to design in vivo models to test whether HAR is abolished when hDAF porcine organs are transplanted into primates. Although RCAs are species specific, it was found that both baboon and cynomolgus monkey complement were downregulated significantly by hDAF, making both these species suitable as recipients for in vivo studies using hDAF transgenic pig organs.

Heterotopic Heart Transplants

An abdominal model of heterotopic heart transplantation was developed in the cynomolgus monkey. The original immunosuppressive protocol consisted of cyclosporin A, cyclophosphamide and steroids. The cyclosporin A was dosed to achieve trough levels of >400ng/ml. The cyclophosphamide dose was titrated against the white cell count, the aim being to prevent the total white count falling below $2x10^9$cells/L. The steroids were commenced at the time of reperfusion of the xenograft at 1mg/kg, and then reduced by 0.05mg/kg/day, to a baseline dose of 0.2mg/kg/day. The choice of cyclophosphamide was based on the findings that, in small animal models of xenotransplantation, it appeared to inhibit the induced xenoantibody response and allow long term graft survival.[13] In addition to monitoring graft function, the amount of antibody lytic for porcine red cells (haemolytic antipig antibody - APA) was measured daily in all recipients in order to assess the degree of antipig reactivity present. Initially 10 heterotopic heart transplants were performed using hDAF transgenic pig hearts. There were no cases of hyperacute rejection. A maximum cardiac xenograft survival of 62 days was achieved.[14] Acute vascular rejection (AVR) was seen in the xenografts that stopped beating and immunohistochemistry revealed deposition of immunoglobulins and complement components in these xenografts. The main limiting factor in this study was the side effects of the drug therapy; the four longest heterotopic heart recipients were euthanased not due to cardiac xenograft dysfunction, but due to severe diarrhoea. Having demonstrated that hDAF transgenic pig hearts are not hyperacutely rejected in primates and that prolonged survival is possible, it was necessary to move to an orthotopic model of cardiac xenotransplantation to see if a pig heart could maintain a primate circulation in addition to surviving the immunological barriers.

Orthotopic Heart Transplants

Orthotopic transplants using hDAF transgenic pig hearts were carried out in baboons due to the larger recipient sizes available. An immunosuppressive protocol based on cyclophosphamide, cyclosporin A and steroids was again employed, but in this model cyclosporin A trough levels of >1500ng/ml (appropriate for baboons) were aimed for.[15] No xenograft underwent HAR and a maximum life-supporting survival of 9 days was achieved.[16] Three hearts were lost on day 5 due to AVR, and all 3 recipients had concomitant rises in their APA levels. Bone marrow suppression in the day 9 orthotopic recipient led to its euthanasia, despite a normally functioning xenograft.

Summary of Preclinical Cardiac Studies

A number of important observations can be made from these in vivo studies. Firstly, it has been demonstrated that hDAF transgenic pig organs are not hyperacutely rejected when transplanted into non-human primates. Secondly, in terms of physiology, pig hearts can support primate life. Thirdly, when rejection does occur, it appears to be vascular in nature and is often accompanied by a rise in the induced xenoantibody level; controlling this appears to be critical in the prevention of AVR.

Future Strategies

There are a number of newer immunosuppressive agents that act relatively selectively on lymphocytes, offering the advantage of fewer systemic side effects. Lymphocytes are dependent on the *de novo* pathway of nucleotide synthesis; drugs that inhibit this cause selective depletion of T and B cells. Agents such as brequinar and leflunomide act on the *de novo* pyrimidine synthesis pathway by inhibiting the enzyme dihydroorotate dehydrogenase, while mycophenolate mofetil inhibits *de novo* purine synthesis by acting on inosine monophosphate dehydroganase.[17] Since inhibition of the induced xenoantibody appears to be important in the prevention of AVR, which is the next immunological hurdle, these newer agents may play an important role in xenotransplantation and are currently being evaluated. It may be that a combined approach using these more selective immunosuppressive agents together with either monoclonal antibodies or tolerance inducing protocols will be necessary. Other future directions include the generation of multiple transgenic pigs that express more that one human RCA, perhaps in combination with lower expression of the gal alpha 1,3, gal epitope. Regular immunoabsorption of the xenoantibody may also have a role to play.

Safety of Xenotransplantation

The potential risks to man from pig pathogens can be evaluated and many microorganisms then eradicated from the herd i.e. the pigs can be bred in specified pathogen free conditions. Thus freedom from many known pathogens can be guaranteed. Concern has focused, however, on two particular issues: the problem of unknown pathogens as well as the risks posed by porcine endogenous retrovirus (PERV). There are a number of strategies being employed at Imutran to assess the risks posed by unknown pathogens. Regular cultural analysis of flora of sentinel pigs is carried out to look for bacteria and parasites. For viruses, co-culture of both sentinel pig tissues and tissues from primate recipients of porcine xenografts, is being carried out with susceptible cell lines (human, primate and pig) to seek non-specific evidence of viral infection. In addition, a study is planned in immunosuppressed pigs to look for unknown viruses using low specificity DNA and RNA primers and viral culture techniques.

Four different types of PERV have been described so far and, although harmless to pigs, two have been shown, in vitro at least, to infect human cell lines.[18] The approach to PERV at Imutran is one of risk assessment for limited clinical trials as well as a longer term strategy. The risk assessment consists firstly of evaluation of infective virion production in pigs in vivo, secondly the evaluation of tissues from primates who have received a pig organ for infection, and, finally, a retrospective evaluation of patients who have previously been exposed to viable pig tissues for the presence of viral DNA, RNA and antibodies. A potential long term strategy is to map the loci of the integration of PERV sequences in both Imutran's pigs and other pig lines and then define an approach to eliminate the important integration sites should this become necessary.

Ethical Considerations

The ethical considerations involved in xenotransplantation can be divided into three broad categories: animal or donor issues, recipient issues and, lastly, issues relating to the general public.

That animals should be killed for human use is a topic that generates intense debate. Most people would agree that a balance needs to be struck between animal suffering and the potential benefits to man.[19] There is widespread although not universal consensus that it would be inappropriate to use primates as donors of organs for human use, predominantly due to their evolutionary "closeness" to humans and their self awareness, as well as the possibility of endangering the species (as in the case of chimpanzees). Pigs, however, are already reared in their millions as a food source. Porcine valves are also used routinely in cardiac surgery. It is would therefore appear be a logical step forward, to most people, to use pig organs as xenografts.[20]

The first recipients of a xenograft will clearly be pioneers in the field. The key issues here are that the recipient is fully informed of the likely outcome of the procedure, the need for intensive postoperative monitoring, and the potential risks posed by infection.

The main issue that affects the general public is that of safety and this has been discussed above.

The Future

A prerequisite of clinical xenografting is regular prolonged life supporting survival of pig organs in primate models. Issues of physiology can also be assessed in more detail as longer survivals are achieved. The question of safety, in particular the potential risk from PERV, also needs to be evaluated fully. A move to the clinic will be appropriate when these immunological, physiological and disease transmission issues have been addressed to the satisfaction of the appropriate regulatory authorities.[21]

Acknowledgments

The authors would like to acknowledge all the staff at Imutran who have been involved in the xenotransplantation programme, in particular Dr. David White, Director of Research. We also wish to thank Dr. Dan Tucker for his contributions and comments.

References

1. Yearly Transplant Statistics for the UK and Republic of Ireland; UKTSSA, 1996
2. United Network of Organ Sharing, 1996
3. Cooper DKC and Ye Y. Experience with Clinical Heart Xenotransplantation. In: Xenotransplantation, The Transplantation of Organs and Tissues Between Species. Eds. Cooper DKC, Kemp E., Reemtsma, White DJG. Springer-Verlag;1991:541/557.
4. Cooper DKC, Ye Y, Rolf JLL, Zuhdi N. The pig as a potential donor for manIn: Xenotransplantation, The Transplantation of Organs and Tissues Between Species. Eds. Cooper DKC, Kemp E. , Reemtsma, White DJG. Springer-Verlag;1991:481-500.
5. Calne RY. Organ transplantation between widely disparate species. Transplant Proc 1970;2(4):550-6.
6. Cooper DKC, Human PA, Lexer G et al. Effects of Cyclosporine and Antibody Adsorption on pig cardiac xenograft survival. J Heart Transplant1988; 7: 238-46.
7. Sandrin MS, Fodor WL, Cohney S et al. Reduction of the major porcine xenoantigen Gal α(1,3) Gal by the expression of α(1,2) fucosyltransferase. Xenotransplantation 1996; 3: 134-40
8. Atkinson JP, Oglesby TJ, White D, Adams EA, Liszewski MK. Separation of self from non-self in the complement: a role for membrane cofactor protein and decay accelerating factor. Clin Exp Immunol 1991; 86(1):27-30.
9. Oglesby TJ, White D, Tedja I et al. Protection of mammalian cells from complement-mediated lysis by transfection of human membrane cofactor protein and decay accelerating factor. Transactions of the Associations of American Physicians CIV. 1991; 164-72.
10. Cozzi E, White DJG. The generation of transgenic pigs as potential organ donors for humans. Nature Med 1995; 1(9): 964-6.
11. Langford GA, Yannoutsos E, Cozzi E et al. Production of pigs transgenic for human decay accelerating factor. Trans Proc 1994; 26(3): 1400-1.
12. Schmoeckel M, Nollert G, Shahmohammadi M et al. Transgenic human decay accelerating factor makes normal pigs function as a concordant species. Heart Lung Transplant 1997 Jul;16(7):758-64.
13. Hasan RI, et al. Prolonged survival of hamster to rat heart xenografts with cyclophosphamide therapy. Transplant Proc 1992 Apr; 24(2): 517-8.
14. Waterworth PD, Cozzi E, Tolan MJ et al. Pig to primate cardiac xenotransplantation and cyclophosphamide therapy. Trans Proc1997;29:899-900.
15. Stark JH, Smit JA, Gridelli B. Sensitivity of baboon lymphocytes to cyclosporin A and FK506: relative resistance of alloactivated cells to CyA. Transplant Int 1994; 7: 372-8.
16. Schmoeckel M, Bhatti FNK, Zaidi A et al. Orthotopic heart transplantation in a transgenic pig to primate model Transplantation 1998; 65(12): 1570-7.
17. Morris RE. Mechanisms of action of new immunosuppressive drugs. Therapeutic Drug Monitoring 1995; 17(6):564-9.
18. Patience C. Takeuchi Y, Weiss RA. Infection of human cells by an endogenous retrovirus of pigs. Nature Med. 1997 Mar; 3(3): 282-6.
19. Smith JA, Boyd KM, Eds. Lives in the Balance. The Ethics of using animals in biomedical research. The Report of a Working Party of the Institute of Medical Ethics. OUP 1991.
20. Report on The Ethics of Xenotransplantation. The Nuffield Council of Bioethics. March 1996.
21. Report by The Advisory Group on the Ethics of Xenotransplantation. Chaired by Professor Ian Kennedy. January 1997.

11. PERMANENT MECHANICAL CIRCULATORY SUPPORT

Tofy Mussivand, Paul J. Hendry, Roy G. Masters, Wilbert J. Keon

Indroduction

Mechanical circulatory support devices have typically been used for temporary support and as a bridge to transplantation. The experience gained with the existing devices, specifically the extended durations of successful support, has led to raised expectations for the more chronic and permanent use of mechanical circulatory devices. [1,-3] While some currently available systems are now being utilized for extended durations outside of the hospital setting, systems are being developed utilizing advanced technologies which will allow for longer term out of hospital, circulatory support.[4,5]

Heart Failure

Circulatory insufficiency caused by the inability of the heart to pump blood to the organs in sufficient amounts to meet the requirements is defined as congestive heart failure (otherwise referred to as heart failure). This pathophysiological condition is caused by a reduction in myocardial contractility (from a variety of disease processes including both chronic ischemia and the cardiomyopathies) ultimately resulting in death.

Cost of Heart Failure

In terms of human suffering and death, the cost of heart failure is overwhelming. In the United States alone, approximately 1% of the adult population are affected by this condition.[6] The estimated patient population and number of deaths related to congestive heart failure for the U.S.A., Canada and the World are shown in Figure 1.[7] In the U.S.A., heart failure is the primary diagnosis of over 900,000 hospitalizations per year with an annual new diagnosis of over 400,000 individuals.[8,9] The estimated cost of heart failure in the U.S.A. for 1998 exceeded $20 Billion.[10] Even with the modern advances in therapies, the five year survival rate after diagnosis is very poor. Survival is less than 50% with a median survival after diagnosis of only 1.7 years for males and 3.2 years for females.[11] Heart failure ultimately results in a slow, painful and costly death.

Therapies

For centuries, therapies for this disease have been the subject of in-depth research. To date, there is no single, effective, widely practiced therapy for heart failure patients. While

Roy Masters (editor), Surgical Options for the Treatment of Heart Failure, 175-186.

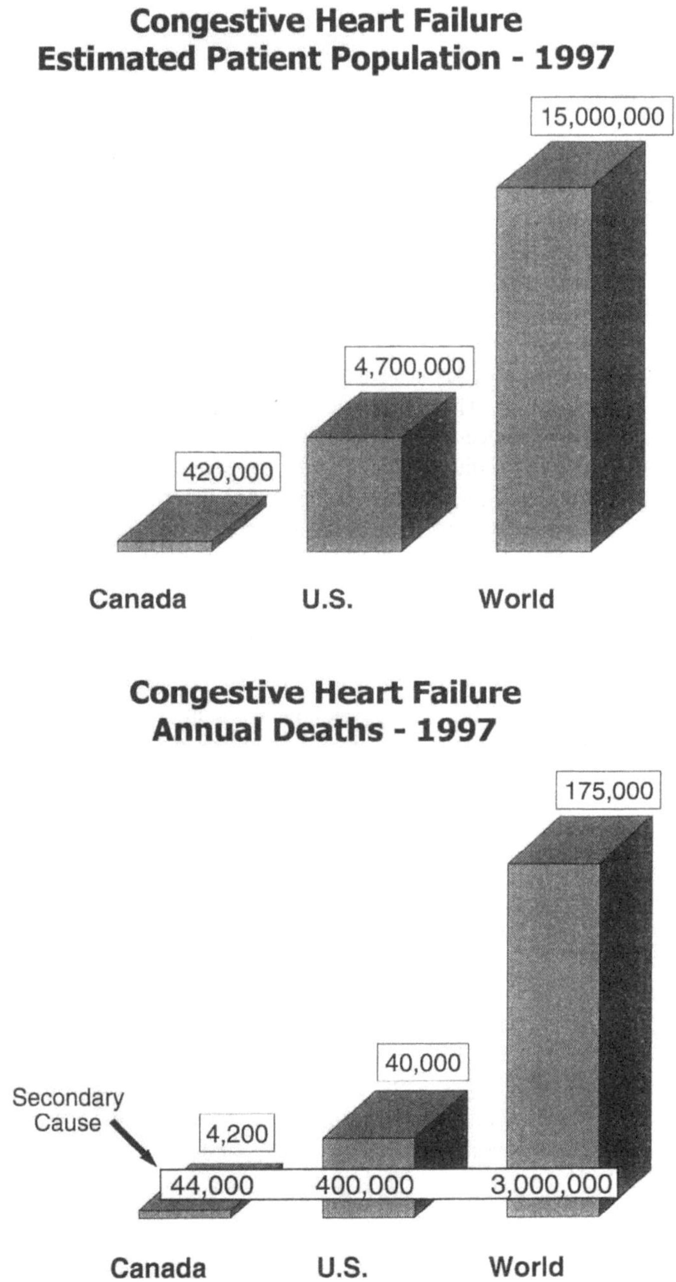

Figure 1. *Estimated patient population and annual deaths due to congestive heart failure.*

heart transplantation is the most effective therapy for end stage heart disease, the limited supply of donors has made mechanical circulatory support a promising alternative at the present time. [12]

Background

Although various mechanical circulatory support devices have been clinically utilized since the late 1960's, the first clinical use of a so-called "permanent" device did not occur until 1982, when a pneumatically actuated Total Artificial Heart (TAH), the Jarvik 7 was implanted as a "permanent" device into Dr. Barney Clark who lived on the device for 112 days. In total, five Jarvik 7's were implanted as "permanent" devices with patients living on the device for 10, 112, 229, 488 and 620 days respectively.[13] Unfortunately, the use of the Jarvik 7 required that the patient be tethered via pneumatic hoses to a large console located beside the patient's bed and required monitoring by skilled personnel, making its use as a so-called "permanent" device costly, while offering a minimal quality of life to the patient. While the device continues to be used at several centers today, it is limited to temporary use as a bridge to transplantation.

Total Artificial Hearts

Total Artificial Hearts (TAHs) are designed to replace the total heart (both ventricles) and require excision of the native heart for placement of the device. At last report, 9 different total artificial hearts had been clinically utilized in 323 patients, between 1969-1997 (Table 1).[14] The vast majority (> 85%) of these implants were performed with Jarvik total artificial heart devices (Jarvik 7, Jarvik 7-70, and CardioWest C-70) which were first introduced in 1982. The CardioWest C-70 (a slightly modified version of the Jarvik 7- 70) is the only currently available TAH for clinical use and continues to be used for select bridge to transplantation cases at several international centers, including the University of Ottawa Heart Institute.

Table 1. Clinical use of Total Artificial Hearts (TAH)

Device	*Country*	*Number of Patients*
Jarvik (Jarvik 7, 7-70, CardioWest C7-70)	U.S.A.	277
Poisk	Russia	16
Unger/Vienna	Austria	10
Berlin	Germany	7
BRNO	Czech	6
Penn State	U.S.A.	4
Phoenix	U.S.A.	1
Akutsu	U.S.A.	1
Liotta	U.S.A.	1

None of the TAHs utilized clinically to date, would serve effectively as a permanent implant due to the requirement that the patient be tethered to a large external driving console, thus confining the patient to the hospital (Figure 2). However, the next generation of TAHs currently being developed will be implantable and actuated electrically, as opposed to pneumatically, thus eliminating the need for a large external driving console and potentially allowing the recipients to be discharged from the hospital.

Ventricular Assist Devices

Ventricular Assist Devices (VADs) are connected in parallel to the native heart and pump all or part of the normal stroke volume. Unlike TAHs, the native heart is left in place allowing for the potential of recovery of native heart function and possible removal of the device, as well as maintaining the native heart neurohormonal control mechanisms. VADs can be classified into two major categories: pulsatile devices and non-pulsatile (or continuous flow) devices.

Clinical use of pulsatile VADs (over 5800 reported cases) has largely surpassed that of TAHs (less than 350 cases) and therefore offers the greatest hope in the near future for permanent use . Not only has there been significant clinical experience with these devices, but certain devices are already being utilized in what could be considered a permanent application (i.e. for extended durations and outside of the hospital). Successful utilization

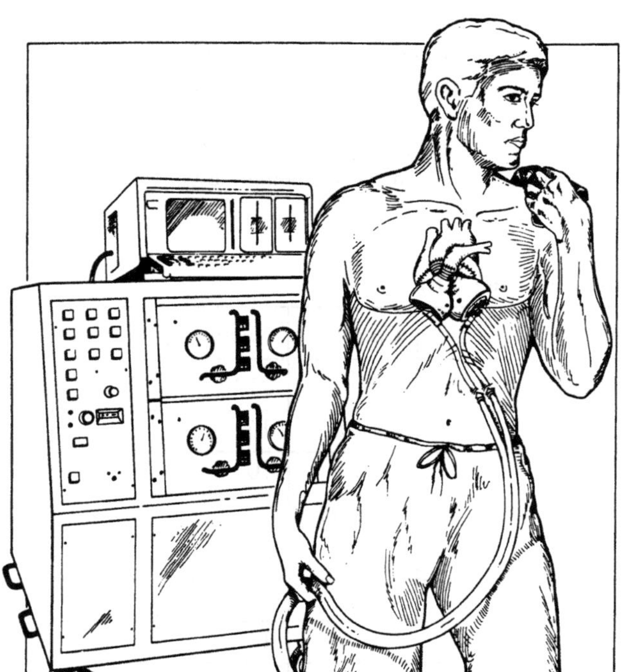

Figure 2. *Artists representation of the Jarvik Total Artificial Heart. (courtesy of CardioWest Technologies, Tucson , AZ, U.S.A..)*

Table 2. Clinical use of Ventricular Assist Devices (VAD)

Device	*Type*	*Number of Patients*	*Maximum Duration*	*FDA Approval Status*
External Devices				
Berlin Heart	Extracorporeal, Console Driven	450		None
Thoratec VAD	Extracorporeal, Console Driven	906	515 days	Bridge to Transplant and Post-Cardiotomy
Abiomed BVS-5000	Extracorporeal, Console Driven	>2500	160 days	Reversible Heart Failure
Implantable Devices				
Novacor LVAS	Electric, Console Driven & Electric Wearable	730	903 days	Bridge to Transplant
TCI Heartmate	Pneumatic, Console Driven & Electric Wearable	>1300	607 days	Bridge to Transplant

of certain devices has also been extended from weeks to months and in some cases even years (Table 2).[15]

It is important to note that until recently the only devices approved for sale in the U.S.A. were the external devices or console driven versions of the implantable devices.[16] Unfortunately these are the devices least suited to the permanent application since, as with the TAH, the patients are tethered to external consoles reducing their mobility, and essentially confining them to hospital. These devices however have demonstrated the potential of the technology for permanent use, as can be seen by the extended periods of support achieved in numerous patients. The devices that come closest to meeting the requirements for permanent use are the so-called implantable wearable systems (Novacor and Thermo Cardiosystems) which have recently received limited regulatory approval for bridge to transplant purposes in the U.S.A.[17] Both of these devices utilize pumps implanted in the abdominal wall with percutaneous power connections and externalized vents. With a portable control and power system they allow some degree of patient mobility (Figure 3) and offer an improved quality of life for patients who are able to leave the hospital and resume fairly normal daily activities.[18 - 21] The experience with these devices, specifically the ability to mobilize patients outside of the hospital setting, has led to the future expectations of permanent devices and the potential widespread use of this lifesaving technology.

Current Status

While the currently available devices have established evidence of improved functional and physiological condition in end-stage heart failure patients several major issues remain to be overcome.[22 - 25] The major clinical complications with circulatory support have been

Wearable N100 LVAS

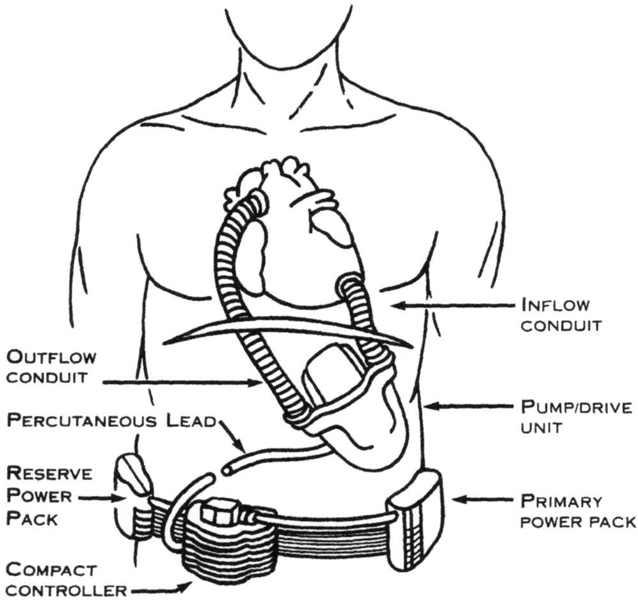

Figure 3. *Novacor N100 LVAS*
courtesy of Novacor Division, Baxter HealthCare Corporation, Oakland, CA, U.S.A..)

well documented and include significant rates of bleeding, infection, renal failure, and thromboembolism, as well as gastrointestinal complications (related to intra-abdominal implantation).[26 - 29] While improved patient selection and management will undoubtedly help to reduce complication rates, improved devices are also needed.[30] One important issue that continues to plague clinical utilization of VADs is the unacceptably high incidence of infection. It has been suggested and is widely acknowledged that a totally implantable system (i.e. one without percutaneous connections) could have a major impact on reducing the incidence of infection which currently affects up to 40-50% of recipients.[31, 32] In addition improved fluid dynamics within the devices and advanced blood contacting interfaces may help to reduce or prevent the formation of thrombus / embolus. Lastly, devices capable of intrathoracic implantation could offer substantial benefits over abdominal implants by: 1) shortening the length of the cannulae (thus reducing the potential for kinking, reducing hydraulic losses thereby improving efficiency, and minimizing the artificial blood contacting surface area); 2) providing a secure anchoring location (i.e. the rib cage) to prevent device migration and 3) eliminating the need for diaphragmatic perforation and extension of the incision into the abdominal area. However, to achieve the goal of intrathoracic implantation, significant efforts dedicated to reducing the size and optimizing the geometrical configuration of these devices are required.

Future Applications

While existing devices have been utilized primarily for bridging to transplantation and for short term support of patients in cardiogenic shock, the future clearly lies in permanent devices as an *alternative* to cardiac transplantation.[33] While, transplantation has long been considered the gold standard for treatment of end-stage heart failure the chronic shortage of donor organs and the need for chronic immunosuppression with its attendant complications severely limits the application of transplantation. However, even if there were sufficient donor hearts available, there are several good reasons why permanent devices may be preferable, including : 1) a shorter hospitalization period 2) no waiting list 3) an unlimited supply 4) no requirement for immune suppression 5) a reduced cost for medication and 6) an improved quality of life.[34-36]

Another potential application for future devices is for myocardial recovery. While sustainable recovery of native heart function after chronic ventricular unloading with ventricular assist devices has long been suggested, only recently has clinical experience with a growing number of patients been available.[37, 38] Most recently, Margulies and colleagues performed studies on myocytes isolated from six VAD supported heart failure patients and found improved contractile properties (magnitude of contraction, time to peak contraction, and time to relaxation) and β-adrenergic responsiveness, compared to non-bridged heart failure patients.[39] Mueller and colleagues previously reported on seven end-stage patients with idiopathic dilated cardiomyopathy in whom substantial recovery was noted, prompting removal of their ventricular assist devices.[40] Previously, both Frazier and McCarthy have also noted substantial histological improvement in patients after chronic mechanical circulatory support.[37, 41] In addition, Levin and colleagues had shown marked improvement and normalization of end diastolic pressure volume relationships after prolonged ventricular unloading by mechanical circulatory support.[38] Farrar and colleagues also noted improved renal and hepatic function during circulatory support, as well as a relationship between organ function improvement and the duration of circulatory support.[42] Given this growing evidence of functional, structural, and histological improvement after mechanical circulatory support, future devices will need to be adaptive for this application. While the potential for recovery of ventricular function is an exciting prospect for the field of circulatory support, it is in its very early stages of investigation, and results and underlying mechanisms are not entirely clear.

The Next Generation of Devices

The next generation of mechanical circulatory devices requires specific technological enhancements to meet the demands of permanent long-term implantation and to overcome the high incidence of clinical complications experienced with existing devices. Development efforts are underway in three major device categories: 1) Total Artificial Hearts 2) Totally Implantable Pulsatile Ventricular Assist Devices and 3) Non-pulsatile Ventricular Assist Devices.

Total Artificial Hearts

The development of next generation TAHs has come about in large part through the long-term funding commitment from the National Heart Lung & Blood Institutes (NHLBI) in the U.S.A.[43] In 1988 four TAH research and development groups were funded to investigate the development of a permanent, tether free, total artificial heart. Additional funding was provided to 3 of the groups between 1993-1996 (Texas Heart Institute/Abiomed, Cleveland Clinic /Nimbus, Penn State/3M) to conduct further in vitro and in vivo experiments. Most recently continued funding was awarded to two of these groups (Texas Heart Institute/Abiomed and Penn State/3M) for the period between 1997-2000 to conduct device readiness testing.[44]

Several other research groups have also made significant progress towards the development of an implantable TAH which could potentially be utilized for permanent implantation, most notably at the Baylor College of Medicine and the Milwaukee Heart Project.[45, 46] It is believed that one or more of these groups will conduct a clinical trial shortly after the turn of the century. However, the initial clinical studies with these devices will probably be for short-term bridge to transplantation to gain valuable experience and to assess the technology. This would follow a similar development and technology adoption path to that of the VAD, one reason why TAH technology development is considered by some to be 8-10 years behind that of the VAD.[47]

Pulsatile Ventricular Assist Devices

Several groups including the joint Cardiovascular Devices Division of the University of Ottawa Heart Institute and the Ottawa-based World Heart Corporation are developing next generation pulsatile ventricular assist devices. Our group has focused its efforts toward the development of an intrathoracically placed, totally implantable VAD without percutaneous connections.[48 - 50] This device, called the HeartSaver VAD (Figure 4), was

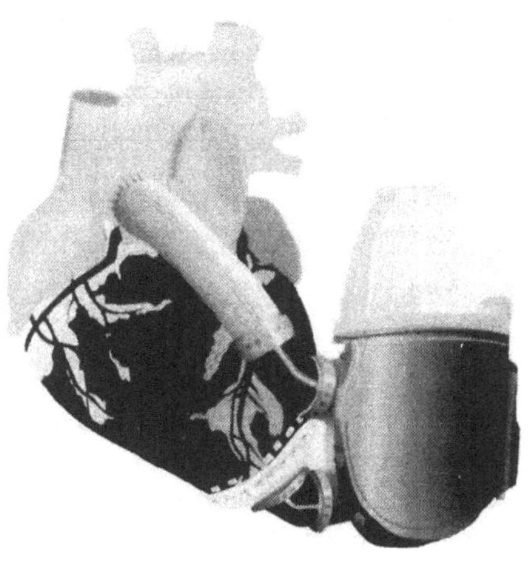

Figure 4. *HeartSaver VAD*
courtesy of WorldHeart Corporation, Ottawa, Canada

designed from the outset for long-term or permanent utilization and combines total implantability with an intrathoracic location, transcutaneous power transfer and remote communication capabilities. This device is designed to be totally implantable (i.e. requiring no percutaneous connections) and is expected to substantially reduce the incidence of infection seen with other devices which utilize percutaneous connections. In addition, the system has the device controls built into the implanted unit allowing the device to operate without external components for short periods of time while utilizing an implanted internal battery. This capability will allow the patient the ability to bathe, shower and undertake activities such as swimming which are not possible with existing devices. The development program has also focused major efforts on the size and anatomical fit of the device to allow implantation in the thoracic cavity which has several clinical benefits as outlined earlier. Based on progress to date, this device is expected to enter clinical trials late in 1999. It is hoped that this type of device, like the many devices that have come before it, will help to contribute to advancing the field of mechanical circulatory support to the next level.

Non-Pulsatile Ventricular Assist Devices

While significant progress is being made in the design and development of non-pulsatile mechanical circulatory support devices, the question of the acceptability of non-pulsatile flow for long-term or permanent support in humans remains to be answered. It is important to note that it took several decades to collect sufficient data on pulsatile devices in humans, to demonstrate their viability and effectiveness. It is therefore reasonable to expect it will take a significant period of time to collect comparable data for non-pulsatile devices. This ongoing debate will certainly continue until the many questions regarding the use of non-pulsatile circulatory support in humans, such as physiological acceptability, potential for blood trauma, blood pressure responses, device durability, and control systems are answered with well designed clinical trials.

Nonetheless there are a large number of research groups developing non-pulsatile VADs with some making substantial progress during in vivo studies in overcoming some of the problems with this design related to blood trauma including hemolysis and thrombosis. Recently the group from Terumo Research and Development Center in Kanagawa, Japan reported an ongoing in vivo experiment of over 650 days with a paracorporeally placed centrifugal pump with a magnetically suspended impeller. [51] In addition, the University of Pittsburgh/Nimbus group has reported on a series of six calf implants with support ranging from 6 to 181 days in duration with minimal hemolysis. [52] Unfortunately, in the University of Pittsburgh/Nimbus study, thrombus in the pump and small renal infarcts were identified in five of the six experiments. Another group achieving significant in vivo progress with a non-pulsatile pump is the Jarvik Research/Texas Heart Institute group who have reported on a series of seven calf implants with support ranging from 40-162 days in duration.[53] Unfortunately five of these experiments were terminated due to device failures (3 for broken wires, 2 for impeller blade/pump housing friction) and thrombus was noted in the pump in one experiment. Each of these groups, together with others, is conducting research to overcome the many difficulties related to the design of the blood contacting impellers and the related blood trauma and to develop suitable physiological control systems.[54]

Conclusions

Since the first utilization of mechanical circulatory support devices in the late 1960's, these devices have evolved from large cumbersome devices capable of very short term support in the ICU to more elegant devices capable of longer term support and even use outside of the hospital setting. During the last three years device utilization has accelerated at an increasingly rapid pace as clinical acceptance of the technology has been gained. To highlight this acceptance over 60 % of all implants of both the Novacor and Thoratec VADs have occurred in the last 3 years, while over 80 % of the Thermo Cardiosystems implants have occurred in this same time period. In addition, devices which had once been utilized only in transplant centers are now beginning to be utilized at non-transplant cardiac centers, further highlighting the rapid clinical acceptance of the technology.

While initial devices required large external consoles to function, effectively tethering the patient to the hospital, advances along the way led to devices with portable controllers that are now in clinical use, and allow patients to leave the hospital. In the very near future, devices with the controllers built right into the implanted devices will enter clinical trials and allow patients unparalleled mobility and quality of life. While the development of devices suitable for permanent support has been the overriding goal for several decades, it appears now that this elusive goal will be achieved in the very near future. However as we strive towards this goal of permanent devices, we must remember that patient acceptance will be vital if the technology is to be used on a widespread basis. Therefore future devices must not simply address the needs of the clinicians and engineers, but must begin to focus on the needs of the patients. Hopefully the next generation of devices will offer not only a valuable medical therapy, but also one which provides the patients the greatest quality of life and places few, if any, limitations on their renewed lifestyles.

References

1. Frazier OH. Long-term ventricular support with the Heartmate in patients undergoing bridge-to-transplant operations. Cardiac Surgery: State of the Art Reviews 1993;7:353-62.
2. McCarthy PM, Young JB, Smedira NG, Hobbs RE, Vargo RL, Starling RC. Permanent mechanical circulatory support with an implantable left ventricular assist device. Ann Thorac Surg 1997;63:1458-61.
3. Oz MC, Argenziano M, Catanese KA, et al. Bridge experience with long-term implantable left ventricular assist devices: Are they an alternative to transplantation? Circulation 1997;95:1844-52.
4. Catanese KA, Goldstein DJ, Williams DL, et al. Outpatient left ventricular assist device support: A destination rather than a bridge. Ann Thorac Surg 1996;62:646-53.
5. Myers TJ, Catanese KA, Vargo RL, Dresslers DK. Extended cardiac support with a portable left ventricular assist system in the home. ASAIO J 1996;42:M576-9.
6. Schocken DD, Arrieta MI, Leaverton PE, Ross EA. Prevalence and mortality rate of congestive heart failure in the United States. J Am Coll Cardiol 1992;20:301-6.
7. The pulse of progress. November 25, 1998. Healthcare and biotechnology research. Scotia Capital Markets.
8. Kannel WB. Epidemiology aspects of heart failure. Cardiol Clin 1989;7:1-9.
9. Massie BM, Packer M. Congestive heart failure: Current controversies and future prospects. Am J Cardiol 1990;66:429-30.
10. 1998 Heart and Stroke Statistical Update. American Heart Association.
11. Ho KKL, Pinsky JL, Kannel WB, Levy D. The epidemiology of heart failure: The Framingham Study. J Am Coll Cardiol 1993:22:6A-13A.
12. Goldstein DL, Oz MC, Rose EA. Implantable ventricular assist devices. N Engl J Med 1998;339:1522-33.
13. Cooley DA. A brief history of heart transplants and mechanical assist devices. In: Frazier OH. Support and replacement of the failing heart. Lippincott Raven, Philadelphia, USA, 1996:5-15.
14. Arabia FA, Copeland JG, Smith RG, et al. International experience with the CardioWest total artificial heart as a bridge to heart transplantation. Eur J Cardiothorac Surg 1997;11:S5-10.
15. Cowen & Company: Cardiovascular Device Update, December 1997.
16. Hunt SA, Frazier OH, Myers TJ. Mechanical circulatory support and cardiac transplantation. Circulation 1998;97:2079-90.
17. Rose EA, Goldstein DJ. Wearable long-term mechanical support for patients with end-stage heart disease: A tenable goal. Ann Thorac Surg 1996;61:399-402.
18. Loisance DY, Deleuze PH, Mazzucotelli JP, Le Besnerais P, Dubois-Rande JL. Clinical implantation of the wearable Baxter Novacor ventricular assist system. Ann Thorac Surg 1994;58:551-4.
19. Frazier OH. Evolution of battery-powered, vented left ventricular assist devices. Ann Thorac Surg 1996;61393-5.
20. Viganó , Scuri S, Cobelli F, et al. Staged discharge out of hospital of the Novacor left ventricular assist system (LVAS) recipients. Eur J Cardiothorac Surg 1997;11:S45-50.
21. Fey O, El-Banayosy A, Arosuglu L, Posival H, Körfer R. Out-of-hospital experience in patients with implantable mechanical circulatory support: present and future trends. Eur J Cardiothorac Surg 1997;11:S51-3.
22. Frazier OH, Rose EA, Macmanus Q, et al. Multicenter clinical evaluation of the HeartMate 1000 IP left ventricular assist device. Ann Thorac Surg 1992;53:1080-90.
23. Levin HR, Chen JM, Oz MC, et al. Potential of left ventricular assist devices as outpatient therapy while awaiting transplantation. Ann Thorac Surg 1994;58:1515-20.
24. Kormos RL, Murali S, Dew MA, et al. Chronic mechanical circulatory support: rehabilitation, low morbidity, and superior survival. Ann Thorac Surg 1994;57:51-8.
25. Miller PJ, Billich TJ, LaForge DH, et al. Initial clinical experience with a wearable controller for the Novacor left ventricular assist system. ASAIO J 1994;40:M465-70.
26. Mehta SM, Aufiero TX, Pae WE Jr., Miller CA , Pierce WS. Combined registry for the clinical use of mechanical ventricular assist pumps and the total artificial heart in conjunction with heart transplantation: sixth official report-1994. J Heart Lung Transplant 1995;14:585-93.
27. Holman WL, Murrah CP, Ferguson ER, Bourge RC, McGiffin DC, Kirklin JK. Infections during extended circulatory support: University of Alabama at Birmingham experience 1989 to 1994. Ann Thorac Surg1996;61:366-71.
28. El-Amir NG, Gardocki M, Levin HR, et al. Gastrointestinal consequences of left ventricular assist device placement. ASAIO J 1996;42:150-3.
29. McCarthy PM, Wang N, Vargo RL. Preperitoneal insertion of the HeartMate 1000 IP implantable left ventricular assist device. Ann Thorac Surg 1994; 57:634-8.

30. Stevenson LW. Patient selection for mechanical bridging to transplantation. Ann Thorac Surg 1996;61:380-7.
31. Pennington DG. Extended support with permanent systems: Percutaneous versus totally implantable. Ann Thorac Surg 1996;61:403-6.
32. McCarthy PM, Schmitt SK, Vargo RL, Gordon S, Keys TF, Hobbs RE. Implantable LVAD infections: Implications for permanent use of the device. Ann Thorac Surg 1996;61:359-65.
33. Watson JT. Innovative ventricular assist systems. ASAIO J 1994;40:M902.
34. Massad MG, McCarthy PM. Will permanent LVADs be better than heart transplantation? Eur J Cardiothorac Surg 1997;11:S11-7.
35. McManus RP, O'Hair DP, Beitzinger JM, et al. Patients who die awaiting heart transplantation. J Heart Lung Transplant 1993;12:159-72.
36. Cloy MJ, Myers TJ, Stutts LA, Macris MP, Frazier OH. Hospital charges for conventional therapy versus left ventricular assist system therapy in heart transplant patients. ASAIO J 1995; 41:M535-9.
37. Frazier OH. First use of an untethered, vented electric left ventricular assist device for long-term support. Circulation 1994;89:2908-14.
38. Levin HR, Oz MC, Chen JM, Packer M,Rose EA, Burkhoff D. Reversal of chronic ventricular dilation in patients with end-stage cardiomyopathy by prolonged mechanical unloading. Circulation 1995;91:2717-20.
39. Dipla K, Mattielo JA, Jeevanandam V, Houser SR, Margulies KB. Myocyte recovery after mechanical circulatory support in humans with end-stage heart failure. Circulation 1998;97:2316-22.
40. Meuller J, Semrau S, Spiegelsberger S, et al. Factors influencing the possibility of weaning from mechanical cardiac support systems in patients with end-stage idiopathic dilated cardiomyopathy. ASAIO Abstracts 1997;26:43.
41. McCarthy PM, Nakatani S, Vargo R, et al. Structural and left ventricular histologic changes after implantable LVAD insertion. Ann Thorac Surg 1995;59:609-13.
42. Farrar DJ, Hill JD. Thoratec Ventricular Assist Device Principal Investigators. Recovery of major organ function in patients awaiting heart transplantation with Thoratec ventricular assist devices. J Heart Lung Transplant 1994;13:1125-32.
43. Report on the workshop on the artificial heart: Planning for evolving technologies. National Heart, Lung, and Blood Institute, National Institutes of Health, U.S. Department of Health and Human Services, 1994.
44. Guy TS. Evolution and the current status of the total artificial heart: The search continues. ASAIO J 1998;44:28-33.
45. Orime Y, Takatani S, Ohara Y, et al. The Baylor-ABI electromechanical total artificial heart. Accelerated endurance testing. ASAIO J 1993;39:M172-6.
46. Gao H, Smith LM, Krymkowski MG, Kohl RJ, Schmidt DH, Christensen CW. In vitro assessment of the Milwaukee Heart and right to left balance. ASAIO J 1992;38:M722-5.
47. Cowen & Company: Industry strategies: Congestive heart failure: Blockbuster potential for emerging therapies, September 1994.
48. Mussivand TV, Masters RG, Hendry PJ, Keon WJ. Totally implantable intrathoracic ventricular assist device. Ann Thorac Surg 1996;61:444-7.
49. Mussivand T, Hendry PJ, Masters RG, Keon WJ. Evaluation of a totally implantable intrathoracic ventricular assist device. Cor Europaeum 1997;6:110-4.
50. Mussivand T, Hendry PJ, Masters RG, Keon WJ. Multi-purpose mechanical circulatory device. Int J Artif Organs 1997;20:217-21.
51. Nojiri C, Kijima T, Horiuchi K, et al. Recent progress in the development of Terumo implantable LVAS (T-ILVAS). ASAIO Abstracts 1998;44:39.
52. Macha M, Litwak P, Yamazaki K, et al. Survival for up to six months in calves supported with an implantable axial flow ventricular assist device. ASAIO J 1997;43:311-5.
53. Macris MP, Parnis SM, Frazier OH, Fuqua JM Jr., Jarvik RK. Development of an implantable ventricular assist system. Ann Thorac Surg 1997;63:367-70.
54. Nishida H, Koyanagi H. Rotary blood pump: paracorporeal, implantable, percutaneous? Artif Organs 1997 Jul;21:589-91.

INDEX

Developments in Cardiovascular Medicine

1. Ch.T. Lancée (ed.): *Echocardiology*. 1979 ISBN 90-247-2209-8
2. J. Baan, A.C. Arntzenius and E.L. Yellin (eds.): *Cardiac Dynamics*. 1980 ISBN 90-247-2212-8
3. H.J.Th. Thalen and C.C. Meere (eds.): *Fundamentals of Cardiac Pacing*. 1979 ISBN 90-247-2245-4
4. H.E. Kulbertus and H.J.J. Wellens (eds.): *Sudden Death*. 1980 ISBN 90-247-2290-X
5. L.S. Dreifus and A.N. Brest (eds.): *Clinical Applications of Cardiovascular Drugs*. 1980 ISBN 90-247-2295-0
6. M.P. Spencer and J.M. Reid: *Cerebrovascular Evaluation with Doppler Ultrasound*. With contributions by E.C. Brockenbrough, R.S. Reneman, G.I. Thomas and D.L. Davis. 1981 ISBN 90-247-2384-1
7. D.P. Zipes, J.C. Bailey and V. Elharrar (eds.): *The Slow Inward Current and Cardiac Arrhythmias*. 1980 ISBN 90-247-2380-9
8. H. Kesteloot and J.V. Joossens (eds.): *Epidemiology of Arterial Blood Pressure*. 1980 ISBN 90-247-2386-8
9. F.J.Th. Wackers (ed.): *Thallium-201 and Technetium-99m-Pyrophosphate. Myocardial Imaging in the Coronary Care Unit*. 1980 ISBN 90-247-2396-5
10. A. Maseri, C. Marchesi, S. Chierchia and M.G. Trivella (eds.): *Coronary Care Units*. Proceedings of a European Seminar (1978). 1981 ISBN 90-247-2456-2
11. J. Morganroth, E.N. Moore, L.S. Dreifus and E.L. Michelson (eds.): *The Evaluation of New Antiarrhythmic Drugs*. Proceedings of the First Symposium on New Drugs and Devices, held in Philadelphia, Pa., U.S.A. (1980). 1981 ISBN 90-247-2474-0
12. P. Alboni: *Intraventricular Conduction Disturbances*. 1981 ISBN 90-247-2483-X
13. H. Rijsterborgh (ed.): *Echocardiology*. 1981 ISBN 90-247-2491-0
14. G.S. Wagner (ed.): *Myocardial Infarction*. Measurement and Intervention. 1982 ISBN 90-247-2513-5
15. R.S. Meltzer and J. Roelandt (eds.): *Contrast Echocardiography*. 1982 ISBN 90-247-2531-3
16. A. Amery, R. Fagard, P. Lijnen and J. Staessen (eds.): *Hypertensive Cardiovascular Disease*. Pathophysiology and Treatment. 1982 IBSN 90-247-2534-8
17. L.N. Bouman and H.J. Jongsma (eds.): *Cardiac Rate and Rhythm*. Physiological, Morphological and Developmental Aspects. 1982 ISBN 90-247-2626-3
18. J. Morganroth and E.N. Moore (eds.): *The Evaluation of Beta Blocker and Calcium Antagonist Drugs*. Proceedings of the 2nd Symposium on New Drugs and Devices, held in Philadelphia, Pa., U.S.A. (1981). 1982 ISBN 90-247-2642-5
19. M.B. Rosenbaum and M.V. Elizari (eds.): *Frontiers of Cardiac Electrophysiology*. 1983 ISBN 90-247-2663-8
20. J. Roelandt and P.G. Hugenholtz (eds.): *Long-term Ambulatory Electrocardiography*. 1982 ISBN 90-247-2664-6
21. A.A.J. Adgey (ed.): *Acute Phase of Ischemic Heart Disease and Myocardial Infarction*. 1982 ISBN 90-247-2675-1
22. P. Hanrath, W. Bleifeld and J. Souquet (eds.): *Cardiovascular Diagnosis by Ultrasound*. Transesophageal, Computerized, Contrast, Doppler Echocardiography. 1982 ISBN 90-247-2692-1
23. J. Roelandt (ed.): *The Practice of M-Mode and Two-dimensional Echocardiography*. 1983 ISBN 90-247-2745-6
24. J. Meyer, P. Schweizer and R. Erbel (eds.): *Advances in Noninvasive Cardiology*. Ultrasound, Computed Tomography, Radioisotopes, Digital Angiography. 1983 ISBN 0-89838-576-8
25. J. Morganroth and E.N. Moore (eds.): *Sudden Cardiac Death and Congestive Heart Failure*. Diagnosis and Treatment. Proceedings of the 3rd Symposium on New Drugs and Devices, held in Philadelphia, Pa., U.S.A. (1982). 1983 ISBN 0-89838-580-6
26. H.M. Perry Jr. (ed.): *Lifelong Management of Hypertension*. 1983 ISBN 0-89838-582-2
27. E.A. Jaffe (ed.): *Biology of Endothelial Cells*. 1984 ISBN 0-89838-587-3
28. B. Surawicz, C.P. Reddy and E.N. Prystowsky (eds.): *Tachycardias*. 1984 ISBN 0-89838-588-1
29. M.P. Spencer (ed.): *Cardiac Doppler Diagnosis*. Proceedings of a Symposium, held in Clearwater, Fla., U.S.A. (1983). 1983 ISBN 0-89838-591-1
30. H. Villarreal and M.P. Sambhi (eds.): *Topics in Pathophysiology of Hypertension*. 1984 ISBN 0-89838-595-4

Developments in Cardiovascular Medicine

31. F.H. Messerli (ed.): *Cardiovascular Disease in the Elderly.* 1984
Revised edition, 1988: see below under Volume 76
32. M.L. Simoons and J.H.C. Reiber (eds.): *Nuclear Imaging in Clinical Cardiology.* 1984
ISBN 0-89838-599-7
33. H.E.D.J. ter Keurs and J.J. Schipperheyn (eds.): *Cardiac Left Ventricular Hypertrophy.* 1983
ISBN 0-89838-612-8
34. N. Sperelakis (ed.): *Physiology and Pathology of the Heart.* 1984
Revised edition, 1988: see below under Volume 90
35. F.H. Messerli (ed.): *Kidney in Essential Hypertension.* Proceedings of a Course, held in New Orleans, La., U.S.A. (1983). 1984 ISBN 0-89838-616-0
36. M.P. Sambhi (ed.): *Fundamental Fault in Hypertension.* 1984 ISBN 0-89838-638-1
37. C. Marchesi (ed.): *Ambulatory Monitoring.* Cardiovascular System and Allied Applications. Proceedings of a Workshop, held in Pisa, Italy (1983). 1984 ISBN 0-89838-642-X
38. W. Kupper, R.N. MacAlpin and W. Bleifeld (eds.): *Coronary Tone in Ischemic Heart Disease.* 1984
ISBN 0-89838-646-2
39. N. Sperelakis and J.B. Caulfield (eds.): *Calcium Antagonists.* Mechanism of Action on Cardiac Muscle and Vascular Smooth Muscle. Proceedings of the 5th Annual Meeting of the American Section of the I.S.H.R., held in Hilton Head, S.C., U.S.A. (1983). 1984 ISBN 0-89838-655-1
40. Th. Godfraind, A.G. Herman and D. Wellens (eds.): *Calcium Entry Blockers in Cardiovascular and Cerebral Dysfunctions.* 1984 ISBN 0-89838-658-6
41. J. Morganroth and E.N. Moore (eds.): *Interventions in the Acute Phase of Myocardial Infarction.* Proceedings of the 4th Symposium on New Drugs and Devices, held in Philadelphia, Pa., U.S.A. (1983). 1984
ISBN 0-89838-659-4
42. F.L. Abel and W.H. Newman (eds.): *Functional Aspects of the Normal, Hypertrophied and Failing Heart.* Proceedings of the 5th Annual Meeting of the American Section of the I.S.H.R., held in Hilton Head, S.C., U.S.A. (1983). 1984 ISBN 0-89838-665-9
43. S. Sideman and R. Beyar (eds.): [3-D] *Simulation and Imaging of the Cardiac System.* State of the Heart. Proceedings of the International Henry Goldberg Workshop, held in Haifa, Israel (1984). 1985
ISBN 0-89838-687-X
44. E. van der Wall and K.I. Lie (eds.): *Recent Views on Hypertrophic Cardiomyopathy.* Proceedings of a Symposium, held in Groningen, The Netherlands (1984). 1985 ISBN 0-89838-694-2
45. R.E. Beamish, P.K. Singal and N.S. Dhalla (eds.), *Stress and Heart Disease.* Proceedings of a International Symposium, held in Winnipeg, Canada, 1984 (Vol. 1). 1985 ISBN 0-89838-709-4
46. R.E. Beamish, V. Panagia and N.S. Dhalla (eds.): *Pathogenesis of Stress-induced Heart Disease.* Proceedings of a International Symposium, held in Winnipeg, Canada, 1984 (Vol. 2). 1985
ISBN 0-89838-710-8
47. J. Morganroth and E.N. Moore (eds.): *Cardiac Arrhythmias.* New Therapeutic Drugs and Devices. Proceedings of the 5th Symposium on New Drugs and Devices, held in Philadelphia, Pa., U.S.A. (1984). 1985
ISBN 0-89838-716-7
48. P. Mathes (ed.): *Secondary Prevention in Coronary Artery Disease and Myocardial Infarction.* 1985
ISBN 0-89838-736-1
49. H.L. Stone and W.B. Weglicki (eds.): *Pathobiology of Cardiovascular Injury.* Proceedings of the 6th Annual Meeting of the American Section of the I.S.H.R., held in Oklahoma City, Okla., U.S.A. (1984). 1985 ISBN 0-89838-743-4
50. J. Meyer, R. Erbel and H.J. Rupprecht (eds.): *Improvement of Myocardial Perfusion.* Thrombolysis, Angioplasty, Bypass Surgery. Proceedings of a Symposium, held in Mainz, F.R.G. (1984). 1985
ISBN 0-89838-748-5
51. J.H.C. Reiber, P.W. Serruys and C.J. Slager (eds.): *Quantitative Coronary and Left Ventricular Cineangiography.* Methodology and Clinical Applications. 1986 ISBN 0-89838-760-4
52. R.H. Fagard and I.E. Bekaert (eds.): *Sports Cardiology.* Exercise in Health and Cardiovascular Disease. Proceedings from an International Conference, held in Knokke, Belgium (1985). 1986
ISBN 0-89838-782-5

Developments in Cardiovascular Medicine

53. J.H.C. Reiber and P.W. Serruys (eds.): *State of the Art in Quantitative Cornary Arteriography.* 1986 ISBN 0-89838-804-X
54. J. Roelandt (ed.): *Color Doppler Flow Imaging and Other Advances in Doppler Echocardiography.* 1986 ISBN 0-89838-806-6
55. E.E. van der Wall (ed.): *Noninvasive Imaging of Cardiac Metabolism.* Single Photon Scintigraphy, Positron Emission Tomography and Nuclear Magnetic Resonance. 1987 ISBN 0-89838-812-0
56. J. Liebman, R. Plonsey and Y. Rudy (eds.): *Pediatric and Fundamental Electrocardiography.* 1987 ISBN 0-89838-815-5
57. H.H. Hilger, V. Hombach and W.J. Rashkind (eds.), *Invasive Cardiovascular Therapy.* Proceedings of an International Symposium, held in Cologne, F.R.G. (1985). 1987 ISBN 0-89838-818-X
58. P.W. Serruys and G.T. Meester (eds.): *Coronary Angioplasty.* A Controlled Model for Ischemia. 1986 ISBN 0-89838-819-8
59. J.E. Tooke and L.H. Smaje (eds.): *Clinical Investigation of the Microcirculation.* Proceedings of an International Meeting, held in London, U.K. (1985). 1987 ISBN 0-89838-833-3
60. R.Th. van Dam and A. van Oosterom (eds.): *Electrocardiographic Body Surface Mapping.* Proceedings of the 3rd International Symposium on B.S.M., held in Nijmegen, The Netherlands (1985). 1986 ISBN 0-89838-834-1
61. M.P. Spencer (ed.): *Ultrasonic Diagnosis of Cerebrovascular Disease.* Doppler Techniques and Pulse Echo Imaging. 1987 ISBN 0-89838-836-8
62. M.J. Legato (ed.): *The Stressed Heart.* 1987 ISBN 0-89838-849-X
63. M.E. Safar (ed.): *Arterial and Venous Systems in Essential Hypertension.* With Assistance of G.M. London, A.Ch. Simon and Y.A. Weiss. 1987 ISBN 0-89838-857-0
64. J. Roelandt (ed.): *Digital Techniques in Echocardiography.* 1987 ISBN 0-89838-861-9
65. N.S. Dhalla, P.K. Singal and R.E. Beamish (eds.): *Pathology of Heart Disease.* Proceedings of the 8th Annual Meeting of the American Section of the I.S.H.R., held in Winnipeg, Canada, 1986 (Vol. 1). 1987 ISBN 0-89838-864-3
66. N.S. Dhalla, G.N. Pierce and R.E. Beamish (eds.): *Heart Function and Metabolism.* Proceedings of the 8th Annual Meeting of the American Section of the I.S.H.R., held in Winnipeg, Canada, 1986 (Vol. 2). 1987 ISBN 0-89838-865-1
67. N.S. Dhalla, I.R. Innes and R.E. Beamish (eds.): *Myocardial Ischemia.* Proceedings of a Satellite Symposium of the 30th International Physiological Congress, held in Winnipeg, Canada (1986). 1987 ISBN 0-89838-866-X
68. R.E. Beamish, V. Panagia and N.S. Dhalla (eds.): *Pharmacological Aspects of Heart Disease.* Proceedings of an International Symposium, held in Winnipeg, Canada (1986). 1987 ISBN 0-89838-867-8
69. H.E.D.J. ter Keurs and J.V. Tyberg (eds.): *Mechanics of the Circulation.* Proceedings of a Satellite Symposium of the 30th International Physiological Congress, held in Banff, Alberta, Canada (1986). 1987 ISBN 0-89838-870-8
70. S. Sideman and R. Beyar (eds.): *Activation, Metabolism and Perfusion of the Heart.* Simulation and Experimental Models. Proceedings of the 3rd Henry Goldberg Workshop, held in Piscataway, N.J., U.S.A. (1986). 1987 ISBN 0-89838-871-6
71. E. Aliot and R. Lazzara (eds.): *Ventricular Tachycardias.* From Mechanism to Therapy. 1987 ISBN 0-89838-881-3
72. A. Schneeweiss and G. Schettler: *Cardiovascular Drug Therapoy in the Elderly.* 1988 ISBN 0-89838-883-X
73. J.V. Chapman and A. Sgalambro (eds.): *Basic Concepts in Doppler Echocardiography.* Methods of Clinical Applications based on a Multi-modality Doppler Approach. 1987 ISBN 0-89838-888-0
74. S. Chien, J. Dormandy, E. Ernst and A. Matrai (eds.): *Clinical Hemorheology.* Applications in Cardiovascular and Hematological Disease, Diabetes, Surgery and Gynecology. 1987 ISBN 0-89838-807-4
75. J. Morganroth and E.N. Moore (eds.): *Congestive Heart Failure.* Proceedings of the 7th Annual Symposium on New Drugs and Devices, held in Philadelphia, Pa., U.S.A. (1986). 1987 ISBN 0-89838-955-0
76. F.H. Messerli (ed.): *Cardiovascular Disease in the Elderly.* 2nd ed. 1988 ISBN 0-89838-962-3
77. P.H. Heintzen and J.H. Bürsch (eds.): *Progress in Digital Angiocardiography.* 1988 ISBN 0-89838-965-8

Developments in Cardiovascular Medicine

78. M.M. Scheinman (ed.): *Catheter Ablation of Cardiac Arrhythmias.* Basic Bioelectrical Effects and Clinical Indications. 1988 ISBN 0-89838-967-4
79. J.A.E. Spaan, A.V.G. Bruschke and A.C. Gittenberger-De Groot (eds.): *Coronary Circulation.* From Basic Mechanisms to Clinical Implications. 1987 ISBN 0-89838-978-X
80. C. Visser, G. Kan and R.S. Meltzer (eds.): *Echocardiography in Coronary Artery Disease.* 1988 ISBN 0-89838-979-8
81. A. Bayés de Luna, A. Betriu and G. Permanyer (eds.): *Therapeutics in Cardiology.* 1988 ISBN 0-89838-981-X
82. D.M. Mirvis (ed.): *Body Surface Electrocardiographic Mapping.* 1988 ISBN 0-89838-983-6
83. M.A. Konstam and J.M. Isner (eds.): *The Right Ventricle.* 1988 ISBN 0-89838-987-9
84. C.T. Kappagoda and P.V. Greenwood (eds.): *Long-term Management of Patients after Myocardial Infarction.* 1988 ISBN 0-89838-352-8
85. W.H. Gaasch and H.J. Levine (eds.): *Chronic Aortic Regurgitation.* 1988 ISBN 0-89838-364-1
86. P.K. Singal (ed.): *Oxygen Radicals in the Pathophysiology of Heart Disease.* 1988 ISBN 0-89838-375-7
87. J.H.C. Reiber and P.W. Serruys (eds.): *New Developments in Quantitative Coronary Arteriography.* 1988 ISBN 0-89838-377-3
88. J. Morganroth and E.N. Moore (eds.): *Silent Myocardial Ischemia.* Proceedings of the 8th Annual Symposium on New Drugs and Devices (1987). 1988 ISBN 0-89838-380-3

Developments in Cardiovascular Medicine

109. J.P.M. Hamer: *Practical Echocardiography in the Adult.* With Doppler and Color-Doppler Flow Imaging. 1990 ISBN 0-7923-0670-8
110. A. Bayés de Luna, P. Brugada, J. Cosin Aguilar and F. Navarro Lopez (eds.): *Sudden Cardiac Death.* 1991 ISBN 0-7923-0716-X
111. E. Andries and R. Stroobandt (eds.): *Hemodynamics in Daily Practice.* 1991 ISBN 0-7923-0725-9
112. J. Morganroth and E.N. Moore (eds.): *Use and Approval of Antihypertensive Agents and Surrogate Endpoints for the Approval of Drugs affecting Antiarrhythmic Heart Failure and Hypolipidemia.* Proceedings of the 10th Annual Symposium on New Drugs and Devices (1989). 1990 ISBN 0-7923-0756-9
113. S. Iliceto, P. Rizzon and J.R.T.C. Roelandt (eds.): *Ultrasound in Coronary Artery Disease.* Present Role and Future Perspectives. 1990 ISBN 0-7923-0784-4
114. J.V. Chapman and G.R. Sutherland (eds.): *The Noninvasive Evaluation of Hemodynamics in Congenital Heart Disease.* Doppler Ultrasound Applications in the Adult and Pediatric Patient with Congenital Heart Disease. 1990 ISBN 0-7923-0836-0
115. G.T. Meester and F. Pinciroli (eds.): *Databases for Cardiology.* 1991 ISBN 0-7923-0886-7
116. B. Korecky and N.S. Dhalla (eds.): *Subcellular Basis of Contractile Failure.* 1990 ISBN 0-7923-0890-5
117. J.H.C. Reiber and P.W. Serruys (eds.): *Quantitative Coronary Arteriography.* 1991 ISBN 0-7923-0913-8
118. E. van der Wall and A. de Roos (eds.): *Magnetic Resonance Imaging in Coronary Artery Disease.* 1991 ISBN 0-7923-0940-5
119. V. Hombach, M. Kochs and A.J. Camm (eds.): *Interventional Techniques in Cardiovascular Medicine.* 1991 ISBN 0-7923-0956-1
120. R. Vos: *Drugs Looking for Diseases.* Innovative Drug Research and the Development of the Beta Blockers and the Calcium Antagonists. 1991 ISBN 0-7923-0968-5
121. S. Sideman, R. Beyar and A.G. Kleber (eds.): *Cardiac Electrophysiology, Circulation, and Transport.* Proceedings of the 7th Henry Goldberg Workshop (Berne, Switzerland, 1990). 1991 ISBN 0-7923-1145-0
122. D.M. Bers: *Excitation-Contraction Coupling and Cardiac Contractile Force.* 1991 ISBN 0-7923-1186-8
123. A.-M. Salmasi and A.N. Nicolaides (eds.): *Occult Atherosclerotic Disease.* Diagnosis, Assessment and Management. 1991 ISBN 0-7923-1188-4
124. J.A.E. Spaan: *Coronary Blood Flow.* Mechanics, Distribution, and Control. 1991 ISBN 0-7923-1210-4
125. R.W. Stout (ed.): *Diabetes and Atherosclerosis.* 1991 ISBN 0-7923-1310-0
126. A.G. Herman (ed.): *Antithrombotics.* Pathophysiological Rationale for Pharmacological Interventions. 1991 ISBN 0-7923-1413-1
127. N.H.J. Pijls: *Maximal Myocardial Perfusion as a Measure of the Functional Significance of Coronary Arteriogram.* From a Pathoanatomic to a Pathophysiologic Interpretation of the Coronary Arteriogram. 1991 ISBN 0-7923-1430-1
128. J.H.C. Reiber and E.E. v.d. Wall (eds.): *Cardiovascular Nuclear Medicine and MRI.* Quantitation and Clinical Applications. 1992 ISBN 0-7923-1467-0
129. E. Andries, P. Brugada and R. Stroobrandt (eds.): *How to Face "the Faces' of Cardiac Pacing.* 1992 ISBN 0-7923-1528-6
130. M. Nagano, S. Mochizuki and N.S. Dhalla (eds.): *Cardiovascular Disease in Diabetes.* 1992 ISBN 0-7923-1554-5
131. P.W. Serruys, B.H. Strauss and S.B. King III (eds.): *Restenosis after Intervention with New Mechanical Devices.* 1992 ISBN 0-7923-1555-3
132. P.J. Walter (ed.): *Quality of Life after Open Heart Surgery.* 1992 ISBN 0-7923-1580-4
133. E.E. van der Wall, H. Sochor, A. Righetti and M.G. Niemeyer (eds.): *What's new in Cardiac Imaging?* SPECT, PET and MRI. 1992 ISBN 0-7923-1615-0
134. P. Hanrath, R. Uebis and W. Krebs (eds.): *Cardiovascular Imaging by Ultrasound.* 1992 ISBN 0-7923-1755-6
135. F.H. Messerli (ed.): *Cardiovascular Disease in the Elderly.* 3rd ed. 1992 ISBN 0-7923-1859-5
136. J. Hess and G.R. Sutherland (eds.): *Congenital Heart Disease in Adolescents and Adults.* 1992 ISBN 0-7923-1862-5
137. J.H.C. Reiber and P.W. Serruys (eds.): *Advances in Quantitative Coronary Arteriography.* 1993 ISBN 0-7923-1863-3

Developments in Cardiovascular Medicine

138. A.-M. Salmasi and A.S. Iskandrian (eds.): *Cardiac Output and Regional Flow in Health and Disease.* 1993 ISBN 0-7923-1911-7
139. J.H. Kingma, N.M. van Hemel and K.I. Lie (eds.): *Atrial Fibrillation, a Treatable Disease?* 1992 ISBN 0-7923-2008-5
140. B. Ostadel and N.S. Dhalla (eds.): *Heart Function in Health and Disease.* Proceedings of the Cardiovascular Program (Prague, Czechoslovakia, 1991). 1992 ISBN 0-7923-2052-2
141. D. Noble and Y.E. Earm (eds.): *Ionic Channels and Effect of Taurine on the Heart.* Proceedings of an International Symposium (Seoul, Korea, 1992). 1993 ISBN 0-7923-2199-5
142. H.M. Piper and C.J. Preusse (eds.): *Ischemia-reperfusion in Cardiac Surgery.* 1993 ISBN 0-7923-2241-X
143. J. Roelandt, E.J. Gussenhoven and N. Bom (eds.): *Intravascular Ultrasound.* 1993 ISBN 0-7923-2301-7
144. M.E. Safar and M.F. O'Rourke (eds.): *The Arterial System in Hypertension.* 1993 ISBN 0-7923-2343-2
145. P.W. Serruys, D.P. Foley and P.J. de Feyter (eds.): *Quantitative Coronary Angio- graphy in Clinical Practice.* With a Foreword by Spencer B. King III. 1994 ISBN 0-7923-2368-8
146. J. Candell-Riera and D. Ortega-Alcalde (eds.): *Nuclear Cardiology in Everyday Practice.* 1994 ISBN 0-7923-2374-2
147. P. Cummins (ed.): *Growth Factors and the Cardiovascular System.* 1993 ISBN 0-7923-2401-3
148. K. Przyklenk, R.A. Kloner and D.M. Yellon (eds.): *Ischemic Preconditioning: The Concept of Endogenous Cardioprotection.* 1993 ISBN 0-7923-2410-2
149. T.H. Marwick: *Stress Echocardiography.* Its Role in the Diagnosis and Evaluation of Coronary Artery Disease. 1994 ISBN 0-7923-2579-6
150. W.H. van Gilst and K.I. Lie (eds.): *Neurohumoral Regulation of Coronary Flow.* Role of the Endothelium. 1993 ISBN 0-7923-2588-5
151. N. Sperelakis (ed.): *Physiology and Pathophysiology of the Heart.* 3rd rev. ed. 1994 ISBN 0-7923-2612-1
152. J.C. Kaski (ed.): *Angina Pectoris with Normal Coronary Arteries: Syndrome X.* 1994 ISBN 0-7923-2651-2
153. D.R. Gross: *Animal Models in Cardiovascular Research.* 2nd rev. ed. 1994 ISBN 0-7923-2712-8
154. A.S. Iskandrian and E.E. van der Wall (eds.): *Myocardial Viability.* Detection and Clinical Relevance. 1994 ISBN 0-7923-2813-2
155. J.H.C. Reiber and P.W. Serruys (eds.): *Progress in Quantitative Coronary Arteriography.* 1994 ISBN 0-7923-2814-0
156. U. Goldbourt, U. de Faire and K. Berg (eds.): *Genetic Factors in Coronary Heart Disease.* 1994 ISBN 0-7923-2752-7
157. G. Leonetti and C. Cuspidi (eds.): *Hypertension in the Elderly.* 1994 ISBN 0-7923-2852-3
158. D. Ardissino, S. Savonitto and L.H. Opie (eds.): *Drug Evaluation in Angina Pectoris.* 1994 ISBN 0-7923-2897-3
159. G. Bkaily (ed.): *Membrane Physiopathology.* 1994 ISBN 0-7923-3062-5
160. R.C. Becker (ed.): *The Modern Era of Coronary Thrombolysis.* 1994 ISBN 0-7923-3063-3
161. P.J. Walter (ed.): *Coronary Bypass Surgery in the Elderly.* Ethical, Economical and Quality of Life Aspects. With a foreword by N.K. Wenger. 1995 ISBN 0-7923-3188-5
162. J.W. de Jong and R. Ferrari (eds.), *The Carnitine System.* A New Therapeutical Approach to Cardiovascular Diseases. 1995 ISBN 0-7923-3318-7
163. C.A. Neill and E.B. Clark: *The Developing Heart: A "History' of Pediatric Cardiology.* 1995 ISBN 0-7923-3375-6
164. N. Sperelakis: *Electrogenesis of Biopotentials in the Cardiovascular System.* 1995 ISBN 0-7923-3398-5
165. M. Schwaiger (ed.): *Cardiac Positron Emission Tomography.* 1995 ISBN 0-7923-3417-5
166. E.E. van der Wall, P.K. Blanksma, M.G. Niemeyer and A.M.J. Paans (eds.): *Cardiac Positron Emission Tomography.* Viability, Perfusion, Receptors and Cardiomyopathy. 1995 ISBN 0-7923-3472-8
167. P.K. Singal, I.M.C. Dixon, R.E. Beamish and N.S. Dhalla (eds.): *Mechanism of Heart Failure.* 1995 ISBN 0-7923-3490-6
168. N.S. Dhalla, P.K. Singal, N. Takeda and R.E. Beamish (eds.): *Pathophysiology of Heart Failure.* 1995 ISBN 0-7923-3571-6
169. N.S. Dhalla, G.N. Pierce, V. Panagia and R.E. Beamish (eds.): *Heart Hypertrophy and Failure.* 1995 ISBN 0-7923-3572-4

Developments in Cardiovascular Medicine

170. S.N. Willich and J.E. Muller (eds.): *Triggering of Acute Coronary Syndromes*. Implications for Prevention. 1995 ISBN 0-7923-3605-4
171. E.E. van der Wall, T.H. Marwick and J.H.C. Reiber (eds.): *Advances in Imaging Techniques in Ischemic Heart Disease*. 1995 ISBN 0-7923-3620-8
172. B. Swynghedauw: *Molecular Cardiology for the Cardiologist*. 1995 ISBN 0-7923-3622-4
173. C.A. Nienaber and U. Sechtem (eds.): *Imaging and Intervention in Cardiology*. 1996 ISBN 0-7923-3649-6
174. G. Assmann (ed.): *HDL Deficiency and Atherosclerosis*. 1995 ISBN 0-7923-8888-7
175. N.M. van Hemel, F.H.M. Wittkampf and H. Ector (eds.): *The Pacemaker Clinic of the 90's*. Essentials in Brady-Pacing. 1995 ISBN 0-7923-3688-7
176. N. Wilke (ed.): *Advanced Cardiovascular MRI of the Heart and Great Vessels*. Forthcoming. ISBN 0-7923-3720-4
177. M. LeWinter, H. Suga and M.W. Watkins (eds.): *Cardiac Energetics: From Emax to Pressure-volume Area*. 1995 ISBN 0-7923-3721-2
178. R.J. Siegel (ed.): *Ultrasound Angioplasty*. 1995 ISBN 0-7923-3722-0
179. D.M. Yellon and G.J. Gross (eds.): *Myocardial Protection and the K_{ATP} Channel*. 1995 ISBN 0-7923-3791-3
180. A.V.G. Bruschke, J.H.C. Reiber, K.I. Lie and H.J.J. Wellens (eds.): *Lipid Lowering Therapy and Progression of Coronary Atherosclerosis*. 1996 ISBN 0-7923-3807-3
181. A.-S.A. Abd-Eyattah and A.S. Wechsler (eds.): *Purines and Myocardial Protection*. 1995 ISBN 0-7923-3831-6
182. M. Morad, S. Ebashi, W. Trautwein and Y. Kurachi (eds.): *Molecular Physiology and Pharmacology of Cardiac Ion Channels and Transporters*. 1996 ISBN 0-7923-3913-4
183. M.A. Oto (ed.): *Practice and Progress in Cardiac Pacing and Electrophysiology*. 1996 ISBN 0-7923-3950-9
184. W.H. Birkenhäger (ed.): *Practical Management of Hypertension*. Second Edition. 1996 ISBN 0-7923-3952-5
185. J.C. Chatham, J.R. Forder and J.H. McNeill (eds.): *The Heart in Diabetes*. 1996 ISBN 0-7923-4052-3
186. J.H.C. Reiber and E.E. van der Wall (eds.): *Cardiovascular Imaging*. 1996 ISBN 0-7923-4109-0
187. A-M. Salmasi and A. Strano (eds.): *Angiology in Practice*. 1996 ISBN 0-7923-4143-0
188. M.W. Kroll and M.H. Lehmann (eds.): *Implantable Cardioverter Defibrillator Therapy: The Engineering – Clinical Interface*. 1996 ISBN 0-7923-4300-X
189. K.L. March (ed.): *Gene Transfer in the Cardiovascular System*. Experimental Approaches and Therapeutic Implications. 1996 ISBN 0-7923-9859-9
190. L. Klein (ed.): *Coronary Stenosis Morphology: Analysis and Implication*. 1997 ISBN 0-7923-9867-X
191. J.E. Pérez and R.M. Lang (eds.): *Echocardiography and Cardiovascular Function: Tools for the Next Decade*. 1997 ISBN 0-7923-9884-X
192. A.A. Knowlton (ed.): *Heat Shock Proteins and the Cardiovascular System*. 1997 ISBN 0-7923-9910-2
193. R.C. Becker (ed.): *The Textbook of Coronary Thrombosis and Thrombolysis*. 1997 ISBN 0-7923-9923-4
194. R.M. Mentzer, Jr., M. Kitakaze, J.M. Downey and M. Hori (eds.): *Adenosine, Cardioprotection and Its Clinical Application*. 1997 ISBN 0-7923-9954-4
195. N.H.J. Pijls and B. De Bruyne: *Coronary Pressure*. 1997 ISBN 0-7923-4672-6
196. I. Graham, H. Refsum, I.H. Rosenberg and P.M. Ueland (eds.): *Homocysteine Metabolism: from Basic Science to Clinical Medicine*. 1997 ISBN 0-7923-9983-8
197. E.E. van der Wall, V. Manger Cats and J. Baan (eds.): *Vascular Medicine – From Endothelium to Myocardium*. 1997 ISBN 0-7923-4740-4
198. A. Lafont and E. Topol (eds.): *Arterial Remodeling*. A Critical Factor in Restenosis. 1997 ISBN 0-7923-8008-8
199. M. Mercury, D.D. McPherson, H. Bassiouny and S. Glagov (eds.): *Non-Invasive Imaging of Atherosclerosis* 1998 ISBN 0-7923-8036-3
200. W.C. De Mello and M.J. Janse (eds.): *Heart Cell Communication in Health and Disease*. 1997 ISBN 0-7923-8052-5

Developments in Cardiovascular Medicine

201. P.E. Vardas (ed.): *Cardiac Arrhythmias Pacing and Electrophysiology.* The Expert View. 1998 ISBN 0-7923-4908-3
202. E.E. van der Wall, P.K. Blanksma, M.G. Niemeyer, W. Vaalburg and H.J.G.M. Crijns (eds.): *Advanced Imaging in Coronary Artery Disease.* PET, SPECT, MRI, IVUS, EBCT. 1998 ISBN 0-7923-5083-9
203. R.L. Wilenski (ed.): *Unstable Coronary Artery Syndromes, Pathophysiology, Diagnosis and Treatment.* 1998 ISBN 0-7923-8201-3
204. J.H.C. Reiber and E.E. van der Wall (eds.): *What's New in Cardiovascular Imaging?* 1998 ISBN 0-7923-5121-5
205. J.C. Kaski and D.W. Holt (eds.): *Myocardial Damage.* Early Detection by Novel Biochemical Markers. 1998 ISBN 0-7923-5140-1
206. M. Malik (ed.): *Clinical Guide to Cardiac Autonomic Tests.* 1998 ISBN 0-7923-5178-9
207. G.F. Baxter and D.M. Yellon (eds.): *Delayed Preconditioning and Adaptive Cardioprotection.* 1998 ISBN 0-7923-5259-9
208. B. Swynghedauw, *Molecular Cardiology for the Cardiologist, Second Edition.* 1998 ISBN 0-7923-8323-0
209. G. Burnstock, J.G. Dobson, Jr., B.T. Liang, J. Linden (eds.): *Cardiovascular Biology of Purines.* 1998 ISBN 0-7923-8334-6
210. B.D. Hoit, R.A. Walsh (eds.): *Cardiovascular Physiology in the Genetically Engineered Mouse.* 1998 ISBN 0-7923-8356-7
211. P. Whittaker, G.S. Abela (eds.): *Direct Myocardial Revascularization: History, Methodology, Technology.* 1998 ISBN 0-7923-8398-2
212. C.A. Nienaber and R. Fattori (eds.): *Diagnosis and Treatment of Aortic Diseases.* 1999 ISBN 0-7923-5517-2
213. J.C. Kaski (ed.): *Chest Pain with Normal Coronary Angiograms: Pathogenesis, Diagnosis and Management.* 1999 ISBN 0-7923-8421-0
214. P.A. Doevendans, R.S. Reneman and M. van Bilsen (eds.): *Cardiovascular Specific Gene Expression.* 1999 ISBN 0-7923-5633-0
215. G. Pons-Lladó, F. Carreras, X. Borrás, M. Subirana and L.J. Jiménez-Borreguero (eds.): *Atlas of Practical Cardiac Applications of MRI.* 1999 ISBN 0-7923-5636-5
216. L.W. Klein and J.E. Calvin, *Resource Ultilization in Cardiac Disease.* 1999 ISBN 0-7923-8509-8
217. R. Gorlin, G. Dangas, P.K. Toutouzas and M.M. Konstadoulaks: *Contemporary Concepts in Cardiology, Pathophysiology and Clinical Management.* 1999 ISBN 0-7923-8514-4
218. S. Gupta and A.J. Camm: *Chronic Infection, Chlamydia and Coronary Heart Disease.* 1999 ISBN 0-7923-5797-3
219. M. Rajskina: *Ventricular Fibrillation in Sudden Cardiac Death.* 1999 ISBN 0-7923-8570-5
220. Z. Abedin and R. Conner: *Interpretation of Cardiac Arrhythmias: Self Assessment Approach.* 1999 ISBN 0-7923-8576-4
221. J.E. Lock, J.F. Keane and S.B. Perry (eds.): *Diagnostic and Interventional Catheterization in Congenital Heart Disease, second edition.* 1999 ISBN 0-7923-8597-7
222. J.S. Steinberg (ed.): *Atrial Fibrillation after Cardiac Surgery.* 1999 ISBN 0-7923-8655-8
223. E.E. van der Wall, A. van der Laarse, B.M. Pluim, A.V.G. Bruschke:*Left Ventricular Hypertrophy.* Physiology versus Pathology. 1999 ISBN 0-7923-6038-9
224. J.F. Keaney, Jr. (ed.): *Oxidative Stress and Vascular Disease.* 1999 ISBN 0-7923-8678-7
225. R.G. Masters (ed.): *Surgical Options for the Treatment of Heart Failure.* 2000 ISBN 0-7923-6130-X

Previous volumes are still available

KLUWER ACADEMIC PUBLISHERS – DORDRECHT / BOSTON / LONDON

MIX
Papier aus verantwortungsvollen Quellen
Paper from responsible sources
FSC® C105338

If you have any concerns about our products,
you can contact us on
ProductSafety@springernature.com

In case Publisher is established outside the EU,
the EU authorized representative is:
Springer Nature Customer Service Center GmbH
Europaplatz 3, 69115 Heidelberg, Germany

Printed by Libri Plureos GmbH
in Hamburg, Germany